Healing with Cannabis

Healing with Cannabis

The Evolution of the Endocannabinoid System and
How Cannabinoids Help Relieve PTSD, Pain, MS, Anxiety, and More

Cheryl Pellerin

Foreword by Jeffrey Y. Hergenrather, MD

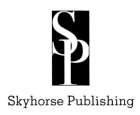

Skyhorse Publishing

Text Copyright © 2020 by Cheryl Pellerin
Foreword copyright © 2020 by Jeffrey Y. Hergenrather

Skyhorse Publishing books may be purchased in bulk at special discounts for sales promotion, corporate gifts, fund-raising, or educational purposes. Special editions can also be created to specifications. For details, contact the Special Sales Department, Skyhorse Publishing, 307 West 36th Street, 11th Floor, New York, NY 10018 or info@skyhorsepublishing.com.

Skyhorse® and Skyhorse Publishing® are registered trademarks of Skyhorse Publishing, Inc.®, a Delaware corporation.

Visit our website at www.skyhorsepublishing.com.

10 9 8 7 6 5 4 3 2 1

Library of Congress Cataloging-in-Publication Data is available on file.

Cover design by Daniel Brount
Cover illustration by Serge Seidlitz

Print ISBN: 978-1-5107-5186-6
Ebook ISBN: 978-1-5107-5190-3

Printed in China

Contents

Foreword ix

Introduction: Lay of the Land xi

   A Critical Biological System No One's Ever Heard Of xv

   Inside *Healing with Cannabis* xv

   Onward xv

Part 1. The Endocannabinoid System 1

Chapter 1. Evolution, Revolution 3

   First, About Cannabis 3

   The Evolution Begins 6

   People and Cannabis Cross Paths 8

Chapter 2. The Endocannabinoid System Discovered 11

   From Fish to People 12

   The Modern Era Begins 13

   Cannabinoid Receptors Discovered 15

   Endocannabinoids Discovered 17

   Enzymes, the Final Element 18

   Raphael Mechoulam: In His Own Words 19

   The Endocannabinoid System Does *What*? 20

   Protective for Brain and Body 24

Chapter 3. The Basic Machinery of Everyday Life 27

   The Endocannabinoids 28

   CB1, CB2, and Other Cannabinoid Receptors 31

   Endocannabinoid Enzymes 46

   "Relax, Eat, Sleep, Forget, and Protect" 47

Chapter 4. Two Main Cannabinoids—THC and CBD 51

   Delta-9-Tetrahydrocannabinol (THC) 52

   Cannabidiol (CBD) 56

Chapter 5. More Cannabinoids, Terpenes, and the Entourage Effect ... 65

   A Few More Cannabinoids 65

The Influence of Cannabis Terpenes   71

Making Cannabinoids and Terpenes   72

The Entourage Effect   76

Chapter 6. The ECS in Balance and Deficiency   **78**

Other Ways to Modulate the Endocannabinoid System   79

Endocannabinoid Deficiency   84

Part 2. Cannabis as Medicine   89

Chapter 7. Medical Cannabis and the Law   **91**

Dominoes Fall   92

Legal in Some States, Illegal in All States   93

Roadblocks for Cannabis Research   94

Chapter 8. Cannabis Medicine: Who Has Access?   **100**

A Big Problem for Public Health   100

Getting Around Barriers to Medical Cannabis   103

Better than Nothing and Maybe Better than That   106

"If This Were Any Other Drug . . ."   108

Chapter 9. Cannabinoids for Inflammation, Stress, and PTSD   **112**

Inflammation: An Immune Response   113

ECS Signaling Collapse: Chronic Stress   115

ECS Signaling Collapse: Chronic Inflammation   117

Cannabinoids, Inflammation, and Mood   118

Posttraumatic Stress Disorder   120

Chapter 10. Cannabinoids for Brain Trauma and Neurodegeneration   **134**

Cannabinoids for Stroke and Brain Trauma   134

Cannabinoids and Other Brain Injuries   137

Cannabinoids and Neurodegeneration   140

Cannabinoids and Alzheimer's Disease   145

Cannabinoids and Parkinson's and Huntington's Diseases   158

Cannabinoids and Amyotrophic Lateral Sclerosis   168

Cannabinoids and Multiple Sclerosis   176

Neurodegenerative Diseases: Future Perspectives   185

Chapter 11. Cannabinoids, Chronic Pain, and Other Inflammatory Disorders   **188**

    Cannabinoids and Chronic Pain   188

    Cannabinoids, Pain, and Arthritis   195

    Cannabinoids, Rheumatoid Arthritis, and Fibromyalgia   202

    Cannabinoids and Inflammatory Bowel Diseases   205

Chapter 12. Cannabinoids, Mood Disorders, and Addiction   **213**

    The Endocannabinoid System in Depression   214

    The Endocannabinoid System and Psychiatric Illness   220

    Cannabinoids and Schizophrenia   225

    Cannabinoids and Addiction   233

    The Endocannabinoid System and Addiction Treatment   236

    Cannabinoids and Alternative Opioid Addiction Treatments   239

Chapter 13. Cannabinoids and Cancer   **242**

    Cannabinoids and Cancer in the Clinic | Dr. Donald Abrams   243

    The Landscape of Medical Cannabis and Cancer   246

    Cannabinoids and Antitumor Effects   248

    Cannabinoids and Other Kinds of Cancers   253

    Cannabinoids in Cancer Treatment   256

    Cannabinoids and Cancer in the Clinic | Dr. Dustin Sulak   258

Resources   **263**

Index   **266**

Foreword

Cannabis is one of the most studied plants of all time. Prohibiting its use, first with the Stamp Act of 1937 and then with the "War on Drugs" in the Nixon era, the United States has attempted to keep cannabis forbidden from the botanical medicine that it has been for thousands of generations. I have been a physician specializing in cannabis medicine for more than twenty years, though for forty years I have considered cannabis a therapeutic option.

Long before we understood the endocannabinoid system (ECS), I followed much of the research designed and funded by the US government through the National Institute on Drug Abuse (NIDA), an organization whose mission is to be the authority on drugs of abuse.

Fortunes have been spent looking for harm and investigating possible therapeutic interventions aimed at those using cannabis. Early research led to the discovery of the ECS, providing insights across nearly all disciplines in biology and medicine. Research findings that suggest harm are inevitably followed by evidence refuting the assertions of harm and even supporting the use of cannabis for many conditions.

Evidence of harm remains elusive and controversial at best. The bias of harm-based research continues to misinform many citizens and lawmakers worldwide who, in turn, shun cannabis as a dangerous and addictive drug. The results of such research are cautions and forbidding its use, as well as punishing users with restrictions, fines, and incarceration. This is the world of cannabis pioneers, both patients and clinicians.

The reference list in this book is truly a Who's Who of the principal investigators and their research in cannabinoid science and medicine for the past few decades. The same tools of the information age that bring us headlines of harm and deceptive information about cannabis also afford unprecedented access to the research into cannabis that occurs worldwide.

The research findings of many of the key contributors to this story are reviewed by Pellerin with skill and balance in a way that simplifies what has proven to be a very complex story. This book is an excellent resource for comprehending cannabinoid science.

While allopathic medicine has been stuck in the reductionist model of designing and marketing single-molecule patentable medicines, cannabinoid scientists are learning that the whole plant outperforms isolated cannabis compounds. The obvious benefit is to focus on modulating the ECS in pursuit of therapies for almost all diseases affecting humans, including pain; seizure disorders; cancer; obesity/metabolic syndrome; diabetes and its complications; autism; neurodegenerative, inflammatory, liver, gastrointestinal, and skin diseases; and psychiatric disorders, among many others.

Research has discovered fascinating details about the effect of cannabis on the ECS. What remains largely unexplored is the fact that all cultivars of cannabis are different from one another; the therapeutic opportunities from the different cannabinoids, terpenes, and flavonoids of cannabis are only beginning to be elucidated. It remains outside of the mission of NIDA to explore the medicinal value of cannabis and to move on to the clinical trials so badly needed to optimize cannabis therapy. Beyond prohibition, we lack the vision and the mandate to study the therapeutic effects of cannabis for the medicine that it is.

Even the enlightened nations that have legalized the adult or medical use of cannabis have failed to appreciate the diversity of cannabis, and, unfortunately, allowed the commercialization of cannabis to limit the chemovars available—not to mention, the costs and taxation putting these medicines out of reach of many in need. Concurrently, the enlightened public has learned by word of mouth of cannabis and its myriad uses for fun, love, laughter, and the serious task of alleviating suffering.

Healing with Cannabis presents this broad foundation of knowledge so the reader can make his or her own decision about this wondrous botanical medicine.

—Jeffrey Hergenrather, MD

Healing with Cannabis is about medical cannabis and a little-known but ancient biological system—the endocannabinoid (en-doe-can-nab-in-noid) system, part of all vertebrates—that allows cannabis to affect body and brain, health and disease. It's also about why medical cannabis can help treat so many illnesses, and how the laws in place nationwide govern—and in many cases constrain—its use.

Through interviews with some of the most knowledgeable cannabinoid scientists, the book describes research and clinical trials that explain what's known so far about how cannabis works to relieve pain, anxiety, stress, and inflammation, and its specific effects in brain trauma, multiple sclerosis, inflammatory bowel disorders, neurodegenerative conditions like Parkinson's disease, and much more. It also describes, in these early days of medical cannabis programs in a growing

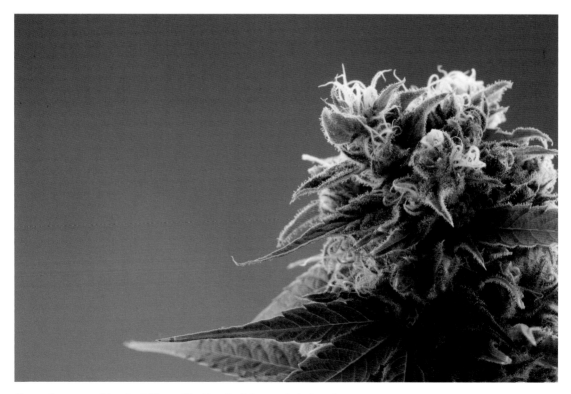

Flowering cannabis plant (From Shutterstock by anointedone)

number of states and US territories, why it's so hard for *everyone* who could benefit from cannabis medicines—not just those who suffer from serious diseases—to access medical cannabis.

For *Healing with Cannabis*, these scientists and healers lent their voices to the story of how cannabis helps treat disorders covered in the book. And I help explain the language of a complex cannabinoid science so most people can understand what medical cannabis does and doesn't do, and where the science stands. Still, some of the words in these sections are long and hard to pronounce (ow).

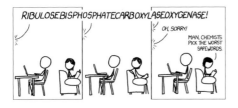

xkcd.com cartoon, RuBisCO 1039 (Courtesy xkcd .com).

But as someone who wants accurate information about medical cannabis, it's worth your time to be familiar with some of the technical terms used in cannabis research and treatment. They will help you understand the research, and why and how to buy and use the products available—especially if you see them on the internet, where scientifically sound medical cannabis information isn't always available and where some not-so-great products are hawked.

Good products—full-spectrum (meaning those that come from the whole plant, with all the cannabinoids and terpenes and flavonoids the plant makes, which all contribute to cannabis health effects) and broad spectrum (like CBD and other extracts that lose some of the original compounds in processing) products—are increasingly available online to anyone who wants them. You'll read more about this later. At the end of the book and on my website (cherylpellerinscience.com), I offer excellent, reliable resources.

In *Healing with Cannabis*, you'll find that a lot of what cannabinoid scientists know, especially about the most serious diseases, is coming from their work in the lab and with animal models of disease. That's because the law that makes cannabis federally illegal has also, for the past fifty years, severely limited research and research funding into the plant's complex biochemistry, pharmacology, and use as a wide-ranging medicine.

In the United States this has hindered the kinds of clinical trials (those with human subjects) that allow cannabis results from the lab and animal models to be confirmed as safe and effective in people. But, like everything else that's changing where cannabis is concerned, a growing number of clinical trials are being conducted for each illness, and a growing body of case reports and recommendations are available from doctors (you'll hear from some of them, too)

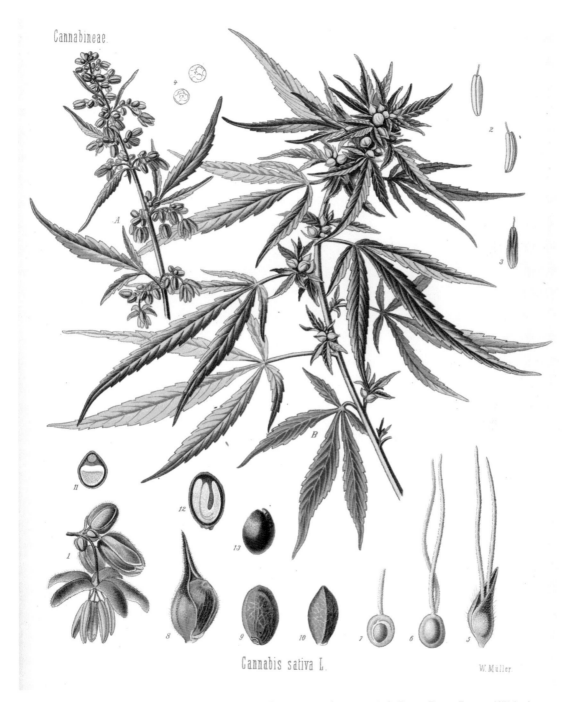

Cannabineae.

A

B

Cannabis sativa L.

W. Müller

Drawing of *Cannabis sativa* by botanist Walther Otto Müller (1833–1887). From Franz Eugen Köhler's *Medizinal-Pflantzen*, published and copyrighted by Gera-Untermhaus, FE Köhler in 1887 (1883–1914). (From Wikimedia Commons. This file is in the public domain)

who use medical cannabis to help their patients.

Medical cannabis, widely available, will change the face of public health. But treating illnesses with cannabinoid medicine can be complicated, and the products don't come with user manuals. Each patient and illness reacts differently to cannabis, its psychoactive (intoxicating) constituent, delta-9 tetrahydrocannabinol (THC), its nonintoxicating constituent, cannabidiol (CBD), and all its other constituents, not all of which have been identified or studied. This complexity, and the drug laws and stigma surrounding cannabis, are keeping medical cannabis from all who would benefit from its therapeutic effects.

The situation won't improve for patients as long as cannabis is legal in some states and federally illegal in all states, and until all jurisdictions—not just the thirty-four states, the District of Columbia, and the US territories of Guam, Puerto Rico, and the US Virgin Islands that have comprehensive public medical cannabis programs—allow access to medical cannabis to anyone who wants or needs it (as California alone does), rather than making it available

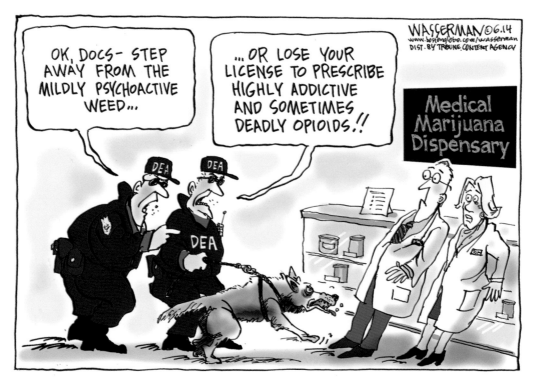

Dan Wasserman editorial cartoon for the *Boston Globe* (Licensed for use in the book by the Tribute Content Agency)

only by doctor's recommendation and only for certain illnesses.

A Critical Biological System No One's Ever Heard Of

The endocannabinoid system (ECS) is why medical cannabis affects so many different illnesses, and cannabis works in the body because ECS elements are everywhere in the body and brain. For hundreds of millions of years, for vertebrates all over the planet, the endocannabinoid system has been balancing health and disease by maintaining homeostasis (balance) among the body's biochemical and physiological systems. But don't feel bad if you've never heard of it. As you'll see, you're not alone.

Despite all the ancient history, scientists only realized in the late 1990s that discoveries they'd been making since 1964 were connected to an ancient biological system that they eventually called the endocannabinoid system. At that time, two researchers in Israel discovered that THC was the intoxicating constituent of cannabis.

Since then, cannabinoid researchers around the world have sought to understand the system, to fully grasp its role in health and disease, and to use the ECS and cannabinoids to help people with health problems twenty-first-century medicine can't safely fix. Yet today the system is all but unknown among most of the nation's population, including many physicians.

Inside *Healing with Cannabis*

Part 1, "The Endocannabinoid System," explains the ECS itself—its origins in the earliest forms of life on Earth, the evolution of its elements, and the discoveries, millions of years later, of more of its elements. These chapters also discuss endocannabinoids—the body's own cannabinoids—and how they work in the body and brain, as well as cannabis and its constituents and the range of health benefits they confer throughout the body and brain.

Part 2, "Cannabis as Medicine," describes state and federal laws that govern medical cannabis and how they affect access to the plant's health benefits. It also details specific illnesses and what researchers say about how medical cannabis works for each one. You'll also hear from doctors who use medical cannabis every day to treat illnesses and what they've learned from that treatment.

At the end of the book you'll find a resources section with recommended medical cannabis organizations, education programs, and websites.

Onward

Like everything else in the realm of medical cannabis, the products and websites and research I've written about here change, mostly for the better, so fast you can't believe it. So if something in the book or in the marketplace doesn't match your needs today, keep searching—you'll find it.

If your state doesn't allow medical cannabis yet, try some of the good broad-spectrum CBD products that are increasingly available online, and follow the cannabis doctors' dosing rule: start low and go slow. Remember that lots of organizations work every day to try to make medical cannabis available to anyone who needs or wants it.

In the meantime, despite the legal and regulatory blockade, researchers continue to learn about this ancient biological system that's been evolutionarily conserved across a billion years, and the singular plant that's vitalizing the medicine of the future.

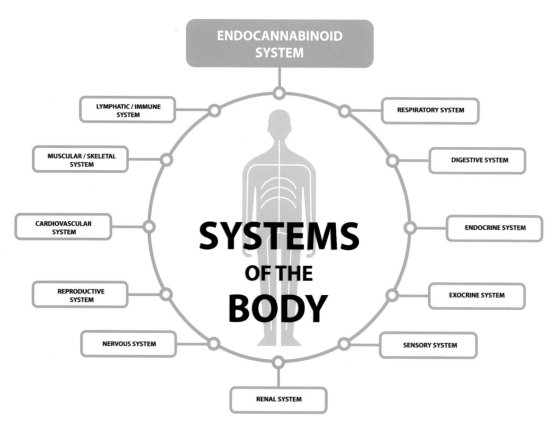

The body's endocannabinoid system (From Shutterstock by Image seller in w)

Part 1
The Endocannabinoid System

In which we learn about the body's endocannabinoid system (ECS). The ECS is how and why cannabis works in the body and brain to treat a range of health problems. We'll explore the system's ancient beginnings, its essential elements, and some of the most well known, so far, of the 565 cannabis constituents and their functions. And we'll also explore the endocannabinoid system's evolutionary emergence as an internal homeostatic regulator of nearly every function in the body and brain.

Chapter 1
Evolution, Revolution

To begin, for those who aren't versed in the complexities of cannabis, the female plant is one whose flower is unlike any other, in more ways than one. The cannabis flower is a biochemical cooperative of working parts that together produce its more than 565 compounds, including the 120 cannabinoids that only cannabis can make.

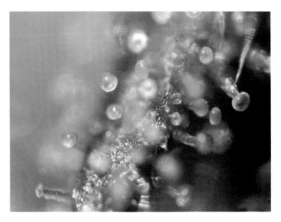

Female cannabis flower with microscopic view of trichomes (From Shutterstock by mikeledray)

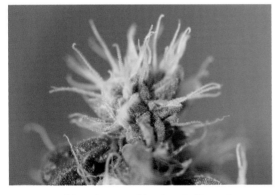

Close-up of female cannabis plant in flowering phase (From Shutterstock by noxnorthys)

First, About Cannabis

On the female cannabis plant, mushroom-shaped glandular trichomes (try-komes) cover the plant's main fan leaves and flowers. Resin spheres are on top of the trichome stalks.

Inside the spheres, the plant's main products—cannabinoids (can-nab-in-noids) and other chemical constituents called terpenes (tur-peens) and flavonoids (flave-on-noids), and others—are manufactured. Terpenes arise in the essential oils of many plants, including pine and citrus trees. Flavonoids are plant chemicals in fruits and vegetables.

Plant biologist Jonathan Page of Anandia Laboratories in Canada, speaking at the 2017 International Association for Cannabis as Medicine Conference in Cologne, Germany, said that cannabis resin, produced in the glandular trichomes of female inflorescences (a plant's flower head, including stems, stalks, and flowers), is the main source

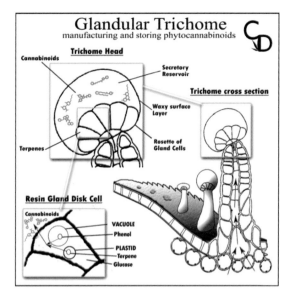

Drawing of a cannabis glandular trichome. (Courtesy Owen Smith)

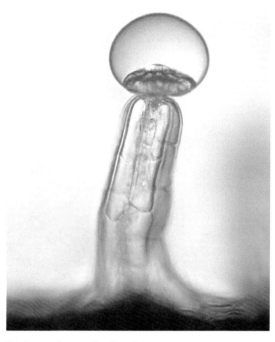

Trichome in profile: For this extreme close-up the trichome was temporarily mounted in glycerol and viewed in transmitted light. (Courtesy ©David Potter 2009)

of cannabinoids, which are unique to the cannabis plant.[1]

Glandular trichomes also produce terpenes, which are responsible for much of the scent of cannabis flowers and contribute to the unique flavor qualities of cannabis products, J. K. Booth and colleagues wrote in a 2017 *PLoS One* paper.[2]

In the cannabis plant, Page said during his presentation, trichomes are specialized epidermal cells, and glandular trichomes produce cannabinoids, terpenes, flavonoids, and other constituents and store them. He added, "Within that glandular head there is a disc of secretory cells, and these are essentially the biochemical factory of the cannabis plant." Page also noted that the secretory cells themselves are not photosynthetic—they don't absorb light and make sugar.[3]

"They're just receiving nutrients and carbon sources up from the leaf or the flower and turning them into

1   Page, J. E. Anandia Laboratories, Vancouver BC, Canada. Presentation at International Association for Cannabis as Medicine, Conference on Cannabinoids as Medicine, Cologne, Germany, September 29–30, 2017.
2   Booth, J. K., J. E. Page, J. Bohmann. 2017. "Terpene synthases from Cannabis sativa." *PLoS One*. 12(3):e0173911 (doi: 10.1371/journal.pone.0173911).
3   Page, J. E.

cannabinoids and terpenes," the plant biologist said. "And then they're pumped out of that secretory disk . . . and . . . into a secretory cavity that's bordered by the cuticle—that's sort of the skin of the plant—and they pump the cannabinoids and terpenes . . . into a cavity beneath the cuticle. So in essence," he said, "[the glandular head is] a balloon full of bioactive metabolites."[4]

To date, researchers have identified 120 cannabinoids (Dr. Mahmoud ElSohly, research professor and professor of pharmaceutics at the University of Mississippi, email communication November 9, 2018), but for now the two main cannabinoids are delta-9 tetrahydrocannabinol (THC, tetra-hydro-can-nab-in-all), the main psychoactive constituent in cannabis, and cannabidiol (CBD, cannab-ih-dye-all), the main nonpsychoactive constituent. Plant cannabinoids also are called phytocannabinoids, *phyto* (fight-o) being from the Greek word for "plant."

Terpenes, according to Ethan Russo, MD, are essential oil components that form the largest group of plant chemicals. He is a board-certified neurologist and founder and chief executive officer of CannabisResearch.org.

More than 200 terpenes have been reported in the plant, Russo wrote, and

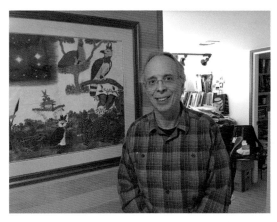

Dr. Ethan Russo, a board-certified neurologist and founder and chief executive officer of credo-science.com. (Courtesy Cheryl Pellerin)

they, not cannabinoids, produce the cannabis aroma. Terpenes like limonene and pinene in cannabis flowers protect the plant from insects, and bitter terpenes like beta-caryophyllene in the lower leaves protect it from grazing animals.[5]

Genetics control terpene composition in the plant, and terpenes are pharmacologically versatile, Russo wrote, adding that they are lipophilic (dissolve in fats) and that they interact with cell membranes, neuron and muscle ion channels, neurotransmitter receptors, G protein-coupled receptors, enzymes, and more. Animal studies indicate that terpenoids (terpenes changed by drying the flowers) may be "relevant to the effects of cannabis."[6]

4   Page, J. E.
5   Russo, E. B. "Taming THC: Potential cannabis synergy and phytocannabinoid-terpenoid entourage effects." *Br J Pharmacol*. 163:1344–1364 (doi10.1111/j.1476-5381.2011.01238.x).
6   Ibid.

In their 2017 *Advances in Pharmacological Science* publication,[7] Russo and biochemist and medical cannabis safety expert Dr. Jahan Marcu wrote in detail about cannabis pharmacology and the contributions to cannabis's physical and medical effects by some of the less-well-known phytocannabinoids and terpenoids.

"Analytical chemistry has revealed a rich and abundant 'pharmacological treasure trove' in the plant," they wrote, quoting Professor Raphael Mechoulam's 2005 *British Journal of Pharmacology* paper, "Plant cannabinoids: A neglected pharmacological treasure trove." Mechoulam, an organic chemist and professor of medicinal chemistry at The Hebrew University of Jerusalem, is known worldwide as the grandfather of modern cannabis research.[8]

Mechoulam and colleagues in Israel kicked off the golden age of cannabis research, Russo and Marcu wrote, by isolating and synthesizing CBD, THC, and other phytocannabinoids, and Mechoulam's work continues. Today, they added, "there are some 100 clinical studies and thousands of articles on the pharmacology and pharmacodynamics of cannabis and its influence on how humans eat, sleep, heal, and learn."[9]

The Evolution Begins

No matter what you know about marijuana, there's a bigger story—ancient and far-reaching. Ultimately it's about the medical use of the flowering plant whose botanical name is cannabis, but this chapter shows what's made it possible, for the past 5,000 years and right up to now, for healers and physicians to use cannabis, in all its forms, to treat in patients a broad and unlikely range of illnesses—maybe all of them.

What's made it possible is the endocannabinoid system, the ancient biological system whose elements—endocannabinoids (cannabinoid-like molecules made in the body's cells), enzymes, and receptors—work throughout the body and brain to balance health and disease. In a recent paper on cannabis pharmacology,[10] Russo and Marcu called the ECS "perhaps the most significant human biological scientific discovery in the last 30 years."

Among the three main endocannabinoid system elements, enzymes are the most ancient, according to Dr. Maurice Elphick, a biologist and professor of physiology and neuroscience in the School of Biological and Chemical Sciences at Queen Mary University–London. It all started well over a billion years ago, when one primordial

---

7   Russo, E. B., and J. Marcu "Cannabis Pharmacology: The Usual Suspects and a Few Promising Leads." *Adv Pharmacol* 80:67–134. (doi: 10.1016/bs.apha.2017.03.004).
8   Ibid.
9   Ibid.
10 Ibid.

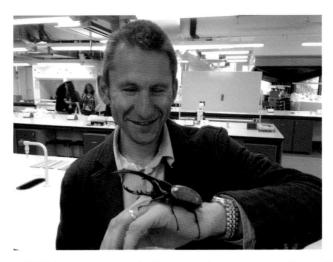

Prof. Maurice Elphick, professor of physiology and neuroscience, Queen Mary University of London, with a Hercules beetle (*Dynastes hercules*). (Photo courtesy Dr. David Hone, senior lecturer and biology program director, Queen Mary University of London.)

enzyme-generated fatty acid arose in the earliest forms of life on Earth, possibly bacteria. Some time later, compounds like the endocannabinoids anandamide and 2-AG evolved out into the world, Elphick said in a May 2017 interview.

"The molecules that we call endocannabinoids, like . . . 2-AG and anandamide, these so-called endocannabinoids themselves are very simple lipid [fatty-acid derivative] molecules, and in principle they could be synthesized in cells of almost any eukaryotic organism—plants, animals, and [single-celled] eukaryotic organisms," Elphick explained. "So there's nothing about their structure which suggests they couldn't in principle be synthesized in most forms of life."

Then, at least 590 million years ago, a primordial cannabinoid receptor evolved out into the world.[11] At first there was only one receptor, and genome-sequencing technology helped present-day researchers up here in the future figure out that only vertebrates, and two kinds of invertebrate, eventually came equipped from the factory with cannabinoid-type receptors.

"If we collectively think of ourselves as being the vertebrates," Elphick said, "being in a family along with fish and reptiles and amphibians, then our closest relatives are marine animals called sea squirts, which belong to a group of animals called chordates, together with an animal called an amphioxus [am-fee-ox-us]."

---

11 Onaivi, E. S., T. Sugiura, and V. Di Marzo, eds. *Endocannabinoids: The Brain and Body's Marijuana and Beyond.* CRC Press, 2005.

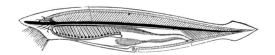

Amphioxus, vintage engraved illustration. La Vie dans la nature, 1890. (From Shutterstock by Morphart Creation)

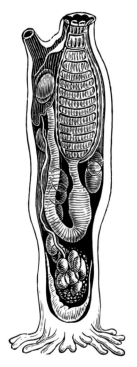

Sea squirt (*Ciona intestinalis*), vintage line drawing or engraving illustration (From Shutterstock by Morphart Creation)

But sea squirts and amphioxus had one receptor, not two as we vertebrates do.

"It's clear what happened is that during evolution that single receptor gene you find in a sea squirt or amphioxus duplicated and gave rise to [the main cannabinoid receptors] CB1 and CB2," Elphick explained. "Some would call it CBX or something like that . . . And when you look at the amino acid sequence, you can see that it's a bit like CB1 and a bit like CB2." For some reason, he said, "this particular receptor protein

acquired the ability to bind the [endocannabinoid] chemicals quite well."

That ability established the interaction between the endocannabinoids and what was the beginning of a cannabinoid receptor, Elphick said.

"Once that interaction occurred," he added, "then it would over time have strengthened and ultimately given rise to this [endocannabinoid] signaling system that's present in the brain but also in other parts of the body."

So, beginning sometime after 590 million years ago, all vertebrates would have come equipped with the endocannabinoids, the cannabinoid receptors, and the specific enzymes that make up the whole endocannabinoid system.

People and Cannabis Cross Paths

Within the past 100 million years or so, flowering plants evolved, Elphick said. But the flowering plant called cannabis, in the family *Cannabaceae*, evolved in a much shorter time, no earlier than about 34 million years ago.[12] Enter early primates around 4.4 million years ago, and then early humans (*Homo sapiens*) about 100,000

12 McPartland, J. M., and J. Nicholson. "Using parasite databases to identify potential nontarget hosts of biological control organisms." *New Zealand J Botany* 41(4):699–706.

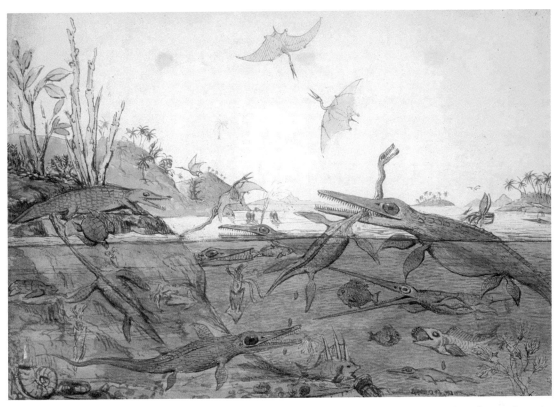

Duria Antiquior, a 1830 watercolor by geologist Henry de la Beche depicting life in ancient Dorset based on fossils found by Mary Anning. (From Wikimedia Commons. This image is in the public domain.)

years ago, and they all came equipped with full-on endocannabinoid systems.

We'll never know what or who among the endocannabinoid-system-endowed vertebrates was first to stumble on cannabis, take a bite or heat up a brew of the interesting-looking flowering plant, and experience THC, the major psychoactive intoxicating cannabinoid in cannabis, in all its glory.

As it relates to cannabis, psychoactivity, for those unfamiliar with it, has been described by Dr. Ken Mackie, of the Department of Psychological and

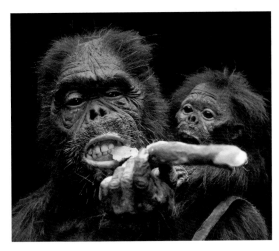

Prehistoric people (From Shutterstock by E.G. Pors)

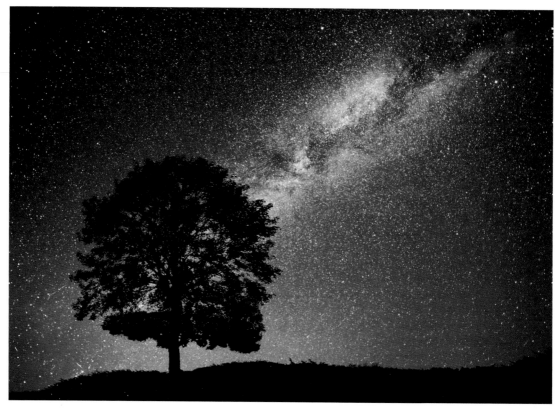

Tree and stars, representing psychoactivity (From Shutterstock by Standret)

Brain Sciences at Indiana University–Bloomington, as "the mild euphoria, altered perceptions, sense of relaxation and sociability that often, but not always, accompany recreational cannabis use."[13]

Because cannabidiol (CBD) isn't intoxicating, no one back then would have known that they also were experiencing the many positive health effects of CBD, the other major cannabinoid in cannabis, and all the other cannabis compounds.

And they wouldn't have known—even up here in the twenty-first century, some people, probably most of us, still don't know—that the only reason cannabis works in the brain and body is because there's an endocannabinoid system that lets it work.

The. Only. Reason.

---

13 Mackie, K. "Understanding cannabinoid psychoactivity with mouse genetic models." *PLoS Biol* 5(10):e280 (doi: 10.1371/journal.pbio.0050280).

Chapter 2
The Endocannabinoid System Discovered

Travel and communication were a challenge 5,000 years ago, but word got around about cannabis, and not just about its unexpected intoxicating effects. Ancient cultures everywhere, each with their own names for the plant, discovered that cannabis was useful in spiritual rites and for a bunch of physical and mental conditions.

The ancient Chinese liked the female cannabis plant's flowers and resin—where cannabinoids and other constituents are made—for menstrual fatigue, rheumatism, malaria, the vitamin B1 deficiency disorder called beriberi, constipation, and absentmindedness. Writers of the Chinese pharmacopeia at that time also noted, maybe in a nod to the plant's psychoactivity, that patients who ate too many cannabis seeds could see demons, and that if anyone consumed cannabis seeds consistently over time they might be able to communicate with spirits.[1]

The Assyrians, who ruled large parts of the Middle East three thousand years ago, also liked cannabis for spiritual rites and medical conditions, and they left hundreds of clay tablets describing its use. *Papaver somniferum*, the opium

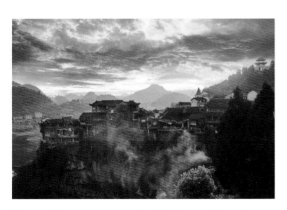

Furong Zhen was an ancient Chinese village in Hunan province. (From Shutterstock by Pavel Dvorak Jr.)

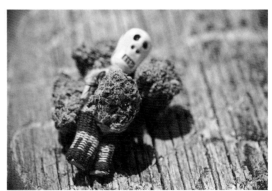

Authors of the Chinese pharmacopeia wrote that patients who ate too many cannabis seeds could see demons. (Shutterstock by Roxana Gonzales)

---

1 Hanus, L. O. "Pharmacological and therapeutic secrets of plant and brain (endo)cannabinoids." *Med Res Rev* 29(2):213–71 (doi: 10.1002/med.20135).

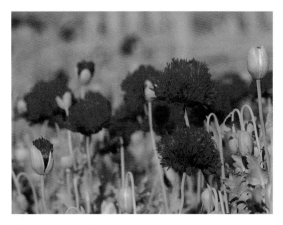

Papaver somniferum, known as poppy tears or *Lachryma papaveris.* (From Shutterstock by Emilio100)

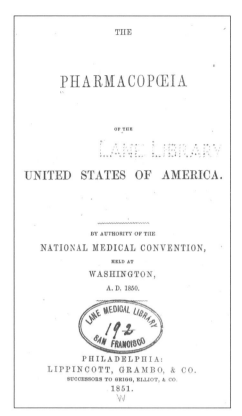

Title page, U.S. Pharmacopeia 1850/1851 (Courtesy U.S. Pharmacopeia)

plant, also was one of their important drugs. In later chapters we'll discuss the links among opioids, cannabis, and endocannabinoids.

Over time, the practice of using cannabis to treat medical and spiritual problems of all kinds spread to the ancient Egyptians, practitioners of the Brahman religion in India, the Persians, northern Mediterranean societies, and many others.[2]

From Fish to People

Thousands of years later, on the other side of the world, using cannabis was briefly not illegal in the United States.

Beginning in 1850, the *US Pharmacopeia* listed cannabis as a treatment for neuralgia, tetanus, typhus, cholera, rabies, dysentery, alcoholism, opioid addiction, anthrax, leprosy, incontinence, gout, convulsive disorders, tonsillitis, insanity, excessive menstrual bleeding, uterine bleeding,[3] and an amazing range of other serious disorders, many of which—you know, opioid addiction, alcoholism, insanity, for example—could benefit today from a plant that has few side effects and a five-thousand-year record of safe medical use.

---

2   Mechoulam, R., and S. Ben-Shabat. "From gan-zi-gun-nu to anandamide and 2-arachidonoyl-glycerol: the ongoing story of cannabis." *Nat Prod Rep* 16(2):131–43.

3   Boire, R. C., and K. Feeny. *Medical Marijuana Law.* Berkeley, CA: Ronin Publishing, 2007.

No one yet knew why or how cannabis worked, but that didn't stop anyone from using it as medicine, or for any other reason.

In 1964—after 600 million years of vertebrates with endocannabinoid systems—the first hint surfaced that something besides getting high and treating a ridiculous range of illnesses was going on with cannabis. Up until then, and for another couple of decades, almost no one had a clue that there might be a network of receptors in the brain and body that, along with the other ECS elements, was responsible for the effects of cannabis on those who smoked it, and for the function of nearly every physiological and biological process in every vertebrate, from fish to people.

The Modern Era Begins

Researchers had been working since the 1930s and '40s to isolate active compounds in the cannabis plant, Dr. Raphael Mechoulam and Dr. Shimon Ben-Shabat wrote in a 1999 *Natural Products Reports* paper.[4] But it wasn't until 1964 and improvements in laboratory technology that Mechoulam and Dr. Yehiel Gaoni at Hebrew University–Jerusalem in Israel "were able to separate numerous new cannabinoids, a term which we suggested then and which has received wide acceptance,"

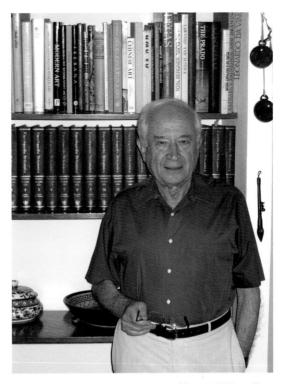

Prof. Raphael Mechoulam, 2009 (From Wikimedia Commons by User:Tzahi, used with permission)

Mechoulam wrote. The work led them to identify one of the cannabinoids as the intoxicating compound in cannabis.

They called it delta-1 tetrahydrocannabinol (THC).[5] Later, because of chemical naming rules, it was changed to delta-9 THC, according to a 2007 published conversation with Mechoulam.[6]

"In a sense," Maurice Elphick said during his May 2017 interview, "that was the beginning of the modern era,

4   Mechoulam, R., and S. Ben-Shabat.
5   Ibid.
6   "A Conversation with Raphael Mechoulam." *Addiction* 102:887–93 (doi:10.1111/j.1360–0443 .2007.01795.x).

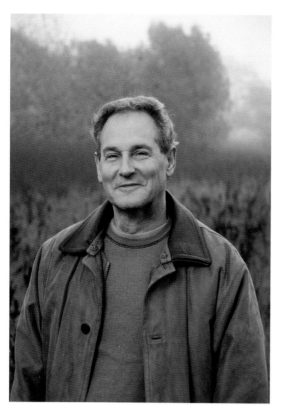

Martin A. Lee, journalist, author, and director of Project CBD. (Courtesy Martin A. Lee). Inset, project CBD logo (Courtesy Martin A. Lee)

wrote, "In the two decades following the identification and synthesis of THC by Mechoulam and his colleague Y. Gaoni in Israel in 1964, scientists learned a great deal about the pharmacology, biochemistry, and clinical effects of cannabis. But no one really knew how it worked— what it actually did inside the brain on a molecular level to alter consciousness, stimulate appetite, dampen nausea, quell seizures, and relieve pain. No one understood how smoked marijuana could stop an asthma attack in seconds, not minutes. No one knew why it lifted one's mood."[7]

It wasn't until around 1984, twenty years later, Elphick said, that researchers began to get indications about what the cannabinoid receptor was like, at least biochemically.

They knew there had to be at least one receptor because that's how drugs or plants or compounds work in the body and brain—through receptors on cell membranes or inside cells.

In the mid-1980s, according to Professor Roger Pertwee in a 2006 *British Journal of Pharmacology* article, Dr. Allyn Howlett and her graduate student William Devane at St. Louis University– Missouri did groundbreaking work that offered conclusive evidence of the existence of a cannabinoid receptor.[8]

inasmuch as once we knew what the psychoactive constituent of cannabis was, it became feasible to start to think about how it works and find molecular components that it's interacting with."

In a 2010 article, author, journalist, and director Martin A. Lee of Project CBD, an expert website dedicated to medical cannabis and cannabinoid science,

---

7   Lee, M. A. "The Discovery of the Endocannabinoid System. The Prop 215 Era." 2010. PDF: http://www.beyondthc.com/wp-content/uploads/2012/07/eCBSystemLee.pdf. Accessed 12/8/2017.
8   Pertwee, R. G. "Cannabinoid pharmacology: the first 66 years." *Br J Pharmacol* 147(Suppl 1):S163–71 (doi: 10.1038/sj.bjp.0706406).

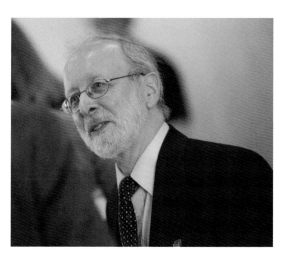
Prof. Roger Pertwee, biochemist and emeritus professor in the School of Medical Sciences, Institute of Medical Sciences, University of Aberdeen-Scotland. (Courtesy Wellcome Trust)

In the period from 1990 onward, Elphick said, researchers gradually discovered the molecular components of the endocannabinoid system.

Cannabinoid Receptors Discovered

One of the receptors was confirmed in 1990, Pertwee wrote, when Dr. Tom Bonner's lab at the US National Institute of Mental Health cloncd a rat cannabinoid receptor, later called CB1. In 1991, Dr. C. M. Gérard and colleagues at the Institute of Interdisciplinary Research in Brussels, Belgium, cloned a human CB1 receptor.[9] Then in 1993, Dr. Sean Munro's lab at the MRC Laboratory of Molecular Biology in Cambridge, England, cloned a second cannabinoid receptor, CB2.[10]

CB1 and CB2 are G protein-coupled receptors (GPCRs), the largest and most diverse group of cell membrane-embedded receptors in eukaryotes, (the domain that includes animals, people, plants, and any other life form whose cells have a membrane-enclosed nucleus that contains genetic material).[11]

GPCRs play a role in many brain and body functions, and at the cell surface they get signals from light energy, peptides, sugars, proteins, and lipids.[12] The two major endocannabinoids are also lipids, and they were discovered within a couple of years of the cannabinoid receptors.

Here's what the *Nature* education website has to say about them: GPCRs

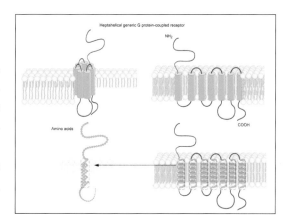
Typical structure of a G protein-coupled receptor, illustration (From Shutterstock by ellepigrafica)

9 Ibid.
10 Ibid.
11 Nature Publishing Group, Scitable: https://www.nature.com/scitable. Accessed 12/8/2017.
12 Ibid.

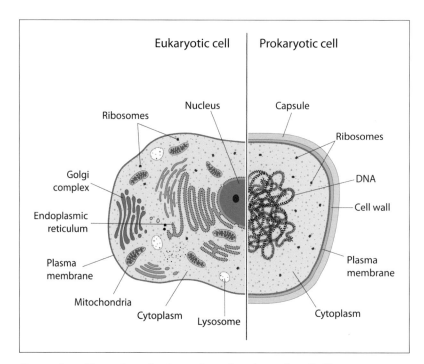

Eukaryotic cell | Prokaryotic cell

Ribosomes
Nucleus
Capsule
Ribosomes
Golgi complex
DNA
Endoplasmic reticulum
Cell wall
Plasma membrane
Plasma membrane
Mitochondria
Cytoplasm
Lysosome
Cytoplasm

Comparison illustration of eukaryotic and prokaryotic cells (From Shutterstock by Aldona Griskeviciene)

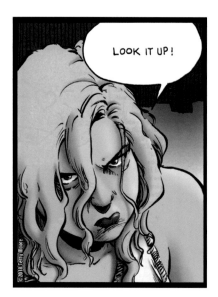

LOOK IT UP!

Terry Moore cartoon, librarian (Courtesy TerryMooreArt.com)

consist of a single polypeptide (a chain of amino acids that form proteins) that's folded into a globular shape and embedded in a cell membrane. These receptors have seven segments that span the cell membrane and have loops inside and outside the cell. The loops outside the cell form part of the pockets where signaling molecules like endocannabinoids bind to the receptor.[13]

Next we'll discuss the names and functions of the endocannabinoid system elements, which include endocannabinoids, enzymes, and receptors. This is where, as I mentioned, some of the words will be long and hard to pronounce (ow).

13 Ibid.

Thankfully, we have acronyms and that's what I'll use afterward throughout the book. Some illustrations of these ECS elements won't make immediate sense unless you're a cannabinoid researcher or a cell biologist, but they're interesting and I figure you might want to see them anyway.

Endocannabinoids Discovered

In 1992, Dr. William Devane, who with Dr. Allyn Howlett in the mid-1980s had found conclusive evidence of a cannabinoid receptor, was working in Raphael Mechoulam's lab at Hebrew University–Jerusalem with Dr. Lumir Hanus when they discovered, in pig brain tissue, the first natural endocannabinoid. It was the fatty-acid derivative arachidonoyl ethanolamide (AEA), which they called anandamide,[14] the Sanskrit word for supreme joy.[15]

In 1995, also in Mechoulam's lab, Devane and Dr. Shimon Ben-Shabat discovered the second natural endocannabinoid, the fatty-acid derivative 2-arachidonoylglycerol (2-AG), which the lab isolated from canine gut tissue.[16] Also in 1994–1995, a research group led by Dr. Takayuki Sugiura at Teikyo University in

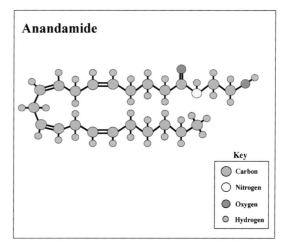

Molecule of the endocannabinoid anandamide (By Ellen Seefelt)

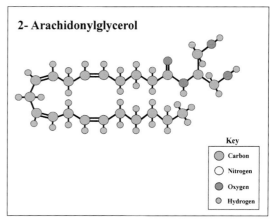

Molecule of the endocannabinoid 2-AG (By Ellen Seefelt)

14 Pertwee, R. G.
15 "A Conversation with Raphael Mechoulam."
16 Mechoulam, R., S. Ben-Shabat, L. Hanuš, et al. "Identification of an endogenous 2-monoglyceride, present in canine gut, that binds to cannabinoid receptors." *Biochem Pharmacol* 50 (1):83–90 (doi:10.1016/0006–2952(95)00109-D).

Japan reported that 2-AG worked at the cannabinoid receptors.[17]

Endocannabinoids have a profile of biological activities similar to that of THC, according to a 2001 *Journal of Cannabis Therapeutics* paper[18] by McPartland and Pruitt, and endocannabinoids explain why people, among other vertebrates, have receptors that are sensitive to cannabis compounds. Plant cannabinoids, they added, are simple mimics of the endogenous (self-produced) cannabinoids.

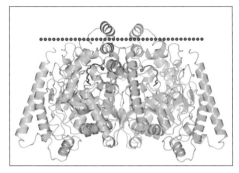

Fatty acid amide hydrolase (FAAH) is the enzyme that degrades anandamide. (Courtesy Orientations of Proteins in Membranes database, Lomize Group, College of Pharmacy, University of Michigan, used with permission)

Enzymes, the Final Element

Soon after 1995—and 1 or 2 billion years after the first enzyme appeared in some of the earliest life on the planet—researchers identified the enzymes involved in synthesizing or degrading the endocannabinoids in the body's cells.

- Fatty acid amide hydrolase (FAAH), which degrades anandamide, its relationship to anandamide reported in 1993.[19]
- Monoglyceride lipase (MAGL or MGL), which degrades 2-AG, its relationship to 2-AG reported in 2002.[20]
- Diacylglycerol lipases (DAGL or DGL alpha and DGL beta), which synthesize 2-AG, their relationship to 2-AG reported in 2003.[21]

---

17 Sugiura, T., S. Kondo, A. Sukagawa, S. Nakane, A. Shinoda, K. Itoh, A. Yamashita, and K. Waku. "2-Arachidonoylglycerol: A possible endogenous cannabinoid receptor ligand in brain." *Biochem Biophys Res Commun* 215(1):89–97 (doi:10.1006/bbrc.1995.2437).

18 McPartland, J. M., and P. Pruitt. "Sourcing the code: Searching for the evolutionary origins of cannabinoid receptors, vanilloid receptors and anandamide." *J Cannabis Ther* 2001:73–103.

19 Deutsch, D. G., and S. A. Chin. "Enzymatic synthesis and degradation of anandamide, a cannabinoid receptor agonist." *Biochem Pharmacol* 46 (5):791–6 (doi:10.1016/0006–2952(93)90486-G).

20 Dinh, T. P., D. Carpenter, F. M. Leslie, T. F. Freund, I. Katona, S. L. Sensi, S. Kathuria, and D. Piomelli. "Brain monoglyceride lipase participating in endocannabinoid inactivation." *PNAS* 160:10819–24 (doi: 10.1073/pnas.152334899).

21 Bisogno, T., F. Howell, G. Williams, A. Minassi, M. G. Cascio, A. Ligresti, I. Matias, A. Schiano-Moriello, P. Paul, E. J. Williams, U. Gangadharan, C. Hobbs, V. Di Marzo, and P. Doherty. "Cloning of the first sn1-DAG lipases points to the spatial and temporal regulation of endocannabinoid signaling in the brain." *J. Cell Biol* 163(3):463–8 (doi:10.1083/jcb.200305129).

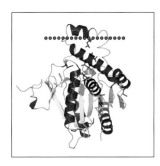

Monoacylglycerol lipase (MAGL) is the enzyme that degrades 2-AG. (Courtesy Orientations of Proteins in Membranes database, Lomize Group, College of Pharmacy, University of Michigan)

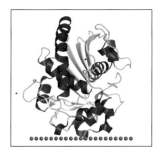

Diacylglycerol lipase (DGL) is the enzyme that biosynthesizes 2-AG. (Courtesy Orientations of Proteins in Membranes database, Lomize Group, College of Pharmacy, University of Michigan)

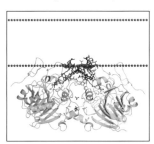

N-acylphosphatidylethanolamine-phospholipase D (just call it NAPE-PLD) is the enzyme that biosynthesizes anandamide. (Courtesy Orientations of Proteins in Membranes database, Lomize Group, College of Pharmacy, University of Michigan)

- N-acylphosphatidyl-ethanolamine-phospholipase D (NAPE-PLD), which synthesizes anandamide, its relationship to anandamide reported in 2004.[22] (And really, don't try to say that.)

All the essential elements of the endocannabinoid system were identified, but a few years passed before the big picture started taking shape.

Raphael Mechoulam: In His Own Words

Throughout this discovery time line of the endocannabinoid system and its elements, Professor Raphael Mechoulam has been at work in his lab at Hebrew University and with colleagues in his lab and around the world. Here, in a June 2019 email, he describes a small part of his body of work.

In 1940, CBD was the second cannabinoid to be isolated after cannabinol (CBN). Mechoulam "re-isolated CBD in 1963 and elucidated its structure," he writes. "In 1964, my colleague Dr. Yehiel Gaoni and I isolated pure THC (I believe for the first time in pure form) and elucidated its structure. We also did that for numerous other plant cannabinoids (cannabigerol, cannabichromene, etc.). We also synthesized most of these molecules.

---

22 Okamoto, Y., J. Morishita, K. Tsuboi, T. Tonai, and N. Ueda. "Molecular characterization of a phospholipase D generating anandamide and its congeners." *J Biol Chem* 279(7):5298–305 (doi:10.1074/jbc.M306642200).

"Over the next few years we worked on the medicinal chemistry, metabolism, pharmacology, and clinical effects (always with colleagues).

"In the early 1990s I invited Bill Devane as a post doc. We first worked on the chemistry needed to possibly identify an endogenous cannabinoid. Together with other workers in my lab and colleagues (in Israel and abroad) we identified the first endogenous cannabinoid (anandamide) in 1992 and a second one in 1995.

"The mammalian body also prepares numerous anandamide-like compounds which are of physiological importance," he concluded. "With colleagues in the US, Canada, Italy, and Israel, we found that one plays a role in brain trauma, another in osteoporosis, a third one in nicotine addiction."

The Endocannabinoid System Does What?

The primordial ECS enzyme didn't appear in bacteria a billion or more years ago just so Mother Nature could be sure that whoever smoked, inhaled, ate, or drank a brew of cannabis a billion years in the future would get high. No. So why was there an evolving endocannabinoid system starting 590 million-ish years before people existed, and about 550 million years before cannabis even appeared on Earth?

"The real turning point came in 2001," Elphick said during his March 2017 interview, "when a group of papers[23] were published that pretty much gave the first indication as to what the physiological role of this endocannabinoid system was in the brain, at least at the level of how cells communicate with each other."

For a hundred years or more, Elphick explained, it had been understood that cells communicated by sending signaling molecules (like neurotransmitters) from one cell to the next, all going in one direction. But, he said, it turned out that endocannabinoids are a class of compounds that communicate mainly backward across the synapse (gap) between cells.

Backward?

I didn't fully appreciate the significance or the purpose of this behavior—what possible reason could endocannabinoids

23 The 2001 retrograde signaling papers were:

—Wilson, R. I., and R. A. Nicoll. "Endogenous cannabinoids mediate retrograde signaling at hippocampal synapses." *Nature* 410:588–92 (doi:10.1038/35069076).

—Kreitzer, A. C., and W. G. Regehr. "Retrograde inhibition of presynaptic calcium influx by endogenous cannabinoids at excitatory synapses onto Purkinje cells." *Neuron* 29:717–27 (doi:10.1016/S0896-6273(01)00246-X).

—Ohno-Shosaku, T., T. Maejima, and M. Kano. "Endogenous cannabinoids mediate retrograde signals from depolarized postsynaptic neurons to presynaptic terminals." *Neuron* 29:729–38 (doi:10.1016/S0896-6273(01)00247–1).

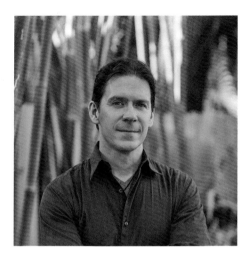

Dr. Greg Gerdeman is a neuroscientist and chief scientific officer with the Colorado-based medical cannabis company United Cannabis (UCANN). (Courtesy Joseph Siciliano) (Courtesy Joseph Siciliano)

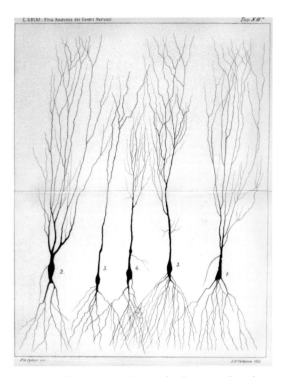

Plate XIII. Ganglion cell types in the convoluted gray layer of the pes hippocampi major. (From Wikimedia commons. Source: Golgi, C. *Sulla fina anatomia degli organi centrali del sistema nervoso.* Reggio-Emilia: S. Calderini e Figlio; 1885. Reprinted in: On the fine structure of the pes hippocampi major (with plates XIII–XXIII). Brain Research Bulletin, 2001, Vol. 54, No. 5, p. 473. This image is in the public domain.)

have to go backward?—until I spoke with Greg Gerdeman, PhD, a neuroscientist and chief scientific officer with the Colorado-based medical cannabis company United Cannabis (UCANN), during a May 2017 interview.

He was one of the researchers involved in discovering that endocannabinoids were retrograde (they go backward) messengers. Gerdeman began his part of the endocannabinoid cell-signaling chronicle by discussing scientists who are now seen as giants in the field of neuroanatomy.

Spaniard Santiago Ramón y Cajal and Italian Camillo Golgi did research in the late nineteenth and early twentieth centuries and shared the 1906 Nobel Prize in Physiology or Medicine for their work on the nervous system's structure, Gerdeman said during a May 2017 interview. Ramón y Cajal traced neurons using tools of the time—stains of static brain cells—and he and Golgi created staining techniques that Gerdeman said "visualized neurons beautifully."

It was only in the 1830s, he added, that scientists Theodor Schwann, Matthias Schleiden, and Rudolph

Virchow developed cell theory, which proposed that all living things are made up of one or more cells, that the cell is the basic unit of life, and that new cells come from existing cells.

But at the turn of the century, Gerdeman said, it was controversial to think that cell theory applied to the brain, which many considered the seat of the soul and way too complex to be broken into individual cells. Ramón y Cajal, because of the staining method he and Golgi worked on, thought the brain was made of cells called neurons connected by gaps that later became known as synapses. Golgi thought the brain was a continuous network.

"It turns out," Gerdeman said, "that modern neuroscience is showing both of them to be right. Neurons are connected by electrical synapses . . . that are the same electrical conduits that connect all the cells in the heart, for example, and allow them to be an electrically continuous tissue." He added, "But it is important for understanding the value of the retrograde [backward!] messenger idea because the gaps between cells were

Cell structure

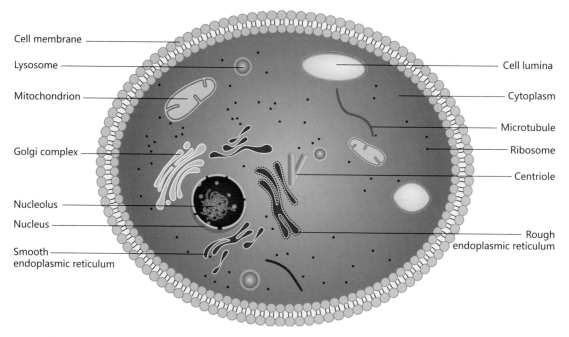

Cell membrane
Lysosome
Mitochondrion
Golgi complex
Nucleolus
Nucleus
Smooth endoplasmic reticulum

Cell lumina
Cytoplasm
Microtubule
Ribosome
Centriole
Rough endoplasmic reticulum

Human cell structure (From iStock by Ivcandy)

part of what [Ramón y] Cajal codified as the neuronal doctrine of the nervous system."

One of the doctrine's tenets was that between neurons are gaps called synapses and the flow of information across the synapses goes one way, Gerdeman said. The thinking, he added, "was that these big broad dendritic trees on neurons were receivers and that the lone axon, a little thin tube that projects oftentimes a great distance, is a transmitting wire, and that the flow of information goes only from one cell, across the synapse, and to the dendrites or cell body of the next cell." For the next century there wasn't a lot of reason to doubt that, and the synapse model became revolutionary in understanding the brain.

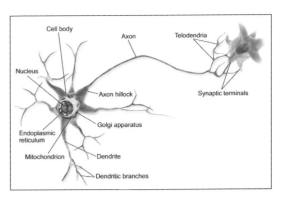

Multipolar neuron (By Bruce Blaus, Blausen. com staff [2014]. Medical gallery of Blausen Medical, 2014 (From WikiJournal of Medicine 1;2, doi:10.15347/wjm/2014.010. ISSN 2002-4436. This file is licensed under the Creative Commons Attribution 3.0 Unported license.)

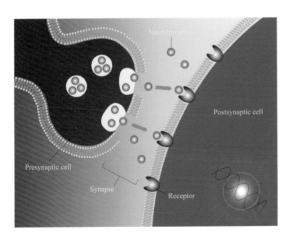

Structure of a typical synapse (From Shutterstock by Designua)

In large ways that's true, Gerdeman said, adding, "The brain is an electrical organ and the most complex structure that we know of in the universe, and those pathways of electrical conductance are largely a matter of dendrite to axon to synapse, and it flows that way."

But, he said, "the ability of the brain to adapt and respond and learn on a cellular and a circuit level is greatly enhanced if information can go the other way as well, and if cells can adjust their own synaptic inputs simply by releasing some sort of feedback molecules, and the endocannabinoids act as feedback, but not *just* feedback."

Gerdeman said the two main endocannabinoids and their retrograde signaling are part of a mechanism of resilience in the brain that's activated in response to trauma like stroke or traumatic brain injury, or electrical activity gone crazy as in epileptic seizures.

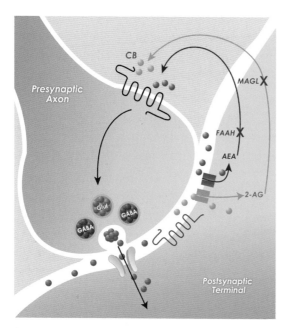

Retrograde signaling (Courtesy Cayman Chemical)

Protective for Brain and Body

This finding, Gerdeman said, was the first indication that the endocannabinoid system is a protective mechanism—protecting brain and body against insults like epilepsy, inflammation, neurodegeneration, brain trauma, and stroke—just like the immune system is protective against viruses, bacteria, and other pathogens.

Over time, and after work by Gerdeman and other researchers in the field, it was established that endocannabinoids were the first really clear example of retrograde signaling, and they were all over the brain.

"There are so many CB1 receptors for the endocannabinoids that this is not a small thing where some brain areas give

negative feedback. It's a huge mechanism by which the brain works, by which postsynaptic cells refine their presynaptic inputs," he explained. "A given neuron in the brain can easily have 10,000 unique synapses. The endocannabinoids are a way that, within that complex dendritic tree on a neuron, some pathways can be tuned down and others can be tuned up. It's like a gain control at a very sophisticated level."

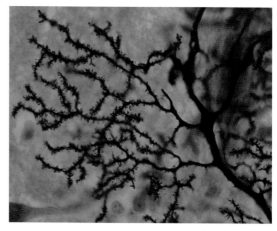

Dendritic tree of a Purkinje neuron stained with the silver Golgi method. The dendrite surface is full of small dendritic spines. (From Shutterstock by Jose Luis Calvo)

Retrograde signaling is important, Gerdeman says, because it has to do with the computational potential of the vast supercomputer of the brain and with tapping this mechanism.

"It's not only a way of feedback—you know, control against overexcitation—but it becomes a mechanism for associative learning because cells have evolved ways where, if you imagine a neuron with a very complex dendritic tree with lots of inputs, inputs from the left side that cause the cell to release endocannabinoids on the right side to dampen those inputs," Gerdeman said. "So it's not just a way to dial the synapses up and down directly, but it allows all kinds of complexity."

For example, he said, "the easiest way to explain this in terms of controlling seizures and neurotoxicity [is that] the transmitter glutamate—which is sort of a primary 'on' switch, an excitatory transmitter in the brain—is toxic when there's too much of it. And one of the primary roles of this endocannabinoid retrograde mechanism may be the context in which it evolved in the first place, in that when a cell receives a very strong onslaught of excitation, [the retrograde mechanism] acts as a simple negative feedback."

The cell is driven so strongly, he said, "that it releases endocannabinoids, which hit the *pre*synaptic terminal's receptors and turn down, or inhibit, the release of glutamate. . . . Too much excitation, turn it down. That is precisely what goes on with epilepsy, with seizure activity in the brain. And we now understand the endocannabinoids to be a sort of primary on-demand defense against excitotoxicity in the brain."

The term *on demand* means that the endocannabinoids—anandamide and 2-AG—aren't stored in the postsynaptic cell

until they're needed for retrograde signaling to the presynaptic cell. Rather, they're biosynthesized by enzymes inside the *post*synaptic cell as they're needed, then released into the synapse to travel backward to the *pre*synaptic cell. There, through CB1 receptors, the endocannabinoids inhibit the release, in this example, of the excitatory neurotransmitter glutamate, and when their job is finished, other enzymes degrade (disassemble) the endocannabinoids.

Ethan Russo gives another example, this one involving how endocannabinoid retrograde signaling helps neuropathic pain (caused by damaged nerves). Neuropathic pain is a common condition associated with multiple sclerosis, diabetes, HIV/AIDS, and other disorders, and "it's notoriously hard to treat with conventional drugs," Russo said.

Glutamate is one of the main stimulatory neurotransmitters, but when it's present in high concentrations it can create neuropathic pain and may even help kill brain cells after a head injury or a stroke, he added. The endocannabinoids anandamide and 2-AG are naturally secreted after such insults and in this case act to inhibit glutamate release, easing nerve-based pain and reducing cell death.[24]

Gerdeman called the endocannabinoids "part of our brain's mechanism of resilience in response to trauma and

24 Russo, E. B., white paper, January 2015, "Introduction to the Endocannabinoid System," corrected version: http://www.phytecs.com/wp-content/uploads/2015/02/IntroductionECS.pdf. Accessed 12/8/2017.

electrical activity gone crazy. We have an electrical organ of unimaginable complexity, in our case, and it can get turned up too high and cause damage."

The endocannabinoid system evolved to turn the system down, scale it down, to protect it, Gerdeman said, adding, "I'm rather convinced that the evolutionary emergence of the endocannabinoid system in this way was a necessary prerequisite for the evolution of the complex brains of vertebrates."

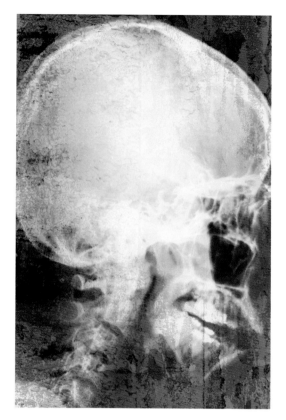

X-ray head of human. (From Shutterstock by Suwan Wanawattanawong)

Chapter 3
The Basic Machinery of Everyday Life

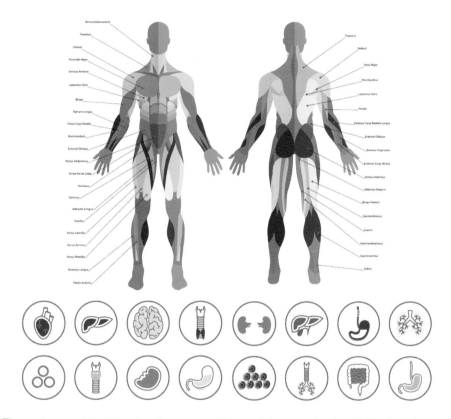

The endocannabinoid system is an essential regulatory mechanism in the body's biochemistry and physiology. (From Shutterstock by NastyaSigne)

Beginning in 1964, driven by the discovery of THC as the psychoactive constituent of cannabis, increasing scientific investigations of the plant led directly to the discovery of the endocannabinoid system (ECS), neurologist Dr. Ethan Russo has said.[1] The ECS, he wrote, "is an essential regulatory mechanism in the body's biochemistry and physiology, the basic machinery of everyday life."[2]

---

1 Russo, E. B. "Beyond cannabis: Plants and the endocannabinoid system." *Trends Pharmacol Sci* 37(7):594–605.
2 Russo, E. B., white paper, January 2015.

Following is a look at the research that describes each ECS element, and that has shown the endocannabinoid system to consist of much more than the initial two endocannabinoids, two cannabinoid receptors, and five enzymes.

The Endocannabinoids

Anandamide and 2-AG are the main players in a large and growing group of endocannabinoids[3] and endocannabinoid-like substances[4] in the brain and body. In a 2015 *Handbook of Experimental Pharmacology* review article,[5] Professor Roger Pertwee wrote that, including anandamide and 2-AG, thirteen of these endogenous biochemicals are probably orthosteric (ortho-stair-ick) endocannabinoids (they bind directly to and activate a cannabinoid receptor) and at least three are allosteric (they bind somewhere else on a cannabinoid receptor and either enhance or reduce the receptor's activation).

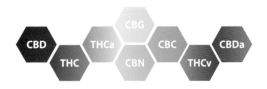

The entourage effect is created by a range of cannabinoids, terpenes, and other constituents that together add to the health effects of cannabis. (From Shutterstock by Image seller in w)

Russo says some of the other endocannabinoids are seemingly inactive molecules when tested on their own, but many experiments have shown that when combined with anandamide and 2-AG, these compounds enhance the overall effects of cannabis on pain, inflammation, and other conditions.[6] This is called an entourage effect, first described in a 1998 *European Journal of Pharmacology* paper by S. Ben-Shabat and colleagues.[7]

In a 2011 *British Journal of Pharmacology* paper,[8] Russo said there was support for the idea that phytocannabinoids (like THC) could have the

3   Ibid.
4   Chiurchiù, V, M. van der Stelt, D. Centonze, and M. Maccarrone. "The endocannabinoid system and its therapeutic exploitation in multiple sclerosis: Clues for other neuroinflammatory diseases." *Prog Neurobiol* 160:82–100 (doi: 10.1016/j.pneurobio.2017.10.007).
5   Pertwee, R. G. "Endocannabinoids and their pharmacological actions." *Handb Exp Pharmacol* 231:1–37 (doi: 10.1007/978-3-319-20825-1_1).
6   Russo, E. B., white paper, January 2015.
7   Ben-Shabat, S., E. Fride, T. Sheskin, T. Tamiri, M. H. Rhee, Z. Vogel, T. Bisogno, L. De Petrocellis, V. Di Marzo, and R. Mechoulam. "An entourage effect: Inactive endogenous fatty acid glycerol esters enhance 2-arachidonoyl-glycerol cannabinoid activity." *Eur J Pharmacol* 353(1):23–31.
8   Russo, E. B. "Taming THC: Potential cannabis synergy and phytocannabinoid-terpenoid entourage effects." *Br J Pharmacol* 163:1344–1364 (doi10.1111/j.1476–5381.2011.01238.x).

same kind of active and seemingly inactive synergists (entourage) as endocannabinoids, as described by Ben-Shabat and colleagues and then refined and qualified by the same group a year later, in 1999:[9] "This type of synergism may play a role in the widely held (but not experimentally based) view," they wrote, "that in some cases plants are better drugs than the natural products isolated from them."

The two most-studied endocannabinoids, anandamide and 2-AG, are the main ECS signaling molecules (also called ligands—lih-gands or lye-gands), which work at the CB1, CB2, and multiple other receptors. Within the endocannabinoid system, they work in a way that's different from regular signaling molecules, remembering the concept of retrograde signaling described in chapter 2.

To review: it's well established among cannabinoid researchers that in the brain and the rest of the nervous system, anandamide and 2-AG act mainly as retrograde messengers. They're created in the *post*synaptic cell when they're needed, and move backward across the synapse to affect CB1 or CB2 receptors at the *pre*synaptic cell.

Also at the presynaptic cell, they modify the release of excitatory or inhibitory neurotransmitters into the synapse, acting as a sort of nervous-system-wide feedback mechanism to tone the system up or down, and in this way protect the brain from, in the glutamate example, neuro-excitotoxicity (nuro-ek-site-o-toxicity)—a pathological process of overactivity that damages or kills neurons. This process also is called, as noted below, modulating synaptic strength.

"It is . . . widely believed that by modulating [increasing and reducing] synaptic strength," Castillo and colleagues wrote in a 2012 *Neuron* paper,[10] "endocannabinoids can regulate a wide range of neural functions, including cognition, motor control, feeding behaviors, and pain." Like nearly every other research team that has studied the endocannabinoid system, they confirm that endocannabinoids are involved in nearly every major process in the body and brain.

"The prevalence throughout the brain [of cannabinoid receptors like CB1 and CB2]," the authors wrote, "suggests endocannabinoids are fundamental modulators of synaptic function."[11]

There's also evidence, they wrote, to suggest that endocannabinoids signal in a non-retrograde way (the regular way, in other words—presynaptic cell to synapse to postsynaptic cell) to affect brain

---

9 Mechoulam, R., and S. Ben-Shabat.
10 Castillo, P. E., T. J. Younts, A. E. Chávez, and Y. Hashimotodani "Endocannabinoid signaling and synaptic function." *Neuron* 76(1):70–81 (doi: 10.1016/j.neuron.2012.09.020).
11 Ibid.

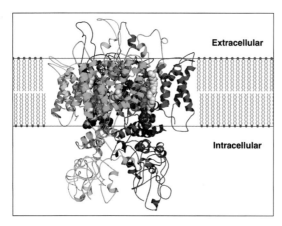

The transient receptor potential vanilloid 1 (TRVP1) model by Boghog2 based on a homology model published in Brauchi S, et al. *Dissection of the components for PIP2 activation and thermosensation in TRP channels.* Natl Acad Sci USA. June 2005;104(24):10246–51. doi:10.1073/pnas.0703420104. (From Wikipedia. This file is in the public domain.)

function and synaptic transmission by engaging a less-studied receptor called transient receptor potential vanilloid receptor type 1 (TRPV1) and CB1 receptors on or in the postsynaptic cell.[12]

TRPV1, Ethan Russo said, is best known as the site of action of capsaicin, the active ingredient of chili peppers. It's also a target of anandamide and CBD, but not THC.[13]

"TRPV1 mediates pain signals through a mechanism distinct from that of the endogenous cannabinoids and opioids, but the receptor is subject to desensitization:

this means that if continuously stimulated, the pathway will eventually slow down or even stop," he added.

"This raises therapeutic possibilities for agents to effectively treat certain kinds of neuropathic pain," Russo wrote, "particularly cannabidiol, which is about equipotent with capsaicin at the TRPV1 receptor and likewise capable of its desensitization. This is particularly exciting as previous attempts to develop synthetic agents to antagonize the receptor have produced profound hypothermia [lowered body temperature] and other side effects that preclude them from further development."[14]

Other recent studies indicate that endocannabinoids also can signal via brain cells called astrocytes to indirectly modulate presynaptic or postsynaptic

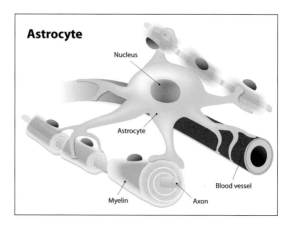

A star-shaped glial cell called an astrocyte, here in association with a blood vessel and neurons. (From Shutterstock by Designua)

---

12 Ibid.
13 Russo, E. B., white paper, January 2015.
14 Ibid.

function.[15] Astrocytes, meaning star-like cells, are the largest and most prevalent kind of glial cell in the central nervous system. Glial cells surround neurons and support and insulate them, and astrocytes help form the blood-brain barrier, maintain balance outside the cell and respond to injury, and affect neuron development and plasticity (adaptability).[16]

So researchers are starting to find a lot of diversity in endocannabinoid signaling, another reason endocannabinoids can be involved in nearly every process in the body and why medical cannabis can affect such a range of illnesses.

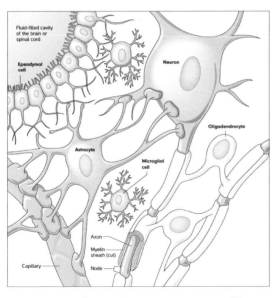

Components of a vertebrate motor neuron (From Shutterstock by Emre Terim)

CB1, CB2, and Other Cannabinoid Receptors

If you haven't studied biology lately, specifically how cells communicate in the brain and body, here are two ways it works. First, cells in the bodies of multi-celled organisms (like us) talk to (signal) each other to coordinate the complex job of interconnecting the biological systems that make life possible.

One form of cell communication happens when a signaling molecule, like one of the endocannabinoids, moves backward or sometimes forward from one cell to another cell, called a target cell, and binds to or somehow affects a specific receptor protein that in many cases is embedded in the cell surface. Another form of cell signaling takes place inside the cell, at the cell nucleus. Some endocannabinoids and cannabinoids can

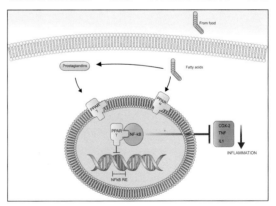

PPAR (peroxisome proliferator-activated receptor) gamma and its actions at a cell nucleus (From Shutterstock by ellepigrafica)

---

15 Castillo, P. E., T. J. Younts, A. E. Chávez, and Y. Hashimotodani.
16 *Nature* https://www.nature.com/subjects/astrocyte. Accessed 11/28/2017.

activate a type of nuclear receptor called a peroxisome proliferator-activated receptor (PPAR) and its subtypes, PPAR alpha, beta, and gamma.

In a 2016 *British Journal of Pharmacology* paper,[17] O'Sullivan wrote that endocannabinoid activation of PPAR alpha and PPAR gamma receptors "mediates some of the analgesic [pain relieving], neuroprotective, neuronal [nerve cell] function modulation, anti-inflammatory, metabolic, antitumor, gastrointestinal, and cardiovascular effects of some cannabinoids."

The researcher noted that this often occurs along with activation of traditional endocannabinoid receptors, CB1, CB2, and TRPV1, and that PPARs also mediate some effects of inhibitors of enzymes involved in endocannabinoid degradation or transport[18] (across a biological membrane).

A signaling molecule can bind directly to receptors only if the molecule has the right shape to fit onto the receptor protein. If it does have that shape, the action of binding changes the receptor's conformation (shape or structure), producing the target cell's response. Some signaling molecules bind strongly to the receptor, and those that do are called agonists (they strongly activate the receptor). Some block an agonist's binding at

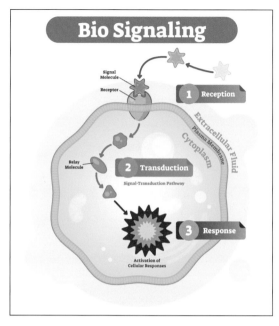

Biological signaling molecule at the cell surface with receptor, transduction, and response activity (From Shutterstock by VectorMine)

the receptor, and these are called antagonists. There are lots of complex variations in this binding activity, but I'll give one more example because it involves THC and CBD.

THC works at an orthosteric binding site on the CB1 receptor, meaning THC has the right shape to bind directly to and activate the CB1 receptor. This is the same orthosteric site where anandamide and 2-AG bind to effect their cellular changes. But THC doesn't bind as strongly as it could, so it's called a partial agonist at CB1. CBD also binds to the CB1 receptor,

17 O' Sullivan, S. E. "An update on PPAR activation by cannabinoids." *Br J Pharmacol* 173:1899–1910 (doi: 10.1111/bph.13497).
18 Ibid.

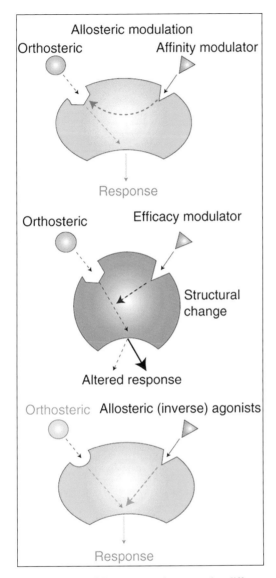

Allosteric modulation

Orthosteric   Affinity modulator

Response

Orthosteric   Efficacy modulator

Structural
change

Altered response

Orthosteric Allosteric (inverse) agonists

Response

CBD acts at the CB1 receptor but at a site different from THC's direct binding site, and CBD's action there when THC is present is called an allosteric effect, meaning it acts somewhere else on the receptor and blocks or otherwise reduces the receptor's activation. (Courtesy CBDpurUS.com)

but at a site different from THC's orthosteric binding site. The CBD binding site is called an allosteric (allo-stair-ick) site, meaning it binds somewhere else on the CB1 receptor and blocks or otherwise reduces the receptor's activation. For its effect on THC at the receptor, CBD is called a negative allosteric modulator.

Dr. Ethan Russo has called a negative allosteric modulator "a fancy way of saying that when THC is present, CBD interferes with its activity, which is a good thing in terms of not wanting too much psychoactivity and limiting side effects like anxiety or rapid heart rate that can be a problem if someone has too much THC."[19]

This allosteric activity of CBD at the CB1 receptor, when THC and CBD are at the receptor at the same time, reduces THC's psychoactivity, which allows medical cannabis patients to take more THC for its therapeutic effects without having to experience its disorienting psychoactivity and other side effects. Physicians call this expanding THC's therapeutic window.

Cannabinoid Receptor 1

The CB1 receptor is best known as the receptor in the brain where THC exerts its effects (as a partial agonist) on short-term memory, pain, emotion, hunger, and more, and, at the right dosage, brings

19 Russo, E. B. Video interview on the endocannabinoid system with Martin A. Lee, director of Project CBD, June 2016.

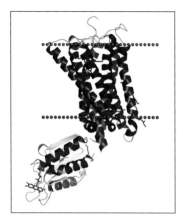

CB1 receptor (From Orientations of Proteins in Membranes database, Lomize Group, College of Pharmacy, University of Michigan, used with permission)

cerebellum, spinal cord, eye, sympathetic ganglia, immune system (bone marrow, thymus, spleen, tonsils), breast cancer cell lines, and other peripheral nervous system sites like the heart, lungs, adrenals, kidneys, liver, colon, prostate, pancreas, testes, ovaries, and placenta.[21]

THC's intoxicating effects to life. In the early days of THC's discovery, researchers thought CB1 receptors were restricted to the brain and the rest of the central nervous system. But more recent studies also have identified CB1 receptors in almost all peripheral (outside the nervous system) tissues and cell types, though at lower densities than in the brain.[20]

In a 2017 *Advances in Pharmacology* paper, Russo and Marcu wrote that CB1 protein (receptors are proteins) is found, for example, in the hypothalamus, motor systems, motor cortex, basal ganglia,

A main result of activating the presynaptic CB1 receptor is inhibiting the release of certain neurotransmitters from that presynaptic neuron, according to a 2013 *Annual Review of Psychology* paper by Mechoulam and Parker. This is how endocannabinoids reduce the excitability or increase the activity (synaptic strength) of neurotransmitters in presynaptic neurons. Along with psychoactivity, CB1 receptor activity in the brain also has effects on cognition, reward, and anxiety.[22]

As discussed in the last chapter, CB1 is a G protein-coupled receptor—in fact, Ethan Russo says it's the most abundant GPCR in the brain, attesting to the receptor's importance in brain function and in health and disease.[23]

In a 2016 *F1000Research* review paper, [24] A. B. Garcia and colleagues wrote that there are lots of CB1 receptors in the

20 Pacher, P., and G. Kunos "Modulating the endocannabinoid system in human health and disease-successes and failures." *FEBS J* 280(9):1918–43 (doi: 10.1111/febs.12260).
21 Russo, E. B., and J. Marcu.
22 Mechoulam, R., and L. A. Parker. "The endocannabinoid system and the brain." *Annu Rev Psychol* 64:21–47 (doi: 10.1146/annurev-psych-113011-143739).
23 Russo, E. B., white paper, January 2015.
24 Garcia, A. B., E. Soria-Gomez, L. Bellocchio, and G. Marsicano. "Cannabinoid receptor type-1: breaking the dogmas." F1000Research 2016, 5(F1000 Faculty Rev):990 Updated: 24 May 2016.

central nervous system (CNS) that control a range of physiological and pathological conditions, including brain development, learning and memory, motor behavior, appetite regulation, body temperature, pain perception, and inflammation, and that the receptors also are involved in some psychiatric, neurological, and neurodevelopmental disorders.

Outside the brain and nervous system, the endocannabinoid system influences the gastrointestinal tract, where CB1 receptors modulate two important aspects of digestion—propulsion (moving food along the digestive tract) and

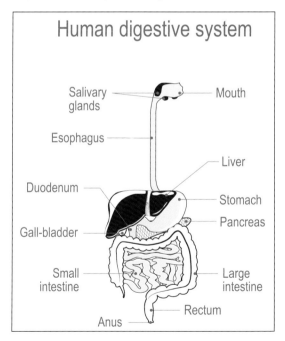

Human digestive system

Salivary glands — Mouth

Esophagus

Liver

Duodenum

Stomach

Pancreas

Gall-bladder

Small intestine — Large intestine

Rectum

Anus

The human digestive system (From iStock by ttsz)

secretion (as in acids involved in the digestive process).[25]

The endocannabinoid system also regulates endocrine (hormone) function and fertility, Russo wrote, and some factors in cell function.[26]

In a 2013 *Annual Review of Psychology* paper, Mechoulam and Parker discussed, among other topics, the CB1 receptor and its effects in people and in animals.[27] In people, the authors wrote, "high CB1 levels in the sensory and motor regions are consistent with the important role of CB1 receptors in motivation and cognition." CB1 receptors also seem to be involved in the activity of the central nervous system's main inhibitory neurotransmitter, gamma-aminobutyric acid (GABA), and the main excitatory neurotransmitter, glutamate. CB1 is present in the earliest phases of human life and is important in nerve cell development and newborn suckling.

CB1 receptors are on presynaptic nerve cells in the central nervous system (brain and spinal cord) and in the peripheral nervous system (everywhere else in the body), Mechoulam and Parker added, where nerves connect the central nervous system to sensory organs like the eye and to other organs, glands, muscles, and blood vessels. CB1 receptors' location on presynaptic nerve cells lets them slow down the release of

25 Ibid.
26 Russo, E. B., white paper, January 2015.
27 Mechoulam, R., and L. A. Parker.

excitatory neurotransmitters like glutamate, "which is one of the major functions of the endocannabinoid system," they added.[28]

Recent advances in understanding the CB1 receptor have been made possible by new imaging and molecular tools, Garcia and colleagues wrote. They report that CB1 receptors can appear on lots of different cell types, including nerve cells and glial cells like astrocytes, as discussed, and in mitochondria, which

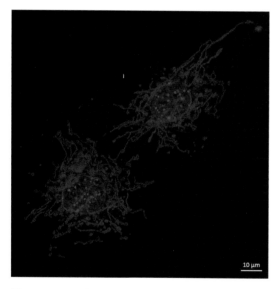

10 µm

Fluorescent microscopy image of the mitochondria (red) and cell nucleus (blue) of two mouse embryonic fibroblast cells. (From Wikimedia Commons by User:Shinryuu, Institute of Molecular Medicine, University of Dusseldorf. This file is licensed under the Creative Commons Attribution 4.0 International license.)

produce about 90 percent of the chemical energy cells need to live.[29]

CB1 receptors don't only respond to endocannabinoids and cannabinoids. CB1 receptors can also be found, among other places, on the neurons that transmit the inhibitory GABA, the excitatory glutamate, and serotonin, whose activity in the central nervous system involves mood, sleep, appetite, and learning and memory. And some kinds of antidepressants may work by raising serotonin concentrations or its activity in the brain. So, they wrote, activated CB1 receptors on GABA neurons can control food intake, running-related behavior, drug addiction, learning and memory processes, and others. Activated CB1 receptors on glutamate neurons control neuroprotection, olfactory (sense of smell) processes, fear memories, social behavior and anxiety, and others. CB1 receptors on serotonin neurons can affect emotional responses.[30]

At the paper's end, Garcia and colleagues called these and other findings new and exciting, and noted, "The better we understand cannabinoid signaling the closer we are to developing specific and local pharmacological drugs that may have importance in brain disorders."[31]

28 Ibid.
29 Garcia, A. B., E. Soria-Gomez, L. Bellocchio, and G. Marsicano.
30 Ibid.
31 Ibid.

CB1 seems so useful that it's hard to imagine living without it. Researchers had the same thought.

"In mice, if you delete the gene that encodes the CB1 receptor," Professor Maurice Elphick said during a 2017 interview, "the mice are completely unaffected by THC, and the same would almost certainly be true of humans." It may even be the case, he added, "that there are humans walking around who don't have a functional set [of cannabinoid receptors], which would be fascinating if we ever found someone because they would presumably have no sensitivity to cannabis whatsoever. And it would be interesting to know what other features they might have as a result of not having a functional cannabinoid receptor."

On that topic, a 1999 *Proceedings of the National Academies of Science* paper[32] listed some of the ways rodents with and without CB1 receptors differed, Dr. Greg Gerdeman said during a May 2017 interview.

"You can genetically remove all of the CB1 cannabinoid receptors and it's not like the animals die *in utero*. They live, and they have very interesting, in some ways surprisingly subtle, phenotypes,"

he said (phenotype means a mix of an animal's observable traits). "They're more anxious, they have different abilities to learn in different assays of learning and memory. . . . They live shorter, more seizure-prone, more inflammation-prone lives," Gerdeman added, noting that the work took place with the first CB1 knockout mice (lab mice in which researchers have inactivated, or knocked out, an existing gene, in this case a gene involving the receptor CB1) created by Andreas Zimmer and colleagues[33] at the National Institute of Mental Health in Bethesda, Maryland.

But THC and its binding at CB1 have adverse effects at higher doses. In a 2017 *Nature Reviews Cardiology*[34] paper, for example, P. Pacher and colleagues wrote that endocannabinoid and CB1 dysregulation has been implicated in certain cardiovascular pathologies. THC "exerts its cardiovascular effects via CB1 activation; at low doses it might have beneficial properties via partial activation of CB1 and CB2 and unrelated mechanisms," they wrote.

"Most synthetic cannabinoids used [recreationally] are full agonists of CB1 [THC is a partial agonist] with up to

32 Zimmer, A., A. M. Zimmer, A. G. Hohmann, M. Herkenham, and T. I. Bonner. "Increased mortality, hypoactivity and hypoalgesia in cannabinoid CB1 receptor knockout mice." *Proc Natl Acad Sci USA* 96(10):5780–5.

33 Ibid.

34 Pacher, P., S. Steffens, G. Haskó, T. Schindler, and G. Kunos. "Cardiovascular effects of marijuana and synthetic cannabinoids: The good, the bad, and the ugly." *Nat Rev Cardiol.* September 2017, advance online publication (doi: 10.1038/nrcardio.2017.130).

several-hundred-fold higher potency and efficacy than THC, causing more dangerous adverse effects," they added. "In parallel with a 10-fold increase in the THC content of marijuana and the widespread availability of synthetic cannabinoids for recreational use, the number of serious cardiovascular adverse effects reported has markedly increased."[35]

Pacher and colleagues added, "Clinicians should be vigilant to recognizing potential cardiovascular effects of marijuana and synthetic cannabinoids; controlled clinical trials should determine the long-term consequences of the use of medical marijuana on cardiovascular morbidity and mortality."[36]

Cannabinoid Receptor 2

The other major cannabinoid receptor, CB2, has been less studied than CB1 but equally important, Dr. Ethan Russo says.

For a long time researchers thought CB2 receptors—where THC acts as a weak partial antagonist (doesn't fully activate the receptor)—were pretty much restricted to immune and hematopoietic (blood-forming) cells, but they're now finding CB2 expression all over the central nervous system under conditions of brain insult or disease, especially in (activated) microglial cells, the brain's major inflammatory cells.[37] Normally these immune

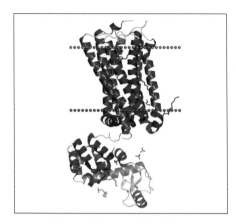

CB2 is one of the main cannabinoid receptors whose activation has a protective effect in many of the body's physiological systems. (From Orientations of Proteins in Membranes database, Lomize Group, College of Pharmacy, University of Michigan, used with permission)

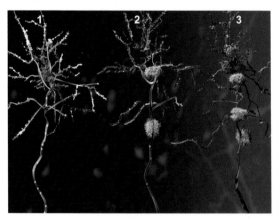

1. Healthy neuron. 2. Neuron with amyloid plaques (yellow). 3. Dead neuron being digested by microglia cells (red). (From iStock by selvanegra)

cells are removers of doomed neurons and other debris, keeping the central nervous system running smoothly.

35 Ibid.
36 Ibid.
37 Russo, E. B.

CB2 receptors also are found in specific brain regions and in heart muscle tissue, the gut, endothelial cells that line the inner surfaces of blood vessels, vascular (blood vessel) smooth-muscle cells, liver cells involved in breaking down red blood cells, the pancreas, bone, reproductive organs and cells, and different kinds of tumors.[38]

Even more CB2 receptors appear on neurons in the brain, created inside the cell itself, on demand, at times of active inflammation from brain injury or neurodegenerative diseases like Alzheimer's, to reduce harm to cells and tissues. In explanation, Professor Raphael Mechoulam (email communication November 2017) wrote, "The brain reacts to the disease or trauma by making its [own] CB2 receptors—nothing basically new. The body reacts to various diseases in different ways. The immune system certainly forms, or enhances the synthesis of, protective entities when needed."

So the receptor enables important signaling molecules with effects on pain and inflammation, and certain areas of the brain express CB2 receptors with the rise of inflammation that follows traumatic injury or in neurodegenerative diseases like Alzheimer's, among others.

Disorders characterized by fibrosis (scar tissue development), like liver cirrhosis and certain heart and kidney disorders, eventually may be targets for drugs that affect the CB2 receptor.[39]

In addition, Mechoulam and Parker say, CB2 receptor agonists (activators) might be expected to become drugs in fields that involve neuropsychiatric, cardiovascular, and liver disease.[40]

"A major consequence of CB2 receptor activation is immunosuppression, which limits inflammation and associated tissue injury," the researchers wrote. "Enhancement of CB2 receptor expression and/or of endocannabinoid levels has been noted in numerous diseases, including CNS-related ones. Thus, a main result of CB2 receptor activation seems to be a protective effect in a large number of physiological systems."[41]

In 2018, B. Bie and colleagues wrote a *Current Opinion in Anesthesiology* review paper summarizing recent work on the CB2 receptor and its potential as a therapeutic target in neuropathic pain (pain from damaged nerves) and neurodegenerative disorders like Alzheimer's, Parkinson's, and Huntington's diseases, multiple sclerosis, AIDS dementia, amyotrophic lateral sclerosis, and others, most

---

38 Pacher, P., and G. Kunos.
39 Russo, E. B., white paper, January 2015.
40 Mechoulam, R., and L. A. Parker.
41 Ibid.

of which have limited or no currently approved therapies.[42]

"Therapeutic target" in this case means that scientists would create CB2-selective drugs to reach CB2 receptors in the central nervous system to affect these diseases and other disorders inside and outside the central nervous system that are helped by CB2 actions.[43]

The CB2 receptor is mainly expressed (on a cell surface) when there is active inflammation, Bie and colleagues wrote, adding that neuroinflammation and something called microglial activation seem to underlie the development of neurodegenerative diseases like those mentioned above.[44]

In normal conditions, as discussed, microglia clean up nerve cell damage by enveloping and destroying the debris and acting as an anti-inflammatory agent. But when microglial cells are activated by damage to the central nervous system, they initiate a pro-inflammatory environment that eventually damages nerve cells. But, the researchers wrote, activating the CB2 receptor system inhibits the neuroinflammatory signaling pathway and helps restore normal microglial function.[45]

In animal models of neuropathic pain, Bie and colleagues said compounds

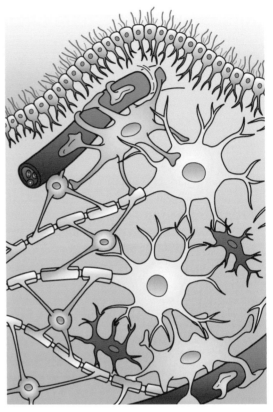

Four kinds of glial cells are found in the central nervous system: Ependymal cells (light pink), astrocytes (green), microglial cells (dark red), and oligodendrocytes (light blue). (From Wikimedia Commons by Holly Fischer. This file is licensed under the Creative Commons Attribution 3.0 Unported license.)

(CB2 agonists) that activate CB2 receptors prevented something called mechanical allodynia—the feeling of pain from something that doesn't usually cause

42 Bie, B., J. Wu, J. F. Foss, and M. Naguib. "An overview of the cannabinoid type 2 receptor system and its therapeutic potential." *Curr Opin Anaesthesiol.* May 22, 2018. doi: 10.1097/ACO.0000000000000616. E-publication ahead of print.

43 Ibid.

44 Ibid.

45 Ibid.

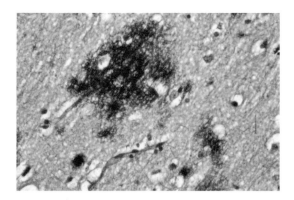

Microscopic photograph of brain tissue demonstrating the characteristics of Alzheimer's disease which include senile plaques, which are extracellular deposits of the amyloid beta-protein. (From iStock by OGphoto)

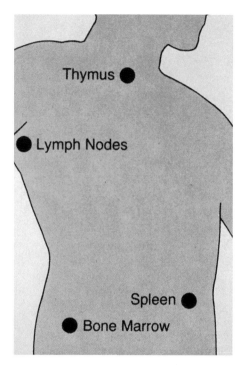

Key organs of the immune system—thymus, lymph nodes, spleen, bone marrow (Courtesy National Cancer Institute)

pain, like a light touch. In animal models of Alzheimer's disease, treatment with CB2 agonists "promoted the clearance of amyloid plaques and recovery of the neuronal synaptic plasticity."[46]

Beta-amyloid is a protein fragment snipped from an amyloid precursor protein. In a healthy brain, the protein fragments are broken down and eliminated. In Alzheimer's disease, the fragments accumulate to form hard, insoluble plaques.[47] Neurofibrillary fibers, amyloid plaques, tau protein clumps, chronic inflammation, and blood vessel issues all are thought to contribute to Alzheimer's disease damage, according to the National Institute on Aging.

In a 2011 *Progress in Lipid Research* paper, Pacher and Mechoulam wrote about endocannabinoids and the CB2 receptor. Endocannabinoids and endocannabinoid-like molecules acting through the CB2 receptor, they wrote, have been reported to positively affect lots of disease conditions, from cardiovascular, gastrointestinal, liver, kidney, lung, neurodegenerative (mentioned above), and psychiatric disorders to pain, cancer,

---

46 Ibid.
47 *Journal of Alzheimer's and Dementia*: http://www.imedpub.com/journal-alzheimers-dementia/. Accessed 8/24/18.

bone, reproductive system, and skin pathologies.[48]

"The mammalian body has a highly developed immune system whose main role is to guard against protein attack and prevent, reduce or repair a possible injury," the researchers wrote. "Protein attack" refers to the immune system's activation by proteins called antigens on the surfaces of bacteria, fungi, and viruses. When the antigens bind to special receptors on immune system defense cells, a series of cell processes begins to protect the body from attackers.[49]

"It is inconceivable that, through evolution, analogous biological protective systems have not developed against non-protein [non-viral, non-bacterial and others] attacks," Pacher and Mechoulam wrote, adding that inflammation and tissue injury trigger rapid rises in local endocannabinoid levels, and these then regulate fast-signaling responses in immune and other cells to modulate their critical functions. The researchers believe that lipid messengers like anandamide and 2-AG signaling through CB2 receptors are part of that biological protective system.[50]

Cannabinoids Outside the Endocannabinoid System

Over the years, researchers have identified lots of different cannabinoid molecular targets that exist outside the original endocannabinoid system and its CB1, CB2, and TRPV1 receptors. These include non-CB1 and non-CB2 G protein-coupled receptors, enzymes, and transporters (proteins involved in moving ions and other molecules across a biological membrane).

S. E. Turner and colleagues described some of these non-ECS therapeutic targets in a 2017 *Progress in the Chemistry of Organic Natural Products* review article about the molecular pharmacology of phytocannabinoids,[51] and below we'll see their findings about actions outside the endocannabinoid system for THC and CBD.

Within the endocannabinoid system, THC binds to and activates the CB1 receptor and, with lower binding affinity, CB2. THC's intoxicating effects are mediated at CB1 by the cannabinoid's partial agonist activity, meaning that it binds to and activates CB1 but with less effectiveness than a full agonist would. Outside the endocannabinoid system, THC has been

---

48 Pacher, P., and R. Mechoulam. "Is lipid signaling through cannabinoid 2 receptors part of a protective system?" *Prog Lipid Res* 50(2):193–211 (doi: 10.1016/j.plipres.2011.01.001).

49 Ibid.

50 Ibid.

51 Turner, S. E., C. M. Williams, L. Iversen, and B. J. Whalley. "Molecular Pharmacology of Phytocannabinoids." *Prog Chem Org Nat Prod* 103:61–101 (doi: 10.1007/978-3-319-45541-9_3).

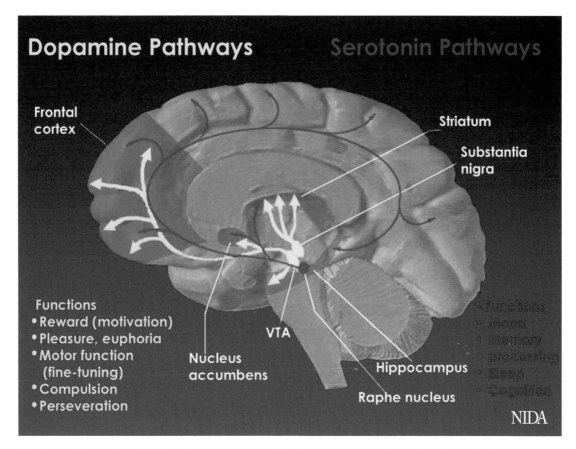

Dopamine Pathways

Serotonin Pathways

Frontal cortex

Striatum

Substantia nigra

Functions
• Reward (motivation)
• Pleasure, euphoria
• Motor function
  (fine-tuning)
• Compulsion
• Perseveration

VTA

Nucleus accumbens

Hippocampus

Raphe nucleus

Functions
• Mood
• Memory processing
• Sleep
• Cognition

NIDA

The dopamine and serotonin pathways are two of the brain systems affected by drugs of abuse. (National Institute on Drug Abuse, in the public domain)

shown to work with the serotonin system, at 5-HT3 receptors (one of fourteen known 5-HT receptors[52]), which along with cannabinoid receptors are involved in controlling pain and vomiting.[53]

Serotonin (chemically, 5-hydroxytryptamine or 5-HT) is a neurotransmitter known to help regulate mood, appetite, sleep, and other important functions, Turner and colleagues wrote. THC also works at glycine (an amino acid) receptors, Turner and colleagues wrote, which are involved in pain transmission and dopamine release from neurons in part of the brain called the ventral tegmental area, one of the major areas for dopamine

52 Malenka, R. C., E. J. Nestler, S. E. Hyman, A. Sydor, and R. Y. Brown, eds. *Molecular Neuropharmacology: A Foundation for Clinical Neuroscience* (2nd ed). 2009, New York: McGraw-Hill Medical. p. 4.
53 Turner SE, Williams CM, Iversen L, Whalley BJ.

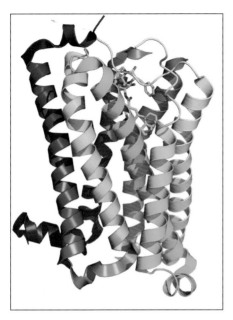

3-D structure model of the 5-HT1B receptor in complex with ergotamine based on crystallographic data for PDB 4IAR [the structural basis for molecular recognition at serotonin receptors] (From Wikimedia Commons by S. Jähnichen. This file is licensed under the Creative Commons Attribution-Share Alike 3.0 Unported license.)

neurons. Because THC works there, it may be important for analgesia (pain relief) and drug addiction, known to involve dopamine. THC activity at cannabinoid receptors also produces pain relief.[54]

THC activates PPAR gamma, located inside the cell at the cell nucleus. THC's effect there has relevance in the cardiovascular system and potentially in cancer treatment, the researchers wrote. PPARG is highly expressed in adipogenesis (a cell-differentiation process that produces adipocytes, cells specialized to store fat), and in type 2 diabetes and gastro-inflammatory disorders. And some scientists consider at least two other G protein-coupled receptors—GPR18 and GPR55—possible cannabinoid receptors, the researchers wrote.[55]

Cannabidiol (CBD) is a nonintoxicating cannabinoid, Turner and colleagues wrote. Within the endocannabinoid system, a recently published study showed, CBD acts as a CB1 negative allosteric modulator (when THC is present, CBD interferes with its activity[56]) but without activating the receptor itself.[57] This is how CBD combined with THC in whole-plant cannabis tones down some of THC's negative effects, like intoxication, anxiety, and impaired memory.

Outside the ECS, E. Aso and colleagues wrote in a 2019 *Molecular Neurobiology* paper,[58] CBD has lots of targets (receptors it can affect) and its activity is different at each one, producing multiple effects. CBD, they wrote, "is a

54 Ibid.

55 Ibid.

56 Project CBD: http://www.projectCBD.org. Accessed 1/2/2018.

57 Turner, S. E., C. M. Williams, L. Iversen, and B. J. Whalley.

58 Aso E., V. Fernández-Dueñas, M. López-Cano, J. Taura, M. Watanabe, I. Ferrer, R. Luján, and F. Ciruela. "Adenosine A2A-Cannabinoid CB1 Receptor Heteromers in the Hippocampus: Cannabidiol Blunts Δ^9-Tetrahydrocannabinol-Induced Cognitive Impairment." *Mol Neurobiol.* January 2019 online (doi: 10.1007/s12035-018-1456-3).

promiscuous compound with activity at multiple targets," including TRPV1 and PPAR gamma (as discussed earlier), and at adenosine receptors, serotonin receptors, glycine receptors, adrenal receptors, dopamine receptors, GABA receptors, and opioid receptors.

Turner and colleagues noted that more than one target (receptor) may control CBD effects, which include anti-inflammatory and immunosuppressive effects. The immunosuppressive effect is important because it limits cellular stress and inflammation, and may explain CBD's ability to improve arthritis and multiple sclerosis symptoms. CBD's

immunosuppressive effects in microglia would have important benefits for neurodegenerative conditions.[59]

At serotonin receptors, studies show that CBD mediates effects like (short-duration) responses to stress, nausea and vomiting, cerebral infarction (an area of dead brain tissue caused by blocked arteries), and antianxiety, anti-panic, and antidepressant effects. It's also reported that glycine (the major inhibitory neurotransmitter in the brainstem and spinal cord) receptors mediate CBD's anti-inflammatory actions and suppress neuropathic pain, Turner and colleagues wrote.[60]

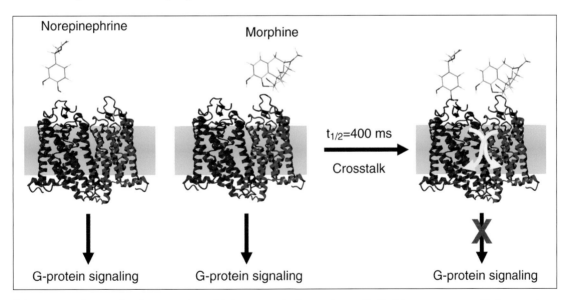

A heteromer is a molecular grouping of interconnected receptor units that form a new multiple-receptor entity that generates new molecular signaling entities. (From Vilardaga JP, Agnati LF, Fuxe K, Ciruela F. *G-protein-coupled receptor heteromer dynamics*. J Cell Sci. 2010 Dec 15;123(24):4215-20 [doi: 10.1242/jcs.063354]. Used with permission)

---

59 Turner, S. E., C. M. Williams, L. Iversen, and B. J. Whalley.
60 Ibid.

Even More Complexity

Briefly—this won't be on the test—just to show you how complex the endocannabinoid system really is, M. S. Aymerich and colleagues wrote that cannabinoid receptors can link up with other G protein-coupled receptors to form something called a heteromer. This is a molecular grouping of interconnected receptor units, forming a new multiple-receptor entity that, the researchers say, "generates new molecular signaling entities that contribute to their diverse responses."[61]

As always with medical cannabis, seriously more research is needed to understand heteromers and determine how to use their effects therapeutically.

Endocannabinoid Enzymes

The final essential component of the endocannabinoid system, along with the endocannabinoids and their receptors, are the cell-based enzymes that synthesize (when needed) or disassemble (after they've had their effects) anandamide and 2-AG. As mentioned in chapter 2, the NAPE-PLD enzyme synthesizes anandamide, DAGL alpha and DAGL beta synthesize 2-AG, FAAH disassembles anandamide, and MGL (also MAGL) degrades 2-AG.

Scientists and drug developers are looking to these enzymes and their effects on anandamide and 2-AG in a search for "new therapeutics that target endocannabinoid signaling," V. Di Marzo wrote in a 2018 *Nature Reviews Drug Discovery* opinion piece.[62]

"Inhibitors of endocannabinoid biosynthesis . . . are in the early stages of development [and] have been investigated in preclinical studies of obesity and inflammatory and neuropathic pain," he wrote. "Recently, the first biologic [biotechnologically made from living organisms] drug in the endocannabinoid field, namacizumab, . . . [which] stabilizes CB1 in an inactive conformation, was submitted for approval to initiate a phase 1a/b clinical trial for nonalcoholic steatohepatitis [liver inflammation and damage from fat buildup], a frequent comorbidity of abdominal obesity."[63]

Importantly, Di Marzo added, "namacizumab, like other biologics, is likely to be peripherally restricted"[64] (meaning it won't be able to cross the blood-brain barrier, so, despite its targeting CB1,

61 Aymerich, M. S., E. Aso, M. A. Abellanas, R. M. Tolon, J. A. Ramos, I. Ferrer, J. Romero, and J. Fernández-Ruiz. "Cannabinoid pharmacology/therapeutics in chronic degenerative disorders affecting the central nervous system." *Biochem Pharmacol*. August 17, 2018. pii: S0006-2952(18)30337-X (doi: 10.1016/j.bcp.2018.08.016) [Epub ahead of print].

62 Di Marzo, V. "New approaches and challenges to targeting the endocannabinoid system." *Nat Rev Drug Discov* 17(9):623–39 (doi: 10.1038/nrd.2018.115).

63 Ibid.

64 Ibid.

it won't have intoxicating or other side effects associated with THC and brain CB1 activation).

Pharmacological blocking of endocannabinoid degradation also has been found to enhance endocannabinoid levels and activate the endocannabinoid system, M. Toczek and B. Malinowska wrote in a 2018 *Life Sciences* review paper,[65] creating a condition researchers call endocannabinoid tone.

Dr. Ethan Russo describes ECS tone as a function of several things—how many endocannabinoid receptors are present and whether they're active or inactive, the activity levels of enzymes that synthesize or degrade the endocannabinoids, and the amounts of available endocannabinoids in the body.[66]

The two main strategies for blocking endocannabinoid degradation, Toczek and Malinowska wrote, are to block endocannabinoid-degrading enzymes, and to block the uptake of endocannabinoids by a cell. Blocking the uptake stops the cell from pulling an endocannabinoid back into the cell from the synapse and leaves more of the molecule to work in the brain.[67]

Both methods, they added, have been found to enhance levels of endocannabinoids and activate the endocannabinoid system. To date, the researchers wrote, "The most investigated compounds are inhibitors of FAAH, the enzyme that degrades the endocannabinoid anandamide." Despite some difficulties and lack of needed studies, Toczek and Malinowska wrote, "Enhancing endocannabinoid signaling is a promising target for drug development not limited to the domain of painkillers."[68]

"Relax, Eat, Sleep, Forget, and Protect"

In a 1998 *Trends in Neuroscience* paper on the endocannabinoid system, Dr. Vincenzo Di Marzo and colleagues wrote about many of the possible neuromodulatory (controlling activity levels of several classes of neurotransmitters) actions of endocannabinoids in the nervous system.[69] Today, Di Marzo is research director at the Institute of Biomolecular Chemistry, National Research Council in Pozzuoli, Naples, Italy, and Canada Excellence Research Chair at University Laval, Quebec City.

---

65 Toczek, M., and B. Malinowska. "Enhanced endocannabinoid tone as a potential target of pharmacotherapy." *Life Sciences* 204:20–45.

66 Russo, E. B. Video interview on the endocannabinoid system with Martin A. Lee, director of Project CBD, June 2016.

67 Toczek, M., and B. Malinowska.

68 Ibid.

69 Di Marzo, V., D. Melck, T. Bisogno, and L. De Petrocellis. "Endocannabinoids: Endogenous cannabinoid receptor ligands with neuromodulatory action." *Trends Neurosci* 1998(12):521–8.

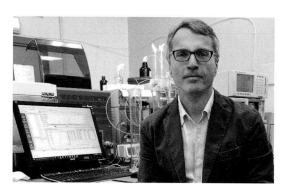

Dr. Vincenzo Di Marzo, director of the Institute of Biomolecular Chemistry at the National Research Council in Naples, Italy, and Canada Excellence Research Chair at University Laval, Quebec City, Canada. (Courtesy Dr. Vincenzo Di Marzo)

In 1998 he and colleagues wrote, "six years of intensive research on endocannabinoids have not yet succeeded in identifying the key physiological function of the endogenous cannabinoid system."[70]

Other studies already had correlated three typical behavioral effects of cannabis smoking—appetite stimulation, anxiety relief, and sedation—with the presence of cannabinoid receptors in the hypothalamus and the limbic system. Researchers had linked the same effects with possible endocannabinoid stimulation of sucrose and ethanol intake, inhibition of anxiety-like responses, and decrease of arousal in rodents.

These and other findings prompted Di Marzo and colleagues to speculate that endocannabinoids might work as stress-recovery factors by relieving typical stress-induced responses in the central and peripheral nervous systems. They wrote that other studies had suggested a neuroprotective role for anandamide.[71]

"Thus," they wrote, "'relax, eat, sleep, forget, and protect' might be some of the messages that are produced by the actions of endocannabinoids, alone or in combination with other mediators." But, they added, "several aspects of endocannabinoid biosynthesis, action and co-localization with other neurotransmitters still need to be investigated, and it will probably take many years of coordinated research among biochemists, neurophysiologists and psychiatrists to critically evaluate this or other hypotheses that relate to the physiological significance of the endogenous cannabinoid system."[72]

A General Strategy of Action

"It was 1998 when I wrote that," Di Marzo said during a 2012 interview in Tucson, Arizona, at the National Clinical Conference on Cannabis Therapeutics.[73] "I was referring to the endocannabinoids [and] what their role could be, their

---

70 Ibid.
71 Ibid.
72 Ibid.
73 Di Marzo, V. CannabisPatientNet, 2012 interview in Tucson, Arizona, at the National Clinical Conference on Cannabis Therapeutics.

general strategy of action. Could they be involved in stress? From what we knew about THC at that time, the answer was yes, and later this prediction was basically confirmed." Definitely, Di Marzo added, endocannabinoid molecules are produced during stressful conditions, at the isolated-cell level but also at the whole-organism level, and they seem to be producing those anti-stress effects.

Of course, he added, "That concept was very simplistic. . . . Now we know more about each of those potential functions—protection, relaxing—activation of this system accompanies the fight-or-flight system and maybe has been evolutionarily conserved to combat the consequences of stress and to recover from stress as quickly as possible. So I would still say this concept is valid, even though it's not so simple as it may have looked in 1998."[74]

Today, many years later, it's known that the endocannabinoid system in the brain primarily influences neuronal synaptic communication and affects biological functions—including eating, anxiety, learning and memory, reproduction, metabolism, growth, and

development—via an array of actions throughout the nervous system.[75]

The endocannabinoid system is very complicated, Di Marzo added during the 2012 interview.[76]

"It's very pleiotropic [produces more than one effect at a time] and works everywhere, and it undergoes changes during nearly every physiological condition," and also during acute (short-duration) pathological and chronic conditions, he said. "We analyze the levels of endocannabinoids and they change during the day, they have seasonal changes. Everything impacts on the endocannabinoid system, both endogenously and exogenously, so it's very complicated to work with but it's also exciting because it's involved in everything." Di Marzo added that the work specifically on plant cannabinoids like THC, CBD, and others also will be exciting.[77]

"Because rather than designing complicated synthetic drugs," he said, "maybe we already have the answer there and it's just a matter of working harder and harder to understand how these compounds work and how the endogenous system works."[78]

---

74 Ibid.
75 Skaper, S. D., and V. Di Marzo. "Endocannabinoids in nervous system health and disease: the big picture in a nutshell." *Philos Trans R Soc Lond B Biol Sci* 367(1607):3193–200 (doi: 10.1098/rstb.2012.0313).
76 Di Marzo, V. CannabisPatientNet.
77 Ibid.
78 Ibid.

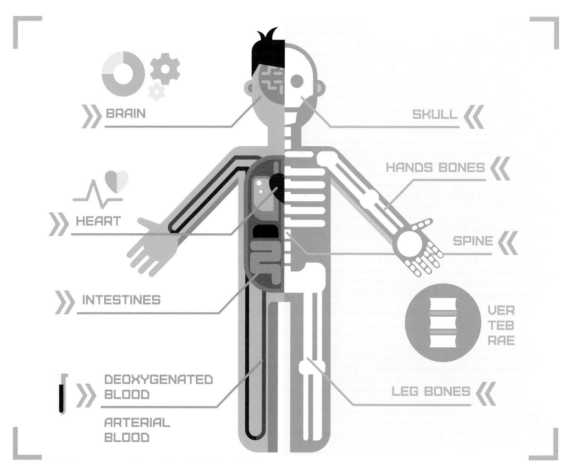

BRAIN

HEART

INTESTINES

DEOXYGENATED
BLOOD

ARTERIAL
BLOOD

SKULL

HANDS BONES

SPINE

VER
TEB
RAE

LEG BONES

Human body anatomy (From iStock by jossdim)

Chapter 4
Two Main Cannabinoids—THC and CBD

Cannabis produces at least 120 plant cannabinoids (ElSohly, email communication November 2018), as far as researchers know right now. The two most studied phytocannabinoids are delta-9-tetrahydrocannabinol (THC), the main intoxicating cannabinoid in cannabis, and cannabidiol (CBD), the main nonintoxicating cannabinoid. But the female plant doesn't synthesize many of these neutral cannabinoids; it mainly makes their acid forms—for example, tetrahydrocannabinolic acid (THCA), cannabidiolic acid (CBDA), and acid forms of the rest of the cannabinoids.[1]

In a 2016 *Cannabis and Cannabinoid Research* paper,[2] M. Wang and colleagues explained that the acidic cannabinoids are thermally unstable and can be decarboxylated when exposed to light or heat through smoking, baking, or refluxing—a form of boiling after which the vapor is returned to the solution. In the chemical process called decarboxylation (dee-car-box-ill-a-shun), a carboxyl group—a

COOH group that acts as a weak acid, for those of us who struggled through organic chemistry—is removed from the raw cannabinoids, and this is important in efficiently producing the active forms of THC, CBD, and other cannabinoids.

"Which is better, CBD or THC?" The question is from the *CBD User's Guide* by Project CBD (see Resources), a California-based nonprofit formed to promote and publicize research into the medical uses of CBD and other cannabis components. The answer, according to the user's guide, is that CBD and THC work best together to boost each other's medicinal effects.

"CBD enhances THC's painkilling and anticancer properties, while lessening THC's psychoactivity," the guide adds. "CBD can also mitigate adverse effects caused by too much THC, such as anxiety and rapid heartbeat. When both compounds are present in sufficient amounts in the same cannabis strain or product, CBD will lower the ceiling on

---

1   Page, J. E.
2   Wang, M., Y. H. Wang, B. Avula, M. M. Radwan, A. S. Wanas, J. van Antwerp, J. F. Parcher, M. A. Elsohly, and I. A. Khan. "Decarboxylation study of acidic cannabinoids: A novel approach using ultra-high-performance supercritical fluid chromatography/photodiode array-mass spectrometry." *Cannabis Cannabinoid Res* 1(1):262–71 (doi.org/10.1089/can.2016.0020).

the THC high while prolonging its duration." CBD, the entry continues, "broadens the range of conditions treatable with cannabis, such as liver, cardiovascular, and metabolic disorders, which may be less responsive to THC-dominant remedies. CBD and THC both stimulate neurogenesis, the creation of new brain cells, in adult mammals."

Delta-9-Tetrahydrocannabinol (THC)

Many phytocannabinoids were discovered throughout the 1960s and early '70s, but most of the research focused on intoxicating THC, which Mechoulam and Gaoni identified in 1964 as cannabis's active cannabinoid.[3]

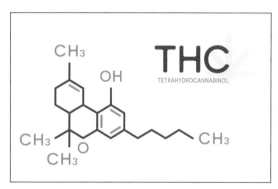

Delta-9 tetrahydrocannabinol (THC) molecule (From Shutterstock by Lifeking)

THC, among more than 100 cannabinoids, is the most common in cannabis drug chemotypes, Russo and Marcu wrote in 2017,[4] and it displays cannabinoid receptor-dependent and -independent mechanisms.

THC interacts efficiently with CB1 and CB2 receptors, they added, and this efficiency underlies its activities in modulating pain, spasticity, sedation, appetite, and mood. THC also is a bronchodilator, a neuroprotective antioxidant, and an anti-itch agent in cholestatic jaundice (decreased bile flow), and it has twenty times the anti-inflammatory power of aspirin and twice that of hydrocortisone.[5]

"It is now well established," Professor Roger Pertwee wrote in a 2008 *British Journal of Pharmacology* paper,[6] "that delta-9 THC is a cannabinoid CB1 and CB2 receptor partial agonist and that, depending on the expression level and coupling efficiency of these receptors, it will either activate them or block their activation by other cannabinoids." Partial agonists bind to and activate receptors but don't produce the maximum response that a full agonist would produce.[7]

3   Russo, E. B.
4   Russo, E. B., and J. Marcu.
5   Ibid.
6   Pertwee, R. G. "The diverse CB1 and CB2 receptor pharmacology of three plant cannabinoids: Δ9-tetrahydrocannabinol, cannabidiol and Δ9-tetrahydrocannabivarin." *Br J Pharmacol* 153(2):199–215 (doi:10.1038/sj.bjp.0707442).
7   Gertsch, J., R. G. Pertwee, and V. Di Marzo. "Phytocannabinoids beyond the *Cannabis* plant—do they exist?" *Br J Pharmacol* 160(3):523–9 (doi: 10.1111/j.1476–5381.2010.00745.x).

Tetrahydrocannabinolic acid (THCA) molecule
(From Shutterstock by pnoiarsa)

Before we talk about THC in research projects, let's discuss tetrahydrocannabinolic acid (tetra-hydro-canna-bin-all-ick, THCA) and its medical effects.

In the cannabis plant, THCA is the immediate precursor to THC.[8] THCA can represent up to 90 percent of total THC content in the plant and has about a 70 percent conversion rate into THC when smoked. THCA can be detected in serum, urine, and oral fluid of cannabis consumers up to eight hours after smoking.

The researchers added that THCA is reported to be a very weak agonist (activator) of CB1 and CB2 receptors compared with THC, but this remains controversial because that activity could be attributable to spontaneous decarboxylation of THCA to THC. THCA also may "inhibit enzymes responsible for the breakdown of endocannabinoids, thus stimulating the ECS by increasing levels of endogenous cannabinoids."[9]

In a basic model of Parkinson's disease, THCA increased cell survival and significantly improved altered neurite (projection from a neuron cell body that is shortened and lacks complexity in some forms of Parkinson's) morphology. THCA reduces the cell viability of various cancer cell lines when administered in vitro (test tube, culture dish), Russo and Marcu added, and "basic research has conclusively shown that THCA can have immunomodulatory, anti-inflammatory, neuroprotective, and antitumor activity."[10] And, according to two research papers,[11,12] THCA recently was shown to be a PPAR-gamma agonist, a receptor at the cell nucleus that affects gene transcription, possibly explaining THCA's role in weight loss, epilepsy, and cancer treatment.

8   Russo, E. B., and J. Marcu.
9   Ibid.
10 Ibid.
11 Nadal, X., C. Del Río, S. Casano, B. Palomares, C. Ferreiro-Vera C. Navarrete, C. Sánchez-Carnerero, I. Cantarero, M. L. Bellido, S. Meyer, G. Morello, G. Appendino, and E. Muñoz. "Tetrahydrocannabinolic acid is a potent PPARgamma agonist with neuroprotective activity." *Br J Pharmacol* 174(23):4263–76.
12 Russo, E. B. "Cannabis therapeutics and the future of neurology." *Front Integr Neurosci* 12:51 (doi: 10.3389/fnint.2018.00051).

THCA also has benefits in clinical practice, according to a tutorial by Dr. Dustin Sulak in his Healer Medical Cannabis Wellness Advisor Training.[13] THCA is the main version of THC produced in raw cannabis flowers, he wrote, and it's nonintoxicating based on animal studies and anecdotal human reports.

"The little research on THCA has demonstrated anti-inflammatory properties via decreased production of tumor necrosis factor alpha [TNF-a, a protein involved in inflammation], stimulation of the PPAR gamma receptor [the cell nucleus receptor discussed earlier], and to a small degree inhibition of the COX-2 enzymes [cyclooxygenase-2 promotes inflammation, pain, and fever], and anti-nausea properties in mice at doses much lower than its neutral counterpart [THC]," Sulak wrote.[14]

He added, "In my clinical practice I have been impressed by the anti-seizure properties of THCA in extraordinarily low doses, as well as its anti-nausea and anti-inflammatory properties."[15]

Now we'll look at THC and the effects it showed in a couple of research studies.

Pain, Opioids, and THC in Whole-Plant Cannabis

In a 2011 *Clinical Pharmacology and Therapeutics* paper on cannabinoid-opioid interactions in chronic pain, D. I. Abrams and colleagues wrote[16] about the results of a clinical trial with twenty-one chronic pain patients on an opioid treatment regimen of twice-daily doses of sustained-release morphine or oxycodone, a semisynthetic opioid. Using a Volcano desktop vaporizer (by Storz and Bickel), patients inhaled vaporized whole-plant cannabis on the evening of day 1, three times a day on days 2 to 4, and in the morning of day 5. The vaporized cannabis didn't significantly affect blood levels of morphine or oxycodone, but pain decreased on average by 27 percent.

The researchers said the small study had some limitations, but they found that the vaporized cannabis boosted pain relief in those who had chronic pain and were on stable doses of sustained-release morphine or oxycodone. They added that pain relief wasn't boosted because cannabis caused higher opioid blood levels, and at the time they didn't know how cannabis helped relieve pain. They called for more research, including testing

---

13 Sulak, D. Healer Certified Online Training Program for medical cannabis. https://healer.com/programs/. Accessed 3/10/19.

14 Ibid.

15 Ibid.

16 Abrams, D. I., P. Couey, S. B. Shade, M. E. Kelly, and N. L. Benowitz. "Cannabinoid-opioid interaction in chronic pain." *Clin Pharmacol Ther* 90(6):844–51 (doi: 10.1038/clpt.2011.188).

different ways of using cannabis (smoke, vape, ingest, others), to find out.[17]

Cannabis seems to slow morphine absorption in the body, so top concentrations for a dosing period are lower, Abrams and colleagues wrote, and "the combination [of opioids and cannabis] may allow for opioid treatment at lower doses with fewer side effects."[18]

THC and Its Effects on Cognition

Other studies show that THC, and THC plus CBD—mainly in animals because of the federal prohibition against THC and other barriers to cannabis research—have positive effects elsewhere. In 2017, for example, two research groups reported a positive THC influence on cognitive effects in older animals.

One of the reports, in *Nature Medicine* by A. Bilkei-Gorzo and colleagues,[19] showed in a series of tests that very low doses of THC in mature and older mice restored learning and memory and social recognition abilities to levels seen in young mice. The treatment also affected molecular processes involved in cell plasticity and cell signaling and positively affected genes involved in extending lifespan and improving cognition, a gene thought to be protective against Alzheimer's disease, and a factor that enhances synapse formation and cognitive functions. The gene-profile changes and cognitive improvements lasted several weeks after the treatment ended, they wrote.[20]

"Cannabis preparations and THC . . . have an excellent safety record and do not produce adverse side effects when administered at a low dose to older individuals," the researchers wrote. "Thus, chronic, low-dose treatment with THC or cannabis extracts could be a potential strategy to slow down or even to reverse cognitive decline in the elderly."[21]

In a 2017 *Neurobiology of Aging* paper,[22] Sarne and colleagues described a study designed to test whether an ultralow THC dose would reverse age-dependent cognitive impairments in old mice, and to examine the effect's possible

---

17 Ibid.

18 Ibid.

19 Bilkei-Gorzo, A, O. Albayram, A. Draffehn, K. Michel, A. Piyanova, H. Oppenheimer, M. Dvir-Ginzberg, I. Rácz, T. Ulas, S. Imbeault, I. Bab, J. L. Schultze, and A. Zimmer. "A chronic low dose of Δ9-tetrahydrocannabinol (THC) restores cognitive function in old mice." *Nat Med* 23(6):782–87 (doi: 10.1038/nm.4311).

20 Ibid.

21 Ibid.

22 Sarne, Y., R. Toledano, L. Rachmany, E. Sasson, and R. Doron. "Reversal of age-related cognitive impairments in mice by an extremely low dose of tetrahydrocannabinol." *Neurobiol Aging* 61:177–86 (doi: 10.1016/j.neurobiolaging.2017.09.025).

biological mechanisms. The researchers reported positive findings, "suggest[ing] that extremely low doses of THC that are devoid of any psychotropic effect and do not induce desensitization [requiring progressively higher doses] may provide a safe and effective treatment for cognitive decline in aging humans."

Together, these studies, if THC eventually shows similar effects in people, could mean that microdosing THC—in, for example, a full- or broad-spectrum, low THC-high CBD cannabis/hemp variety or capsule—would be a safer, nonintoxicating alternative to current drugs, if any, for cognitive problems of the elderly and neurodegenerative diseases.

Cannabidiol (CBD)

CBD is the main nonintoxicating cannabinoid in cannabis plants and its popularity is growing nationwide as a medicine for a range of medical problems.

Cannabidiol (CBD) molecule (From Shutterstock by Lifeking)

In mid-2019, a Google search for CBD returns 230 million links, and there will be more each year. A search of CBD on PubMed.gov—a US National Library of Medicine website that offers access to more than 28 million citations for biomedical literature from MEDLINE (Medical Literature Analysis and Retrieval System Online)—returns 6,372 research papers and reviews. A PubMed search of the word "cannabis" returned 19,667 papers; medical cannabis 7,016; endocannabinoid system 4,846; cannabinoids 16,220; THC 9,859. More results will be available each year.

A section on the expert Project CBD website (projectcbd.org)—established in 2010 and headed by journalist and author Martin A. Lee—called "What is CBD?" says preclinical and clinical research, much of it sponsored by the US government, underscores CBD's potential as a treatment for conditions or symptoms of conditions including arthritis, diabetes, alcoholism, multiple sclerosis, chronic pain, schizophrenia, posttraumatic stress syndrome, depression, antibiotic-resistant infections, and epilepsy, among others.[23]

CBD has effects that protect against some kinds of illnesses and injuries in the brain and nervous system, and academic research centers in the United States and around the world are investigating CBD's anticancer properties, Project CBD says,

---

23 Project CBD.

noting that evidence from recent studies suggests the CBD varieties and forms used in the studies were safe even at high doses.[24]

For decades, only high-THC cannabis was available in North America and elsewhere—who wanted cannabis that wouldn't get you high? But Lee and others involved in Project CBD devoted years of effort to educating growers and the public about the health benefits of CBD. Today, CBD-rich strains and products are available to medical users, Lee said (author interview July 27, 2017), at least those in states and countries that have approved the use of medical cannabis for certain medical conditions.

Over the past few years, the online availability of broad-spectrum CBD to anyone who wants it has grown and products have improved, although buyers should research sellers and buy products only from companies that provide good information about their products and have good customer reviews. CBD is available as oil, tinctures, capsules, edibles, crystals, and many other forms. According to Russo and Marcu,[25] CBD can produce a wide range of pharmacological activity, including

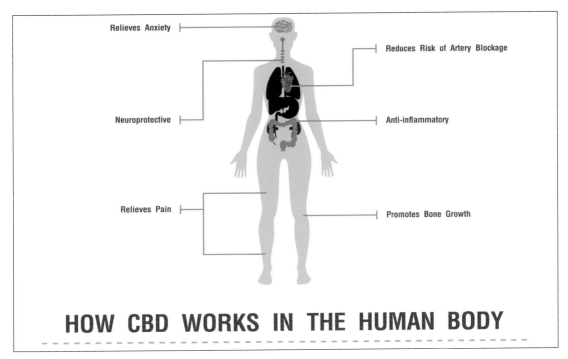

How CBD works in the body. (From Shutterstock by Image seller in w)

24 Ibid.
25 Russo, E. B., and J. Marcu.

anticonvulsant, anti-inflammatory, antioxidant, and antipsychotic effects.

"These effects underlie the neuroprotective properties of CBD and support its role in the treatment of a number of neurological and neurodegenerative disorders," the researchers wrote, "including epilepsy, Parkinson disease, amyotrophic lateral sclerosis, Huntington disease, Alzheimer disease, and multiple sclerosis." CBD has the unique ability to counteract the intoxicating and adverse effects of THC in cannabis, like anxiety, tachycardia, hunger, and sedation in rats and people.[26]

Recently, Russo and Marcu wrote, "CBD demonstrated its strong anti-inflammatory and immunosuppressive properties in a phase II study on graft-versus-host disease [GvHD],"[27] which the Cleveland Clinic website describes as "a condition that might occur after an allogeneic transplant [in which matching-donor stem cells are transplanted]. In GvHD, the donated bone marrow or peripheral blood stem cells view the recipient's body as foreign, and the donated cells/bone marrow attack the body." In the study, they added, 300 mg per day of CBD starting a week before the procedure was associated with lower mortality and fewer complications.[28]

CBD's medical benefits and lack of intoxication, according to Project CBD,[29] "makes it an appealing option for patients looking for relief from inflammation, pain, anxiety, psychosis, seizures, spasms, and other conditions without disconcerting feelings of lethargy or dysphoria," dysphoria meaning a feeling of unease.

In 2018, Project CBD launched an interactive research survey for CBD users who will be able to share their CBD experiences. Survey results are available at projectcbd.org/reports/cbd-survey-results.

"Figuring out how to maximize the therapeutic benefits of cannabis is still a work in progress," Project CBD writes. "This effort is the driving force behind the great laboratory experiment in democracy known as medical and recreational cannabis that's been unfolding state-by-state and around the world in recent years. Big Pharma can have their overpriced, single-molecule meds. Whole-plant cannabis is the people's medicine and always will be. Let's crowdsource our therapeutic knowledge and share what we've learned. Let's democratize the data by taking the Project CBD survey and asking your friends, colleagues, or memberships to do so. The Project CBD data collection platform will track CBD's

---

26 Ibid.
27 Ibid.
28 Ibid.
29 Project CBD.

impact on a range of conditions and provide real-time results as a public resource for those who might benefit from cannabis therapeutics."[30]

As with the relationship of THCA to THC, CBD is produced in cannabis plants mainly as cannabidiolic acid (canna-bih-dye-all-ick, CBDA). According to Russo and Marcu, CBDA shares CBD's ability to enhance the serotonin subtype 5-HT1A receptor activation, but the acidic compound doesn't interact efficiently with CB1 receptors as an agonist or antagonist. CBDA's affinity at 5-HT1A is greater than an order of magnitude higher compared to CBD. Evidence from animals shows significant CBDA antiemetic (prevents vomiting and nausea) effects.[31]

Cannabidiolic acid (CBDA) (From Shutterstock by pnoiarsa)

According to Dr. Dustin Sulak's Healer.com wellness advisor training website,[32] scientists haven't thoroughly explored the physiologic effects or therapeutic potential of CBDA, but it has shown anti-nausea properties in mice at very low doses and anti-inflammatory effects by inhibiting the COX-2 enzyme—the same mechanism of action as the arthritis drug Celebrex.

Adding to the Cannabis Medicine Chest

A turning point for public awareness about CBD came in 2013 when CNN began airing a three-part documentary called *Weed*, created by its chief medical correspondent and neurosurgeon Dr. Sanjay Gupta. The latest documentary in the series, *Weed 4: Pot vs. Pills*, streamed live for subscribers on April 29, 2018, and examined the potential of medical cannabis and especially CBD as an alternative to opioids for treating pain and helping to end opioid addiction.

At Project CBD, during his interview, Lee calls CBD a "very important addition to the medical marijuana medicine chest. It really has opened up the whole world—not only drawing in a lot of people who might not otherwise be open to the notion of trying medical marijuana . . . it has expanded the whole

---

30 Ibid.
31 Russo, E. B., and J. Marcu.
32 Sulak, D.

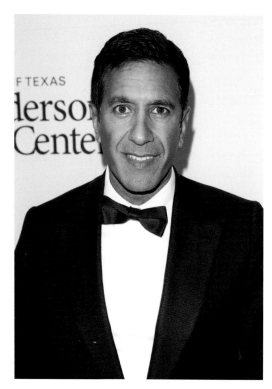

Dr. Sanjay Gupta attends the launch of the Parker Institute for Cancer Immunotherapy, a collaboration among leading immunologists and cancer centers on April 13, 2016, in Los Angeles, California. (From Getty Images by Jesse Grant)

cannabinoid compound over another but to challenge the idea that cannabis equals THC. THC is a remarkable molecule in its own right, but THC is not the whole plant, and neither is CBD. Project CBD defends and supports whole-plant cannabis therapeutics."[33]

During a 2016 interview[34] with Lee at the northern California offices of Project CBD, Ethan Russo called CBD "really distinct" from THC, although the cannabinoids offer benefits when taken together.

"In its own right cannabidiol is an endocannabinoid modulator," Russo said. "In other words, when given chronically it actually increases the gain of system, which is, at its core, a homeostatic regulator. To explain that: homeostasis is a state of balance. Many diseases interfere with balance in a given system and, if we can bring that balance back to where it should be, there'll be improvement in the overall condition." This is one reason CBD is such a versatile medicine, he added, because so many disorders operate on that level.[35]

"If there's too much activity in a system, homeostasis requires that it be brought back down. If there's too little, it's got to come up. And that's what cannabidiol can do as a promoter of endocannabinoid tone," Russo said.[36]

audience, the participating community, for medical marijuana because of the lack of psychoactive [effects], at least not psychoactive like THC."

The following statement appears on the Project CBD website along with a range of other information: "We emphasize CBD not to privilege one

33 Project CBD.
34 Russo, E. B., video interview.
35 Ibid.
36 Ibid.

CBD Medicine

CBD and THC differ in another way, Russo added.[37] "We can think of THC as acting directly on the cannabinoid receptors. In contrast, CBD . . . doesn't tend to bind directly to what's called the orthosteric site where THC binds. Rather, it binds on what's called an allosteric site, another site on the receptor, and it alters the binding of both THC and the endogenous cannabinoids, the endocannabinoids."

CBD is what's called a negative allosteric modulator, Russo added, meaning that when THC is present, CBD interferes with its activity. This reduces THC's psychoactivity and limits its side effects like anxiety or rapid heart rate at higher doses.[38]

Russo notes that CBD is very good for treating a variety of conditions. One is epilepsy. "CBD as an anticonvulsant has a broad spectrum of activity. In other words, it works on many different kinds of seizures and has the possibility of doing this without any of the liability that THC might produce, both in terms of side effects but also legal constraints. That's a big advantage," he said.[39]

On June 25, 2018, GW Pharmaceuticals' Epidiolex became the first Food and Drug Administration (FDA)-approved pharmaceutical formulation of the purified, plant-derived (and non-intoxicating) cannabinoid CBD, and the first in what probably will be a new category of anti-epileptic drugs. This was a huge breakthrough for CBD, and Russo explained it in the following way (email communication June 27, 2018).

"The approval of Epidiolex by the FDA represents a landmark as the first American recognition of a cannabis-derived pharmaceutical. Unfortunately, it follows by almost 15 years the approval of oromucosal (mouth spray) cannabis-based medicine in Canada (GW's Sativex, called nabiximols in the United States), a medicine that has been accepted in more than 30 other countries around the world, but not in the USA," he wrote. "Epidiolex has the approved indications as an adjunctive [used with a primary treatment] treatment of Dravet and Lennox-Gastaut syndromes, two severe forms of epilepsy. It remains to be seen whether [Epidiolex], an extract of cannabidiol, will be more extensively utilized as a treatment for various other possible diagnoses: schizophrenia, rheumatoid arthritis, inflammatory bowel diseases, and others."

---

37 Ibid.
38 Ibid.
39 Ibid.

But now anyone with a doctor's prescription will be able to find out, because on April 6, 2020, the Drug Enforcement Administration removed Epidiolex—the only highly purified plant-derived CBD medicine approved by FDA—from its list of controlled substances. The change took place immediately, according to a statement by GW. Epidiolex was launched in the United States on November 1, 2018, to treat seizures from Lennox-Gastaut Syndrome or Dravet syndrome in young patients. The company is implementing the change at the state level and through the Epidiolex distribution network, after which doctors will be able to prescribe the new medicine for patients.

More Help for CBD: The 2018 Farm Bill

On December 20, 2018, the Agriculture Improvement Act of 2018,[40] the 2018 Farm Bill, was signed into law. The new law removed industrial hemp from the Controlled Substances Act and moved oversight of hemp production, marketing, research, and other functions from the Drug Enforcement Administration (DEA) to the US Department of Agriculture (USDA) to regulate hemp growing, and to the FDA for oversight of hemp-derived products. The bill defines hemp as cannabis and cannabis derivatives (like CBD) that contain no more than 0.3 percent (of the plant's dry weight) THC.

Also on December 20, 2018, FDA Commissioner Scott Gottlieb, MD, issued a statement[41] about the agency's regulation of cannabis and cannabis-derived products, describing the processes required going forward for hemp-derived products like broad-spectrum CBD. The Farm Bill didn't change everything, though.

Gottlieb wrote in his statement: "Congress explicitly preserved the [FDA's] current authority to regulate products containing cannabis or cannabis-derived compounds under the Federal Food, Drug and Cosmetic Act and section 351 of the Public Health Service Act. . . . This allows the FDA to continue enforcing the law to protect patients and the public while also providing potential regulatory pathways for products containing cannabis and cannabis-derived compounds."[42]

---

40 GovTrack.us, H.R. 2: Agriculture Improvement Act of 2018. https://www.govtrack.us/congress/bills/115/hr2. Accessed 12/22/18.

41 US Food and Drug Administration, December 20, 2018, statement from FDA Commissioner Scott Gottlieb MD on the Agriculture Improvement Act, https://www.fda.gov/NewsEvents/Newsroom/PressAnnouncements/ucm628988.htm. Accessed 12/22/18.

42 Ibid.

On March 5, 2019, Gottlieb resigned for his own reasons, and was replaced by the former National Cancer Institute Director Dr. Ned Sharpless as acting FDA commissioner. Despite the uncertainty of a new commissioner, getting approval for research using high-CBD/low-THC hemp should be less complicated for scientists now because hemp is legal, they won't need special permissions and storage approvals, and they won't have surprise DEA visits disrupting their laboratories.

That's good news, for CBD and the other nonintoxicating cannabinoids in hemp, anyway. So far, THC is still on the DEA's Schedule 1. But CBD is as close to legal as it takes for CBD companies to get their products approved by the FDA, at least according to the rules as they stand in 2020.

CBD-Rich Cannabis Extracts vs. Purified CBD

We've already discussed the idea that whole-plant, full-spectrum cannabis and CBD are more effective medicine (because of the entourage effect) than isolated or synthesized THC or CBD. A 2018 *Frontiers in Neurology* clinical study by F. A. Pamplona and colleagues shows just how two kinds of CBD differ. The researchers analyzed observational clinical studies on treating refractory epilepsy with cannabidiol-based products. They were trying to establish the products' safety and effectiveness, but they also investigated whether there was evidence of a difference in effectiveness between CBD-rich (broad-spectrum) extracts and purified (CBD alone) CBD products.[43]

The researchers said two-thirds (64 percent) of patients reported reduced seizure frequency. Similar reports came from patients treated with CBD-rich extracts (71 percent) than from patients treated with purified CBD (36 percent). Still, when the standard clinical threshold of a "50 percent reduction or more in the frequency of seizures" was applied, only 39 percent of the patients were considered responders (to the therapy) and in this group there was no real difference between treatments with CBD-rich extracts (38 percent) and purified CBD (42 percent). But patients treated with CBD-rich extracts reported a much lower average dose (6.1 mg per kilogram per day) than those using purified CBD (27.1 mg/kg/day). And reports of mild and severe adverse effects were more frequent in products containing purified CBD than in CBD-rich extracts.[44]

---

43 Pamplona, F. A., L. R. da Silva, and A. C. Coan. "Potential clinical benefits of CBD-rich cannabis extracts over purified CBD in treatment-resistant epilepsy: Observational data meta-analysis." *Front. Neurol* 9:759 (doi: 10.3389/fneur.2018.00759).
44 Ibid.

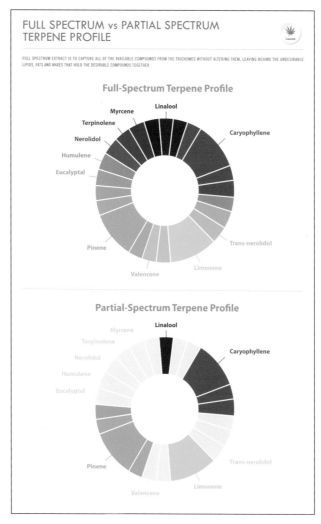

FULL SPECTRUM vs PARTIAL SPECTRUM
TERPENE PROFILE

FULL SPECTRUM EXTRACT IS TO CAPTURE ALL OF THE AVAILABLE COMPOUNDS FROM THE TRICHOMES WITHOUT ALTERING THEM, LEAVING BEHIND THE UNDESIRABLE
LIPIDS, FATS AND WAXES THAT HOLD THE DESIRABLE COMPOUNDS TOGETHER.

Full-Spectrum Terpene Profile

Partial-Spectrum Terpene Profile

An example of the entourage effect. (From iStock by About time)

"CBD-rich extracts seem to present a better therapeutic profile than purified CBD, at least in this population of patients with refractory epilepsy," Pamplona and colleagues wrote. "The root of this difference is likely due to synergistic effects of CBD with other phytocompounds [entourage effect], but this remains to be confirmed in controlled clinical studies."[45]

45 Ibid.

Chapter 5
More Cannabinoids, Terpenes, and the Entourage Effect

More than 560 constituents have been identified in cannabis, according to ElSohly and colleagues in a 2017 *Progress in the Chemistry of Organic Natural Products* paper on the plant chemistry (phytochemistry) of cannabis.[1]

"The recent discoveries of the medicinal properties of cannabis and the cannabinoids, in addition to their potential applications in the treatment of a number of serious illnesses, such as glaucoma, depression, neuralgia [nerve pain], multiple sclerosis, Alzheimer's, and alleviation of symptoms of HIV/AIDS and cancer," the researchers wrote, "have given momentum to the quest for further understanding the chemistry, biology and medicinal properties of this plant."[2]

A Few More Cannabinoids

Cannabinol was the first cannabinoid to be isolated and identified from cannabis, and this led to speculation that the psychotropically active constituents of cannabis could be tetrahydrocannabinols, according to Thomas and ElSohly in 2016.[3] The non-psychotropic compound CBD was later isolated from Mexican cannabis and the structure determined, and Gaoni and Mechoulam determined the structure of THC after isolating and purifying the compound.

Since then, the number of cannabinoids and other compounds isolated from cannabis has continually increased, with 565 now reported, 120 of them phytocannabinoids, according to Dr. Mahmoud ElSohly (email communication, August 4, 2019).

---

1   ElSohly, M. A., M. M. Radwan, W. Gul, S. Chandra, and A. Galal. "Phytochemistry of *Cannabis sativa* L.," *Prog Chem Org Nat Prod* 103:1–36 (doi: 10.1007/978-3-319-45541-9_1).
2   Ibid.
3   Thomas, F., and M. ElSohly. "The Analytical Chemistry of Cannabis," in *Emerging Issues in Analytical Chemistry Elsevier*, 2016.

But most recently, in a December 2019 Nature.com Scientific Reports paper ([2019] 9:20335 | https://doi.org/10.1038/s41598-019-56785-1), Italian scientists C. Citti and colleagues announced their identification of two new cannabinoids. Tetrahydrocannabiphorol (THCP) has the same structure as THC but with an extra chemical sidechain. Cannabidiphorol (CBDP) has the same structure as CBD but with the same kind of chemical sidechain. More work must be done on these new phytocannabinoids for researchers to fully understand their properties. This means 122 phytocannabinoids have been identified, and more are doubtless are coming, and more speedily than in the past.

Between the isolation and structural elucidation of THC in 1964 and 1980, sixty-one phytocannabinoids were isolated and reported. Only nine new ones were characterized between 1981 and 2005, but thirty-one were reported between 2006 and 2010.[4]

These are descriptions of some of the best-studied cannabinoids.

Cannabinol (CBN)

Cannabinol (can-na-bin-all) was identified and isolated from cannabis in 1899 and is a by-product of THC, usually an artifact found after the cannabis has been stored for a long time, Russo and Marcu

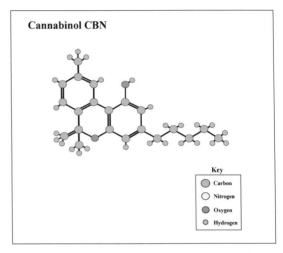

The cannabinoid cannabinol (By Ellen Seefelt)

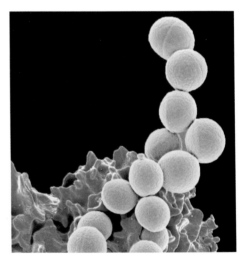

Neutrophil (blue) ingests methicillin-resistant *Staphylococcus aureus* (yellow). (Courtesy NIH National Institute for Allergy and Infectious Diseases)

wrote, adding, "CBN can be sedative, anticonvulsant in animal and human studies, and has demonstrated significant

---

4 Ibid.

properties related to anti-inflammatory, antibiotic and anti-MRSA," referring to methicillin-resistant *Staphylococcus aureus*. In topical form CBN also may be able to treat psoriasis and burns, and because of its actions related to bone marrow stem cells, it could promote bone formation.[5]

Russo wrote in a personal communication (June 3, 2019), "CBN is a non-enzymatic breakdown product of THC that appears spontaneously as cannabis ages or is exposed to air and light. This process also purges the material of lower-molecular-weight monoterpenoids [like limonene] and favors retention of oxygenated sesquiterpenoids [like beta-caryophyllene], that combination producing a more sedating mixture. CBN displays about 25 percent of the intoxicating potency of THC but otherwise is not particularly advantageous as a development target. Its current popularity in the marketplace may actually represent a marketing ploy to utilize a great deal of old cannabis that might otherwise be discarded."

Cannabigerol (CBG)

Cannabigerol (can-na-bih-jair-all) was purified from cannabis in 1964, the same year as THC. It's chemically related to THC but has no intoxicating effects. It's usually present in trace amounts

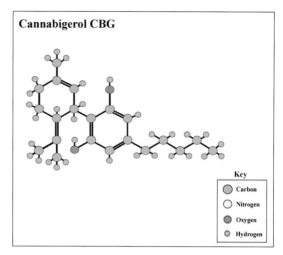

Cannabigerol CBG

Key
- Carbon
- Nitrogen
- Oxygen
- Hydrogen

The cannabinoid cannabigerol (CBG) (By Ellen Seefelt)

in cannabis and "displays fascinating pharmacology in its own right," Ethan Russo wrote in a 2015 white paper. This includes antidepressant-like effects in rodent studies, pain relief, chemotherapeutic benefits, antibiotic effects including against MRSA, and other benefits.[6]

Russo also noted[7] that in the lab CBG has, at high doses, proven to kill human cancer cells, and that after CBD it's the next most effective phytocannabinoid with effects against breast cancer. It's also mildly effective against high blood pressure and may be useful against psoriasis, prostate cancer, and bladder pain.

In 2017, Russo and Marcu wrote that CBG also may stimulate a range of receptors important for pain, inflammation and heat sensitization, and has possible

---

5   Russo, E. B., and J. Marcu.
6   Russo, E. B., white paper, January 2015.
7   Russo, E. B.

application in prostate cancer and effects on detrusor (the muscle that stays relaxed to let the bladder store urine) overactivity. CBG also had significant antidepressant effects in tests with rodents, is mildly effective against high blood pressure and may have use against psoriasis, a skin condition that speeds up the skin-cell life cycle.[8]

In his lab's work on cannabinoid science, Professor Roger Pertwee said in an interview (July 18, 2017) that he and colleagues had discovered that CBG could block the serotonin receptor 5-HT1A, and that CBG also can activate a receptor where the neurotransmitter noradrenaline (norepinephrine) acts as an agonist, the alpha-2 adrenergic receptor.

"The fact that cannabigerol can activate this receptor suggests it might be good to relieve pain. And we were able to show, in a collaboration with an Italian scientist who could do preclinical pain studies, that in fact it did relieve pain in an animal model," Pertwee said. "So it's possible in the future that cannabigerol might be developed as a medicine for pain relief. That's yet one more example of a potential new plant cannabinoid medicine."

Cannabichromene (CBC)

Cannabichromene (can-na-bih-crow-meen) was isolated in 1966 by two different research groups. It represents about 0.3 percent of constituents from confiscated cannabis, but commercial and medical preparations occasionally have much higher content, Russo and Marcu wrote. CBC-rich cannabis strains are the result of selecting for the inheritance of a recessive gene, achievable through extensive crossbreeding. It has shown anti-inflammatory and pain-relief activity, an ability to reduce THC intoxication in mice, antibiotic and antifungal effects, and an observed ability to kill cells in certain cancer-cell lines.[9] Also, Russo wrote in 2011,[10] a CBC extract has displayed

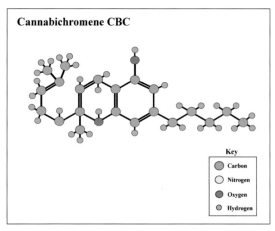

The cannabinoid cannabichromene (CBC) (By Ellen Seefelt)

8 Russo, E. B., and J. Marcu.
9 Ibid.
10 Russo, E. B.

pronounced antidepressant-like effects in rodent research models.

In a 2016 review of major and minor phytocannabinoids, Marcu wrote that CBC could be one of the most abundant nonintoxicating cannabinoids found in cannabis varieties. CBC can also have strong anti-inflammatory effects in animal models of edema (swelling), and its effects can be boosted when co-administered with THC.[11] An early study[12] of the biological activity of CBC and related molecules found that it had strong antibacterial activity and mild-to-moderate antifungal effects.

Tetrahydrocannabivarin (THCV)

Tetrahydrocannabivarin (tetra-hydro-cannab-ih-vair-in) is chemically related to THC and most often occurs as a small percentage of dried cannabis plant material. One pharmaceutical company has developed plants that are 16 percent THCV by dry weight.[13] THCV can act as an agonist and an antagonist at CB1 receptors depending on its concentration,[14] and it binds strongly to CB2 receptors. Because of the CB2 activation, THCV was able to

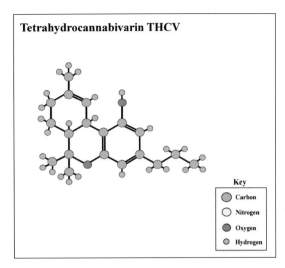

Tetrahydrocannabivarin THCV

Key
- Carbon
- Nitrogen
- Oxygen
- Hydrogen

The cannabinoid tetrahydrocannabivarin (By Ellen Seefelt)

suppress hyperalgesia (increased sensitivity to pain), inflammation, and pain in tests with mice.[15]

In 2016, K. A. Jadoon and colleagues performed the first-ever investigation of the effects of CBD and THCV on dyslipidemia (abnormally high cholesterol or fats in the blood) and glycemic control in people with type 2 diabetes. Earlier studies had shown effects on lipid (derived from fatty acid) and glucose metabolism in animal models. Results from sixty-two people over thirteen weeks showed that,

11 Marcu, J. "An overview of major and minor phytocannabinoids." 2016:672–78 (doi: 10.1016/B978-0-12-800213-1.00062–6).

12 Turner, C. E., and M. A. ElSohly. "Biological activity of cannabichromene, its homologs and isomers." *J Clin Pharmacol* 21(8–9 Suppl):283S–91S.

13 Marcu, J.

14 Russo, E. B., and J. Marcu.

15 McPartland, J. M., M. Duncan, V. Di Marzo, and R. G. Pertwee. "Are cannabidiol and Δ9-tetrahydrocannabivarin negative modulators of the endocannabinoid system? A systematic review." *Br J Pharmacol* 172(3):737–53 (doi:10.1111/bph.12944).

compared with placebo, THCV significantly decreased fasting plasma glucose and improved pancreatic beta-cell function, adiponectin (a protein hormone involved in regulating glucose levels), and apolipoprotein A (a protein carried in cholesterol high-density lipoprotein [HDL]). This led the researchers to conclude that THCV could become a new therapeutic agent in glycemic control for people with type 2 diabetes.[16]

In 2015, M. G. Cascio and colleagues published a THCV study in the *British Journal of Pharmacology*.[17] They found that THCV can boost activation of the serotonin receptor 5-HT1A, and that some of the receptor's apparent antipsychotic effects may depend on THCV enhancement. They concluded that THCV has therapeutic potential for easing some of the negative, cognitive, and positive (the three symptom categories) symptoms of schizophrenia.

Also in 2015, in a *Handbook of Experimental Pharmacology* paper,[18] J. Fernández-Ruiz and colleagues called THCV "an interesting compound to be

DIABETES MELLITUS

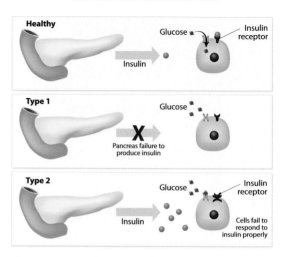

The two types of diabetes (From iStock by ttsz)

used therapeutically in Parkinson's disease, alone or in combination with CBD," because of its combination of effects. A future cannabinoid-based neuroprotective therapy for PD, they wrote, would need antioxidant activity exerted by cannabinoid receptor-independent mechanisms (as CBD and THCV provide), maybe involving activation of receptors that work at the cell nucleus, PPARs, discussed earlier, that have shown benefits in experimental parkinsonism.

16 Jadoon, K. A., S. H. Ratcliffe, D. A. Barrett, E. L. Thomas, C. Stott, J. D. Bell, S. E. O'Sullivan, and G. D. Tan. "Efficacy and safety of cannabidiol and tetrahydrocannabivarin on glycemic and lipid parameters in patients with type 2 diabetes: A randomized, double-blind, placebo-controlled, parallel group pilot study." *Diabetes Care* 39(10):1777–86 (doi.org/10.2337/dc16-0650).

17 Cascio, M. G., E. Zamberletti, P. Marini, D. Parolaro, and R. G. Pertwee. "The phytocannabinoid, delta-9-tetrahydrocannabivarin, can act through 5-HT1A receptors to produce antipsychotic effects." *Br J Pharmacol* 172(5):1305–18 (doi:10.1111/bph.13000).

18 Fernández-Ruiz, J., J. Romero, and J. A. Ramos. "Endocannabinoids and Neurodegenerative Disorders: Parkinson's Disease, Huntington's Chorea, Alzheimer's Disease, and Others." *Handb Exp Pharmacol* 231:233–59 (doi: 10.1007/978-3-319-20825-1_8).

Parkinson's therapy also would need to activate CB2 receptors, control neuroinflammatory events, and blockade CB1 receptors to improve akinesia (impaired voluntary movement) and reduce motor inhibition (suppression of sensory cues or stimuli that trigger movement). THCV has such a profile, Fernández-Ruiz and colleagues wrote, and this "highlights the need for a formulation that can be further evaluated in patients."[19]

The Influence of Cannabis Terpenes

In their 2017 paper, Russo and Marcu wrote that fifty cannabis terpenes (from Giese, Lewis, Giese, and Smith 2015[20]) are routinely found in North American chemovars (chemical varieties), of which seventeen are most common, and eight of these form terpene super classes: myrcene, terpinolene, ocimene, limonene, alpha-pinene, humulene, linalool, and beta-caryophyllene. Cannabis samples from a single California cannabis dispensary over the course of a year (from Fischedick 2017[21]) identified five terpene groups based on predominant content: myrcene, terpinolene, myrcene/limonene, beta-caryophyllene, and bisabolol.[22]

We will discuss beta-caryophyllene, myrcene, linalool, and limonene.

Lots of plants, including cannabis, biosynthesize terpenes, all of which contain the 5-carbon skeleton of a common organic compound called isoprene, the main component of natural rubber. Terpenes are characterized by the number of 5-carbon isoprene units present in their molecular structures, so those with two isoprene units (ten carbons total) are called monoterpenes and those with three isoprene units (fifteen carbons total) are called sesquiterpenes. There are also diterpenes (twenty carbons) and triterpenes (thirty carbons).

At the 2017 International Association for Cannabis as Medicine Conference on

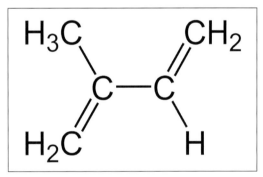

All terpenes contain the 5-carbon skeleton of isoprene, a common organic compound. (From Wikimedia Commons by Jag123. This file is in the public domain)

19 Ibid.
20 Giese, M. W., et al. "Development and Validation of a Reliable and Robust Method for the Analysis of Cannabinoids and Terpenes in Cannabis." *J AOAC Int* 98(6):1503–22.
21 Fischedick, J. "Identification of terpenoid chemotypes among high (-)-trans-delta nine-tetrahydrocannabinol-producing Cannabis sativa L. cultivars." *Cannabis Cannabinoid Res* 2.1:34–47.
22 Russo, E. B., and J. Marcu.

Cannabinoids as Medicine in Germany, plant biologist Dr. Jonathan Page said[23] cannabinoids occur along with terpenes in cannabis—terpenes like myrcene, linalool, limonene, and beta-caryophyllene, and other metabolites like flavonoids (plant chemicals found in nearly all fruits and vegetables) and polyketides (natural products with a range of biological activities and pharmacological properties). But cannabinoids and terpenes, Page said, "really drive the biological activity" in cannabis. Cannabinoids are best studied in terms of their pharmacology, Page said, including "the synergy between a mixture of cannabinoids and terpenes giving rise to psychoactivity, and maybe the influence of terpenes on that psychoactivity, but also the analgesic [pain relieving] properties, the antispasticity, [and] all the useful medical properties. It's the chemical factory of the cannabis plant that's driving this interesting pharmacology."[24]

Making Cannabinoids and Terpenes

Differences in the pharmaceutical properties of cannabis varieties, Page said, have been attributed to interactions between cannabinoids and terpenes. For example, beta-caryophyllene interacts with mammalian cannabinoid receptors.

As a result, medicinal compositions have been proposed to incorporate different blends of cannabinoids and terpenes. Terpenes may contribute to the antianxiety, antibacterial, anti-inflammatory, and sedative effects of cannabis.[25]

Following are descriptions of some of the most well-known terpenes.

Beta-caryophyllene

Beta-caryophyllene (bayta-carry-o-fyeleen), a sesquiterpene, is the most common terpenoid in cannabis extracts and is nearly ubiquitous in food in the food supply.[26] It has "extensive potent and various pharmacological activities and a wide therapeutic index, safety, and low toxicity."

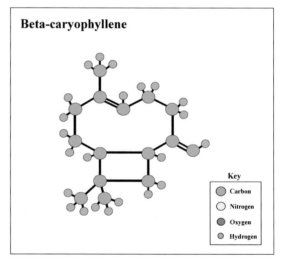

Beta-caryophyllene molecule (by Ellen Seefelt)

---

23 Page, J. E.
24 Ibid.
25 Ibid.
26 Russo, E. B., and J. Marcu.

Beta-caryophyllene targets the CB2 receptor and acts as a full agonist there, meaning that it fully activates the receptor, and it's a major compound in cannabis essential oil, Gertsch and colleagues wrote in a 2010 *British Journal of Pharmacology* review paper.[27] Beta-caryophyllene also is found in many other plants. According to other studies, it has anti-inflammatory effects through CBD, gastric protective actions through THC, and antimalarial effects, and may be able to treat severe skin itching and addiction.[28]

Ethan Russo has called it a very safe agent. Beta-caryophyllene is in black pepper, for example. "It's called GRAS by the government . . . Generally Recognized As Safe as a food additive, so this is something with the government's seal of approval. It's in our diet but more of this

would certainly have a positive influence on health, particularly for people with arthritis or other kinds of chronic pain, and it's without any liability in terms of having unwanted side effects."[29]

Orally administered beta-caryophyllene produces strong anti-inflammatory and pain-relieving effects in rodents, and ongoing studies show that it works through the CB2 receptor to effectively reduce neuropathic pain. Therefore, Gertsch and colleagues wrote, "The FDA-approved food additive b-caryophyllene has the potential to become an attractive candidate for clinical trials targeting the CB2 receptor."[30]

Russo and Marcu said that basic experiments have shown strong evidence that beta-caryophyllene is protective for the heart, liver, gastrointestinal tract, kidneys, immune response, and brain cells, and acts against free radicals, inflammation, and harmful microorganisms. Thus, they wrote, "it has shown potent therapeutic promise in neuropathic pain and neurodegenerative and metabolic diseases . . . and protection from alcoholic steatohepatitis [fatty liver disease] via anti-inflammatory effects" and helping to ease metabolic disturbances.[31]

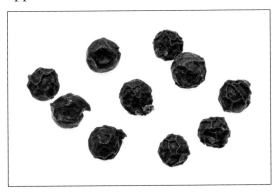

Black peppercorn (From Getty by Akepong Srichaichana / EyeEm)

---

27 Gertsch, J., R. G. Pertwee, and V. Di Marzo.
28 Russo, E. B.
29 Russo, E. B., Video interview.
30 Gertsch, J., R. G. Pertwee, and V. Di Marzo.
31 Russo, E. B., and J. Marcu.

Russo says[32] beta-caryophyllene is present to some degree in almost all cannabis varieties, "but if you have, say in a dispensary, the ability to have a good assay for the cannabinoid content and you're able to select for one that is high in caryophyllene, we would expect that to be much better at treating pain and inflammation."

Beta-caryophyllene also may provide supplemental support in addiction, Russo wrote in 2011.[33] In a clinical trial, "48 cigarette smokers inhaling vapor from an essential oil of black pepper ([beta-caryophyllene-containing] *Piper nigrum*), a mint-menthol mixture, or placebo, black pepper essential oil reduced nicotine craving significantly . . . an effect attributed to irritation of the bronchial tree, simulating the act of cigarette smoking but without nicotine or actual burning of material. Rather, might not the effect have been pharmacological? The terpenoid profile of black pepper suggests possible candidates . . . especially caryophyllene via CB2 agonism [activation] and a newly discovered putative [reputed] mechanism of action in addiction treatment."

Myrcene

Myrcene (mer-seen), a monoterpene, is the most prevalent terpene in modern

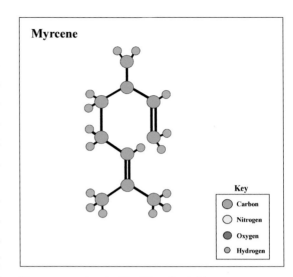

Myrcene molecule (By Ellen Seefelt)

cannabis chemovars in the United States and Europe, Russo and Marcu wrote, and is likely most responsible for the sedative effects of many cannabis preparations on the market, a result termed "couch lock." It's also anti-inflammatory, blocks the cancer-causing effects of aflatoxin (produced by fungi) in the liver, and in mice has pain-relieving and muscle-relaxant effects. Tests in the lab indicate it might be able to help those with osteoarthritis. In rats myrcene showed notable effects against peptic ulcers, and in mice it prevented oxidative injury. This activity, the authors wrote, "suggests the possibility of synergistic benefits with the neuroprotective antioxidant effects of THC and CBD."[34]

32 Russo, E. B., Video interview.
33 Russo, E. B.
34 Russo, E. B., and J. Marcu.

Linalool

Linalool (lin-ah-lool), also a monoterpene, is commonly extracted from lavender, rose, basil, and neroli oil (from the flowers of the bitter orange tree).[35] It also has established sedative, antidepressant, anxiolytic (anxiety reducing), and immune potentiating effects, and can be a significant part of cannabis essential oil. Recent reports "support the possibility that small concentrations found in certain cannabis chemovars may exert anticonvulsant benefits in human patients." In traditional aromatherapy, "linalool is the likely suspect in the remarkable therapeutic capabilities of lavender essential oil to alleviate skin burns without scarring."[36]

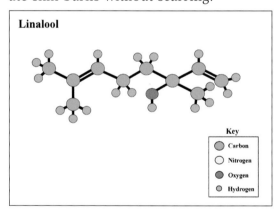

Linalool molecule (By Ellen Seefelt)

Limonene

Limonene (lim-oh-neen) is a monoterpene common to citrus rinds and common in nature but only irregularly found

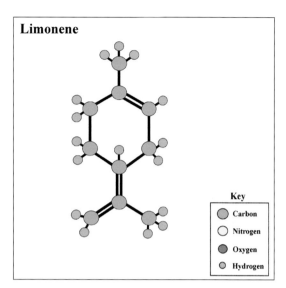

Limonene molecule (By Ellen Seefelt)

in cannabis. Limonene is the parent compound of the entire family of cannabis monoterpenes, and experiments in mice confirm that it strongly reduces anxiety. A study in Japan showed that depressed patients—nine of twelve hospitalized patients—exposed to citrus scent were eventually able to stop taking antidepressants. Researchers also have shown limonene to stimulate the immune system, act as an antidote to adverse intoxicating events produced by THC, improve gastroesophageal reflux (a commercial capsule is available for this), induce cell death in some forms of cancer, and reduce inflammation in rats and older people. It may also be useful in obesity treatment.[37]

35 Ibid.
36 Ibid.
37 Ibid.

The Entourage Effect

The synergy or boosting of cannabis effects because of an ensemble of ingredients is called the entourage effect.[38] For cannabis, the entourage includes endocannabinoids and endocannabinoid-like molecules, the range of cannabinoids and terpenes made in the plant's resin, and other constituents, some maybe undiscovered so far.

S. Ben-Shabat and colleagues introduced the term in a 1998 *Journal of European Pharmacology* paper. Based on data from research on the subject with mice, they wrote that related endogenous substances called 2-acyl-glycerols, which alone showed no significant activity in any of their tests, potentiated (increased) the apparent binding of the endocannabinoid 2-AG to the cannabinoid receptors CB1 and CB2.[39]

"This 'entourage effect' may represent a novel route for molecular regulation of endogenous cannabinoid activity," they wrote, noting that this information might be important for those who study biologically active natural products from plants or animals, most of which contain chemically related but (seemingly) biologically inactive constituents.[40]

"Very seldom is the biological activity of the active constituent assayed together with the inactive entourage compounds," the scientists wrote. In view of those results, "investigations of the effect of the active component in the presence of its 'entourage' compounds may lead to observations of effects closer to those in nature than investigations with the active component only."[41]

THC and CBD in the whole plant exist with all the natural entourage compounds and are called full-spectrum products. CBD extracted from the whole plant is called broad spectrum because processing removes some of the whole-plant constituents.

A recent article about the entourage effect at Project CBD[42] says that "whole plant extractions typically include CBD, THC, and more than 400 trace compounds. Many of these compounds interact synergistically to create what scientists refer to as an 'entourage effect' that magnifies the therapeutic benefits of the plant's individual components—so that the medicinal impact of the whole plant is greater than the sum of its parts." The article notes that in considering effects reported in animal studies, "100

---

38 Russo, E. B., Video interview.
39 Ben-Shabat, S., E. Fride, T. Sheskin, T. Tamiri, M. H. Rhee, Z. Vogel, T. Bisogno, L. De Petrocellis, V. Di Marzo, R. Mechoulam. *Eur J Pharmacol* 353:23–31.
40 Ibid.
41 Ibid.
42 Project CBD.

mg of synthetic single-molecule CBD is not equivalent to 100 mg of a CBD-rich whole plant cannabis extract."

Quoting researcher Dr. John McPartland, the article adds, "Cannabis is inherently polypharmaceutical [contains many medicine-related constituents], and synergy arises from interactions [among] its multiple components."[43]

---

43 Ibid.

Chapter 6
The ECS in Balance and Deficiency

The endocannabinoid system can be thought of as a key mediator of physiological homeostasis (balance), ensuring that all systems in the body and brain work "within tight parameters with neither a deficiency nor excess of activity," Dr. Ethan Russo wrote in a 2015 white paper.[1]

"Just as the immune system deals with invasive proteins from bacteria and viruses, Professor Raphael Mechoulam has hypothesized that the endocannabinoid system serves an analogous role in the body to neutralize and rectify non-protein insults such as trauma or oxygen lack." When the endocannabinoid system itself is out of balance, recent discoveries have shown how endocannabinoid levels that were too high or too low would affect the body, Russo added.[2]

Ideally, he wrote, if the endocannabinoid system is functioning normally, a person would have a normal mental state, live without pain, and have good digestive function, among other things.

On the other hand, "morbid obesity is accompanied by a metabolic syndrome with increased inflammation, insulin resistance and even diabetes, [and] the endocannabinoid system has been observed to be hyperactive in such states. Similarly, an excess of CB1 activity can be associated with hepatic (liver) fibrosis." When endocannabinoid levels are too low, "it has been theorized and shown in subsequent research that numerous mysterious disorders fit the description of clinical endocannabinoid deficiency." Among these are migraine, fibromyalgia, and irritable bowel syndrome (IBS, or spastic colon).[3]

Given the endocannabinoid system's broad involvement "in nervous system development, homeostasis, dysfunction and energy balance," Skaper and Di Marzo wrote in 2012,[4] "the more we know of the endocannabinoid system, the better are prospects for capitalizing on endocannabinoid-based therapies" in health and disease.

---

1   Russo, E. B., white paper, January 2015.
2   Ibid.
3   Ibid.
4   Skaper, S. D., and V. Di Marzo.

Other Ways to Modulate the Endocannabinoid System

Few clinical trials have assessed interventions that upregulate (boost activity of) the endocannabinoid system, but many preclinical (lab and animal) studies identify potential approaches. In a 2014 *PLOS One* paper,[5] J. M. McPartland and colleagues wrote about their "systematic review of clinical interventions that enhance the endocannabinoid system— ways to upregulate cannabinoid receptors, increase endocannabinoid synthesis or inhibit endocannabinoid degradation." They added, "Human trials are needed to explore . . . [the following] promising interventions."

Pharmaceutical Drugs

Some nonsteroidal anti-inflammatory agents (NSAIDs), including aspirin and ibuprofen, have been shown in preclinical studies to inhibit FAAH, the enzyme that degrades anandamide, and enhance the activity of endocannabinoids, phytocannabinoids, and synthetic cannabinoids.[6]

In preclinical studies with rodents, acetaminophen enhances endocannabinoid and synthetic cannabinoid activity.

Researchers don't know yet why acetaminophen doesn't have cannabimimetic (cannabis-like) effects in people. Acetaminophen-cannabinoid drug interactions may be species-specific, McPartland and colleagues wrote.[7]

Preclinical studies and clinical trials indicate that acute (short-duration) opiate (morphine, heroin, oxycodone) administration enhances endocannabinoid, phytocannabinoid, and synthetic cannabinoid activity. Acute opiates also may upregulate CB1 receptor expression. But chronic (long-term) opiate administration may damage the endocannabinoid system.[8]

The effects of antidepressant drugs or treatments on the endocannabinoid system aren't definitive, McPartland and colleagues wrote, but likely result in CB1 upregulation, at least in some brain regions. Antipsychotic drugs have not affected the THC high in human clinical studies, but they dampen dysphoria (unease, discontent) and worsen verbal recall and distractibility.[9]

In the case of anxiolytics, sedatives, and anesthetics, diazepam (Valium) is used to treat anxiety, insomnia, muscle spasms, and seizure disorders. In mice,

5   McPartland, J. M., G. W. Guy, and V. Di Marzo. "Care and Feeding of the Endocannabinoid System: A systematic review of potential clinical interventions that upregulate the endocannabinoid system." *PLOS One* 9(3) (doi: 10.1371/journal.pone.0089566).

6   Ibid.

7   Ibid.

8   Ibid.

9   Ibid.

strong elevation of brain endocannabinoid levels accompanied chronic and especially acute administration of diazepam. A CB1 receptor blocker reduced the anxiety-reducing and sedative effects of sedatives (like Xanax), but CB1 knockout mice had weakened anxiolytic (anxiety-reducing) responses to the antianxiety drugs buspirone (BuSpar) and bromazepam (Lectopam).

In people, the beta-adrenergic blocking agent (beta blocker) propranolol causes mild sedation, but in a small clinical trial, pretreatment with propranolol blocked cannabis-induced cardiovascular effects and learning impairment. General anesthesia (with drugs like Versed) caused decreased serum anandamide in patients stressed by upcoming cardiac surgery.[10]

For anticonvulsants, in a human the drug tiagabine (Gabitril) works by inhibiting the reuptake into cells of the neurotransmitter GABA (gamma-aminobutyric acid). Researchers found that inhibited GABA reuptake boosted THC discrimination (being able to tell THC from another drug) and enhanced THC effects in other outcomes.[11]

Dietary Supplements

For polyunsaturated fatty acids (such as fish oil and krill oil), dietary omega-3 fatty acids seemed to act as homeostatic (balancing) regulators of the endocannabinoid system. In obese rodents fed a high-omega-6 diet, omega-3s significantly decreased endocannabinoids, especially 2-AG, particularly in tissues that become dysregulated in obesity, like adipose (fat) and liver tissues. Also in obese people, omega-3-rich krill oil reduced plasma endocannabinoid levels. Little change in endocannabinoid levels was seen in normal-weight individuals who weren't fed a high-omega-6 diet and, the researchers wrote, dietary omega-3s are needed for proper endocannabinoid signaling.[12]

Probiotics are endosymbiotic (organisms living inside another organism) microorganisms that benefit human health. Fermented foods like yogurt and kimchi contain probiotics. The best-known organisms are *Lactobacillus acidophilus* and *Bifidobacterium* species. Prebiotics like oligofructose (an insoluble fiber that survives the first part of the digestion process) are carbohydrates that feed probiotic organisms and some of the microorganisms that constitute our intestinal flora, the so-called gut microbiota. Human intestine cells incubated with *L. acidophilus* produced more CB2 mRNA. Feeding *L. acidophilus* to mice and rats increased CB2 mRNA expression in cells from the colon, and mice fed *L. acidophilus*

---

10 Ibid.
11 Ibid.
12 Ibid.

showed less pain behavior after painful events than control mice did.[13]

Probiotics and prebiotics also modulate CB1 expression, McPartland and colleagues wrote. Pathologically obese mice expressed elevated levels of colon CB1 mRNA, and when fed prebiotics like oligofructose they expressed less CB1 mRNA, produced less of the endocannabinoid anandamide, and gained less fat mass.[14] Based on these data, a Canada Excellence Research Chair was created in 2017 at University Laval, Quebec City, to study the gut microbiome-endocannabinoidome (the expanded endocannabinoid system) axis, directed by Dr. Vincenzo Di Marzo.

Early-Life Dietary Considerations

Human breast milk has small amounts of anandamide and high 2-AG levels, but researchers don't yet know the biological significance. Giving anandamide and especially 2-AG orally to rats calms them. Mouse breast milk also contains endocannabinoids, and newborn mice fed a CB1 receptor blocker stop suckling and die.[15]

Mind and Body Medicine

Chronic stress harms the endocannabinoid system by lowering anandamide and 2-AG levels, and CB1 expression is more changeable. Managing stress may reverse the effects of chronic stress on endocannabinoid signaling, but few studies have been performed that explore this possibility. Clinical anecdotes suggest that stress-reduction techniques like meditation, yoga, and deep-breathing exercises create mild cannabis-like effects. In rats, social play increased CB1 phosphorylation (a marker of CB1 activation) in the brain and enhanced anandamide levels in the amygdala and nucleus accumbens.[16]

Acupuncture reduced stress-related behavior in a rat model of stress and normalized corticosterone release (hormone secreted by the adrenal cortex) induced by the hypothalamic-pituitary-adrenal axis. Electroacupuncture (a small electric current passed between acupuncture needles) reduced hyperalgesia (heightened pain sensitivity) and allodynia (feeling pain from stimuli that doesn't usually hurt) in a rat model of pain, and it raised anandamide levels in skin tissue.[17]

Electroacupuncture also upregulated CB2 receptor expression in skin tissue; McPartland and colleagues wrote that CB2 activation in the skin likely stimulates release of beta-endorphin (a pain-blocking opioid peptide), which

---

13 Ibid.
14 Ibid.
15 Ibid.
16 Ibid.
17 Ibid.

then acts on peripheral nervous system mu-opioid receptors to inhibit nociception (pain sensors detecting harmful stimuli).[18]

Human studies have shown that massage and osteopathic manipulation of participants with no symptoms increased blood serum anandamide 168 percent over pretreatment levels, with no change in 2-AG. Those who received sham manipulation (treatment with no effects) showed no changes. Osteopathic manipulation of participants with lower back pain increased serum PEA (palmitoylethanolamide, a fatty acid amide made in the body that rodent studies have shown to be anti-inflammatory and help with chronic pain) 1.6-fold over pretreatment levels, with no change in anandamide. Those receiving sham manipulation showed no changes.[19]

Lifestyle Modifications

Dozens of animal and human studies have shown that diets rich in fats and sugars alter levels of anandamide, 2-AG, their metabolic enzymes, and CB1, McPartland and colleagues wrote. And lots of studies have shown that CB1 agonists (activators) stimulate fat and sugar consumption. Rewarding food

properties are reduced when the CB1 receptor is blocked and in CB1 knockout mice. Weight loss by calorie restriction or fasting modulates the endocannabinoid system. In summary, they wrote, increased food intake, adiposity (severe overweight), and elevated anandamide and 2-AG levels apparently spiral in a feed-forward mechanism. Weight loss from caloric restriction breaks the cycle, possibly by reducing CB1 expression and endocannabinoid levels.[20]

On the effects of exercise, human serum anandamide levels doubled over baseline in male subjects after thirty minutes or more of running, and increased significantly in male subjects after biking (increasing anandamide usually is positive for the body). Serum 2-AG levels didn't significantly increase.[21]

Another researcher reported similar findings in male cyclists—serum anandamide levels increased significantly during exercise, but 2-AG concentrations were stable. Anandamide levels rose incrementally at 55 percent maximum work output (Wmax), at 75 percent Wmax, and during a fifteen-minute recovery period. Beta-endorphin levels had a different trajectory—they didn't increase until 75 percent Wmax, and

---

18 Ibid.
19 Ibid.
20 Ibid.
21 Ibid.

dropped significantly during the recovery period.[22]

In summary, McPartland and colleagues wrote, medium- to high-intensity voluntary exercise in cursorial mammals (those, including people, who can run a long way to find food), increases endocannabinoid signaling through higher serum anandamide levels (but not 2-AG), and possibly increased CB1 expression. Runner's high may be an endocannabinoid-induced reward for exercise.[23]

Acute (short-duration) ethanol drinking may enhance endocannabinoid release and signaling, but it varies by brain area and synapse, and this complexity requires further testing. Two studies suggested that ethanol dampens endocannabinoid system effects. Chronic ethanol consumption and binge drinking likely desensitize or downregulate CB1 and impair endocannabinoid signaling, except maybe in areas involved in reward and motivation to self-administer alcohol.[24]

On smoking, in a human randomized controlled trial, nicotine augmented the THC-induced high and heart rate. CB2 is also involved. In the brain, acute nicotine also produced marked increases in anandamide in the amygdala, hypothalamus, and prefrontal cortex, but decreased levels in the hippocampus; 2-AG variations were less pronounced.[25]

Chronic nicotine increased anandamide levels in the limbic forebrain and increased anandamide and 2-AG in rat brainstem, but decreased anandamide and 2-AG in the hippocampus, striatum, and cerebral cortex. Chronic nicotine also increased CB1 density in the prelimbic prefrontal cortex, ventral tegmental area, and hippocampus, and kept tolerance from developing to THC antinociceptive (inhibits pain sensation) and hypothermic (lowers body temperature) effects.[26]

In people, acute (single-dose or short-duration) caffeine administration reduced headache pain, but exposure to chronic high doses, 300 or more mg a day, may worsen chronic pain.[27]

In their conclusions, McPartland and colleagues wrote that many of the randomized controlled trials identified in their review were conducted on lifestyle modifications like exercise, maintaining ideal body weight, and complementary and alternative medical interventions like stress modification, acupuncture, massage, and osteopathic manipulation.

---

22 Ibid.
23 Ibid.
24 Ibid.
25 Ibid.
26 Ibid.
27 Ibid.

In their opinion, "these [rather than drugs] are sensible methods of enhancing the endocannabinoid system."[28]

Endocannabinoid Deficiency

The concept of endocannabinoid deficiency is based on endocannabinoid tone, which Dr. Ethan Russo says reflects a person's levels of anandamide and 2-AG activity, their production and metabolism, and the relative abundance and states of the cannabinoid receptors, among them CB1 and CB2. If this tone is reduced because endocannabinoid activity drops, illness results.[29]

Russo presented the concept of clinical endocannabinoid deficiency in two 2001 publications[30,31] and discussed it in more detail in a 2004 *Neuroendocrinology Letters* paper.[32] His latest information on the topic[33] was published in a 2016 *Cannabis and Cannabinoid Research* paper.

The notion that such a deficiency could cause illness came from the understanding that brain disorders often are associated with neurotransmitter deficiencies—for example, the up-to-90-percent drop in acetylcholine in Alzheimer's disease,[34] the loss of dopamine-producing brain cells in Parkinson's disease,[35] and the reduced activity of serotonin and norepinephrine in depression.[36] Russo thought that a comparable deficiency in endocannabinoid levels could work similarly in disorders that had predictable clinical features because of the deficiency and that resisted treatment with traditional medicines.

When he first proposed the condition of clinical endocannabinoid deficiency

---

28 Ibid.

29 Russo, E. B., white paper, January 2015.

30 Russo, E. B. "Hemp for headache: an in-depth historical and scientific review of cannabis in migraine treatment." *J Cannabis Ther* 1:21–92.

31 Russo, E. B. *Handbook of psychotropic herbs: a scientific analysis of herbal remedies for psychiatric conditions*. Binghamton, NY: Haworth Press, 2001.

32 Russo, E. B. "Clinical endocannabinoid deficiency (CECD): Can this concept explain therapeutic benefits of cannabis in migraine, fibromyalgia, irritable bowel syndrome and other treatment-resistant conditions?" *Neuroendocrinol Lett* 25(1–2):31–9.

33 Russo, E. B. "Clinical endocannabinoid deficiency reconsidered: current research supports the theory in migraine, fibromyalgia, irritable bowel and other treatment-resistant syndromes." *Cannabis Cannabinoid Res* 1(1):154–65 (doi: 10.1089/can.2016.0009).

34 Williams College, Williamstown, MA website: "Clinical Application: Acetylcholine and Alzheimer's Disease": https://web.williams.edu/imput/synapse/pages/IA5.html. Accessed 11/22/17.

35 National Institutes of Health, National Institute of Neurological Disorders and Stroke, Parkinson's Disease information page: https://www.ninds.nih.gov/Disorders/All-Disorders/Parkinsons-Disease-Information-Page. Accessed 11/22/2017.

36 Moret, C., and M. Briley. "The importance of norepinephrine in depression." *Neuropsychiatr Dis Treat* 7(Suppl 1):9–13 (doi: 10.2147/NDT.S19619) 2016.0009).

(CED) in 2001, there was no objective proof or formal clinical trial data. But now, Russo said in his 2016 paper, researchers have documented statistically significant differences in cerebrospinal-fluid anandamide levels in those with migraine, and advanced imaging studies have shown decreased endocannabinoid system function in posttraumatic stress disorder (PTSD). Other clinical data has shown evidence for decreased pain, improved sleep, and other benefits with cannabinoid treatment and lifestyle approaches like diet and exercise that affect the endocannabinoid system.[37]

If the ECS is functioning normally, Russo wrote in a 2015 white paper on the endocannabinoid system, a person might have a normal mental state, have no pain, and have good digestive function and other signs of health. But if endocannabinoid function is decreased, a person could have a lower pain threshold and problems with digestion, mood, and sleep, among the almost universal physiological symptoms involving the ECS. CED theory says such deficiencies could arise for genetic or hereditary reasons, or be acquired due to an injury or illness.[38]

The Best Evidence for Clinical Endocannabinoid Deficiency

Russo says the best evidence for CED is present for migraine, fibromyalgia, irritable bowel syndrome (IBS), and other treatment-resistant disorders.[39]

According to the Mayo Clinic,[40] a migraine can cause severe throbbing pain or a pulsing sensation, usually on one side of the head, often with nausea, vomiting, and extreme sensitivity to light and sound. A migraine attack can cause pain for hours to days and can be so severe that it is disabling. Warning symptoms, known as aura, may occur before or with the headache. These can include flashes of light, blind spots, or tingling on one side of the face or in an arm or leg. Medications can help prevent some migraines and make them less painful.

Fibromyalgia patients can have widespread musculoskeletal pain along with issues of fatigue, sleep, memory, and mood. Researchers think fibromyalgia can amplify painful sensations by affecting the way the brain processes pain signals. Symptoms can accumulate over time, or can begin after physical trauma, surgery, infection, or serious psychological stress.[41]

---

37 Russo, E. B. "Clinical endocannabinoid deficiency reconsidered . . ."
38 Russo, E. B., white paper, January 2015.
39 Russo, E. B. "Clinical endocannabinoid deficiency reconsidered. . ."
40 Mayo Clinic: http://www.mayoclinic.org. Accessed 11/24/2017.
41 Ibid.

Irritable Bowel Syndrome

Normal

Villus

Microvillus

Diseased

Inflammation

Irritable bowel syndrome (From Shutterstock by joshya)

IBS is a chronic condition that affects the large intestine. Symptoms include cramping, abdominal pain, bloating and gas, and diarrhea, constipation, or both. Only a small number of IBS patients have severe symptoms. Some people can control symptoms by managing diet, lifestyle, and stress. More severe symptoms can be treated with medication and counseling.[42]

About CED, Russo says a strong case can be made for unifying trends in the three conditions:[43]

- All arise with increased sensitivity to pain and must be clinically diagnosed based on subjective criteria because they lack characteristic tissue pathology or easily accessible objective lab findings.
- All are diagnoses of exclusion —reached by a process of elimination—that can generate many negative diagnostic workups.
- Patients show an increased incidence of anxiety and depression, and at one time or another skeptical clinicians have called all the disorders psychosomatic or worse.

---

42 Ibid.
43 Russo, E. B. "Clinical endocannabinoid deficiency reconsidered . . ."

- Patients with any one of the conditions often have two or more of the conditions at the same time, called comorbidity. In cited studies, primary headaches co-occurred in 97 percent of 201 fibromyalgia patients, 35.6 percent of 101 chronic daily headache subjects also fit clinical fibromyalgia criteria, 31.6 percent of IBS subjects could be diagnosed with fibromyalgia, and 32 percent of fibromyalgia patients also fit for IBS.
- Some patients suffer from one syndrome, but lifetime risk is common for developing another syndrome or all three.

These disorders affect millions of otherwise healthy people who are plagued by chronic pain and other symptoms, leading to extensive medical tests and treatment attempts, often with limited benefit.[44]

Benefiting from Cannabinoid Treatment

All three disorders are characterized by "central sensitization," the concept that normal sensations in the brain are magnified to the point of becoming painful, when they wouldn't be painful to a person free from the affliction. And all three, according to patient testimonials, benefit from treatment with cannabinoids. Data confirm that the target organs—brain, gut, musculoskeletal system—seem to express lower-than-normal levels of anandamide, bolstering the concept that they would benefit from treatments that would upregulate, or raise, ECS activity back to normal tone.[45]

Russo also writes that similar theoretical deficiencies have been highlighted in the ECS for other conditions, including intractable depression, PTSD, neuropathic pain conditions like complex regional pain syndrome, causalgia (burning pain in a limb caused by an injured peripheral nerve), post-herpetic neuralgia (a shingles complication in which burning pain lasts long after rash and blisters disappear), interstitial cystitis (painful bladder syndrome), and even certain forms of infertility and early miscarriage.[46]

---

44 Ibid.
45 Russo, E. B., white paper, January 2015.
46 Russo, E. B. "Clinical endocannabinoid deficiency reconsidered . . ."

Part 2
Cannabis as Medicine

In which we skim the surface of the legal blockades that brutally limit cannabis research and make cannabis medicine federal if not state crimes, and watch as the dominoes stacked against the 5,000-year-old medicine continue to fall. We'll also hear from scientists whose work has made medical cannabis possible and what they're learning about how cannabis helps the many illnesses it's been used to treat. We'll discuss how hard it is, still, for patients who don't have certain serious illnesses to access medical cannabis (despite the growing number of states that now allow its use), and how to use it for best effect and find the right products. And we'll see what potential patients can do to help themselves while the nation decides whether to keep treating cannabis as a dangerous drug or finally to recognize its centuries of medical value and its future as a safe and effective treatment for almost any illness you can name.

Chapter 7
Medical Cannabis and the Law

The history of medical cannabis stretches across at least 5,000 years, and its mechanism for interacting with every biological and physiological process—the endocannabinoid system (ECS)—is a 590-million-year-old internal biological network responsible for homeostasis and neuroprotection in every vertebrate, including people, on Earth.

Before 1937, at least twenty-seven cannabis-containing medicines were legally available in the United States, according to a briefing paper[1] on the website of the Marijuana Policy Project (MPP) in Washington, DC. Respected pharmaceutical firms like Parke, Davis and Co. (now

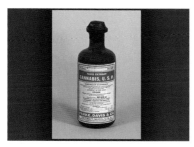

Cannabis fluid extract (80 percent alcohol), USP, Parke Davis & Co., 1933. (Courtesy National Museum of American History and displayed by the National Library of Medicine, Pick Your Poison Exhibition, in the public domain.)

Pfizer subsidiary Parke-Davis), Squibb (now Bristol-Myers Squibb), and Eli Lilly produced many of those medicines.

And yet.

In 1937, MPP says, US legislators used the Marijuana Tax Act to federally prohibit cannabis. Dr. William C. Woodward of the American Medical Association opposed the act and testified before Congress that prohibition ultimately would prevent the medical uses of cannabis—as it has, and still does, in many states.

Then, beginning in 1969, the Federal Bureau of Narcotics, which evolved into the Drug Enforcement Administration (DEA), created the Comprehensive Drug Abuse Prevention and Control Act of 1970. This act, also called the Controlled Substances Act, categorized cannabis along with LSD, mescaline, ecstasy, heroin, methamphetamine, and other drugs under Schedule I—meant for drugs with no currently accepted medical use, a high potential for abuse, and a lack of accepted safety for use under medical supervision.

And they're all still there, under Schedule I, the most restrictive category

---

1   Marijuana Policy Project, medical marijuana briefing paper, https://www.mpp.org/issues/medical-marijuana/medical-marijuana-briefing-paper/. Accessed 12/18/2017.

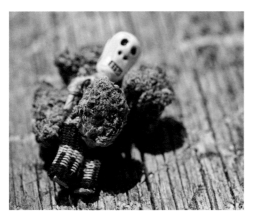

Authors of the Chinese pharmacopeia wrote that patients who ate too many cannabis seeds could see demons. (Shutterstock by Roxana Gonzales)

of illegal substances in the United States, and too dangerous to study.

No currently accepted medical use? With a 5,000-year history of safe treatments for every disease you can think of, on nearly every continent on Earth? Well, except for that demon thing noted 5,000 years ago in the Chinese pharmacopeia. And even now, with legalized (sort of) hemp and an FDA-approved medicine made from the major cannabis constituent CBD?

For cannabis and its long history of safety and broad applications, listing it on Schedule I as a drug (it's a plant) with no currently accepted medical treatment in the United States is ridiculously harsh and, you know, wrong.

Dominoes Fall

Despite the legal constraints, Oregon became the first state to decriminalize small amounts of cannabis in 1973, and in 1996 California voters passed a statewide initiative called Proposition 215, the Compassionate Use Act, making it the first state to approve the use of medical cannabis.[2] Under the initiative, some California patients could use medical cannabis even though it was untested by the FDA and illegal under the federal Controlled Substances Act.

Since 1996, according to the National Conference of State Legislators (NCSL),[3] thirty-four states, the District of Columbia, and US territories Guam, Puerto Rico, and the US Virgin Islands have enacted comprehensive public medical cannabis and cannabis programs. Approved efforts in twelve more states allow the use of low-THC products for medical reasons in limited situations or as a legal defense (oh great).

Among the medical cannabis states and territories, fourteen states and territories—including the District, Alaska, California, Colorado, Illinois, Maine, Massachusetts,

---

2   NORML.org, the National Organization for the Reform of Marijuana Laws. http://norml.org, marijuana law reform timeline http://norml.org/shop/item/marijuana-law-reform-timeline. Accessed 1/4/2018.

3   National Conference of State Legislators, State Medical Marijuana Laws section. http://www.ncsl.org/research/health/state-medical-marijuana-laws.aspx. Accessed 7/15/2018.

Nevada, Oregon, Washington, and Vermont—have legalized small amounts of marijuana for adult use.[4]

So the dominoes are falling for medical cannabis and increasingly for cannabis-use legalization for adults.

In the United States, according to an April 2019 CBS News poll, 65 percent of Americans think cannabis should be legal, showing a steady increase over the past decade and more than double what it was in 2000 (31 percent).

National polls consistently show that most Americans support letting seriously ill patients use cannabis as medicine with their doctors' approval, the Marijuana Policy Project says, but because Congress and the DEA have failed to make medical cannabis legal, states have enacted their own laws to protect patients.[5] Still, even now, doctors can't write prescriptions for medical cannabis because cannabis is federally illegal, but they're allowed to recommend its use in writing to qualified patients in medical cannabis states.

Legal in Some States, Illegal in All States

The legal status of medical cannabis has long been contentious, and now, says Gerald Caplan, a law professor and dean emeritus of Pacific McGeorge School of Law in Sacramento, California, it's also a legislative oddity, "because state governments authorize cannabis possession and use in clear violation of federal criminal law." Medical cannabis, he wrote, "is simultaneously legal in 28 states [34 states and territories in July 2019], and illegal in all 50 states, the District and US territories. And nearly a third of the US population live in jurisdictions" whose legislation or ballot initiatives authorize cannabis as a medical treatment, also "in direct opposition to federal law."[6]

The federal law against cannabis is the main reason doctors can't prescribe but can only recommend medical cannabis to patients, and it's the reason it's so hard for scientists to get funding for and conduct cannabis research. The too-dangerous-to-study plant actually is simply too-against-federal-law to study, especially for universities and other research institutions whose scientists depend on federal funds to do their important work.

Researchers who do meet the many requirements needed to study cannabis in the lab or in animal models of disease, and receive government approval to do so, have to obtain the cannabis from the National Institute on Drug Abuse (NIDA) Drug Supply Program, which gets its cannabis from one source,

---

4   NORML.org.
5   MPP, legalization: https://www.mpp.org/issues/legalization/. Accessed 12/18/2017.
6   Caplan, G. "Medical Marijuana: A Study of Unintended Consequences." 2012. Pacific McGeorge School of Law.

the University of Mississippi School of Pharmacy's National Center for Natural Products Research. But there are two problems with that. One is that much of the approved research focuses on drug-abuse questions rather than on therapeutics (cannabis medicine), and the other is that for federally funded research there is only one source of cannabis.

Roadblocks for Cannabis Research

What's really needed, Ethan Russo said in a 2017 interview, is for private enterprise to be able to grow cannabis and standardize the products for medical use.

"Roadblocks for doing research are still substantial . . . [including] the idea that everything's funneled through NIDA," Russo said. "It has to be their cannabis, and, with apologies to my friends at [the University of] Mississippi, the cannabis is neither representative nor suitable for what I would require to do *bona fide* clinical studies aimed toward developing cannabis as medicine."

To be fair, Russo said, "the problem does not lie with the University of Mississippi, which is populated with excellent scientists who are well equipped. Rather, they are also victims of the system who have been straitjacketed by the federal constraints. The Drug Enforcement Administration has prohibited them from importing any new

cannabis genetics or performing any crossbreeding that might improve the stock. The lack of standardization of the material means that even a successful clinical trial with NIDA-supplied cannabis cannot be followed up with identical materials, thus making any commercial development of a cannabis-based pharmaceutical impossible since it is the only legal domestic source. This explains why I have worked for foreign companies for the majority of the last couple of decades."

One company he worked for was GW Pharmaceuticals, the British company whose Epidiolex product the FDA approved in June 2018 and whose Sativex drug is approved for use in more than thirty countries, but not the United States, where Sativex is called nabiximols.

Sativex was the first cannabis-based medicine, Di Marzo and colleagues wrote in a 2015 *Nature Reviews Neuroscience* paper,[7] and the medical use of cannabis extracts in multiple sclerosis patients was approved in June 2010 by ten European countries. The researchers wrote that the drug was "prepared by combining botanical extracts from two varieties of *Cannabis sativa* plants, one producing mainly . . . THC . . . and the other producing mainly CBD . . . with a ratio of approximately 1:1. Thus, despite the medicinal uses of THC for the treatment of emesis and cachexia

---

7   Di Marzo, V., N. Stella, and A. Zimmer. "Endocannabinoid signaling and the deteriorating brain." *Nat Rev Neurosci* 16(1):30–42 (doi:10.1038/nrn3876).

in patients with cancer undergoing chemotherapy, and for promoting appetite in patients with AIDS, cannabis extracts were finally given *bona fide* therapeutic status after a decade of clinical trials dedicated to the testing of a combination of THC and CBD on untreatable spasticity, one of the typical and most widespread symptoms of the neurodegenerative disease multiple sclerosis."

In contrast to the protracted and undesirable US process for studying cannabis, Russo continued in his 2017 interview, "GW Pharmaceuticals could cultivate, process, and manufacture cannabis medicines with the full backing of the British Home Office and export it around the world, including to the USA, to do full-scale phase 2 and phase 3 clinical trials."

First and foremost, Russo said,[8] "we need to better understand the role of the endocannabinoids in our lives and our health status. That's been ignored, possibly because of its name—having the term [marijuana] in the name and that pejorative connotation has impeded education, even in medical school."

Basically, he said, medical education about cannabis and the endocannabinoid system hardly exists. Consider that "there are more cannabinoid receptors in the brain than there are for all the neurotransmitters put together. . . . Recognizing that

fact, why would one ignore this system? Why isn't this being taught? Our public needs to know about this, and how lifestyle and diet affect this system, and how it could be brought to bear to improve their life conditions."

Teaching the Endocannabinoid System

It's been nearly two decades since researchers discovered the existence of the endocannabinoid system, and still this system that's critical to balancing health and disease is all but unknown among most of the nation's population, sadly including many physicians and those who oversee medical school curricula.

In a 2013 survey of US medical schools, Dr. David Allen, a retired cardiothoracic and vascular surgeon, found that only 21 of 157 schools surveyed, or 13.3 percent, offered any course that mentioned the ECS. No school had a department of endocannabinoid science; none taught about the ECS as an organized course. But one medical school happened to have one of the world's leading cannabinoid scientists working as an adjunct (part-time) associate professor as early as 1999—the Medical College of Virginia (MCV) in the Department of Pharmacology and Toxicology at Virginia Commonwealth University in Richmond.

---

8   Russo, E. B., Video interview.

It was Dr. Vincenzo Di Marzo, the same researcher who wrote with colleagues in 1998[9] about the "relax, eat, sleep, forget, and protect" messages produced in the body by the actions of endocannabinoids. Over the years he's written about endocannabinoids and pain, obesity, and glycemic control; their role in neurological disorders, endometriosis, multiple sclerosis, diabetic neuropathy, and neurodegenerative disorders; exercise and its activation of the endocannabinoid system; and many more research topics.

In an email (April 23, 2018), Di Marzo wrote that he lectured on cannabinoid science at the university in 1999 and again in 2008. His MCV lectures are rare occurrences in medical schools, but things are changing (see the example below in the commonwealth of Pennsylvania). Others are assuming responsibility for training physicians and other health-care professionals on the endocannabinoid system and medical cannabis.

- **Healer.com**
  Dr. Dustin Sulak has created a doctor-developed, Healer.com-certified online medical-cannabis training program for industry professionals, allied health-care providers, and consumers. The site offers "reliable, accurate and practical online training and education based on proven protocols, peer-reviewed science, and Sulak's clinical experience."

- **The Medical Cannabis Institute (TMCI) themedicalcannabisinstitute.org**
  TMCI has created an eLearning website with courses to help educate a growing global community of health-care professionals, caregivers, and patients who want to learn about the science and clinical data behind medical cannabis.

- **Americans for Safe Access (ASA) safeaccessnow.org**
  ASA's mission is to ensure safe and legal access to cannabis (marijuana) for therapeutic use and research. ASA and The Answer Page Inc. have created the Cannabis Care Certification program to help medical professionals, patients, and their caregivers better understand the endocannabinoid system and cannabis therapeutics. ASA is based in Washington, DC.

- **International Cannabis and Cannabinoids Institute (ICCI) icci.science/en/**
  The Czech Republic–based ICCI identifies, coordinates, and supports global research

---

9   Di Marzo, V., D. Melck, T. Bisogno, and L. De Petrocellis.

priorities to advance cannabis and cannabinoid treatments through a multidisciplinary, evidence-based approach that incorporates innovative tools and methods. ICCI has partnered with The Answer Page for accredited education on the endocannabinoid system, medical cannabis, opioid prescribing, pain medicine, and country-specific information initially for Germany, the Czech Republic, the Netherlands, the United Kingdom, Ireland, and Canada.

- **International Association for Cannabis as Medicine (IACM) cannabis-med.org/**
  IACM's aim is to advance knowledge on cannabis, cannabinoids, the endocannabinoid system, and related topics, especially with regard to their therapeutic potential. Their journal and annual conferences bring patients and doctors together to learn about and discuss the latest research, and the organization legally fights restrictive practices against medical cannabis in many countries. IACM is based in Steinheim, Germany.
- As I write this, the Colorado nonprofit cannabis patient support organization, Realm of Caring (RoC) Foundation, is launching an accredited online continuing medical education course with cannabinoid researchers from Johns Hopkins University in Maryland and the University of Pennsylvania and Thomas Jefferson University in Pennsylvania.

Pennsylvania Revolts

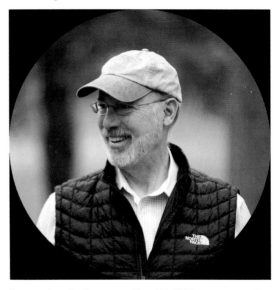

Pennsylvania Governor Tom Wolf (From pa.gov, in the public domain)

Pennsylvania's medical cannabis program, approved by the legislature and signed into law by Governor Tom Wolf in April 2016, is doing something that no other medical cannabis state has done. It added a cannabis research program to its legislation, and in May 2018 the Wolf administration approved eight

Pennsylvania universities as certified medical cannabis academic clinical research centers, calling it the "first step toward clinical research to commence in the commonwealth."

Mike Adams, author of a May 15, 2018, *Forbes* article,[10] put it another way: "Pennsylvania is determined to lead the nation in medical marijuana research. The state has already taken a bold leap, sticking its middle finger in the face of Uncle Sam's bureaucratic labyrinth of red tape when it comes to examining Schedule I drugs, to become a driving force behind the discovery of how the

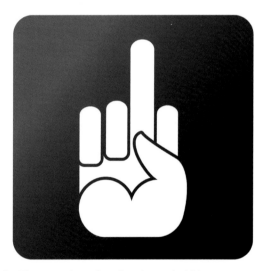

"...The state has already taken a bold leap, sticking its middle finger in the face of Uncle Sam's bureaucratic labyrinth of red tape when it comes to examining Schedule I drugs. . ." Written by Mike Adams, *Forbes*, May 15, 2018. (Image from Shutterstock by MaryValery)

cannabis plant can benefit the masses in the realm of safe and effective medicine."

The certified centers are Drexel University College of Medicine, Lake Erie College of Osteopathic Medicine, Lewis Katz School of Medicine at Temple University, Penn State College of Medicine–Hershey, Perelman School of Medicine at the University of Pennsylvania, Philadelphia College of Osteopathic Medicine, Sidney Kimmel Medical College at Thomas Jefferson University, and University of Pittsburgh School of Medicine with University of Pittsburgh Medical Center.

A June 20, 2019, press release said the Pennsylvania Department of Health had launched a first-in-the-nation research program for medical cannabis by announcing the first three approved clinical registrants that will work with approved universities to conduct clinical research on any of the twenty-one serious medical conditions that Pennsylvania's medical cannabis program allows.

"Pennsylvania is on the forefront of clinical research on medical marijuana," Secretary of Health Dr. Rachel Levine said. "This research is essential to providing physicians with more evidence-based research to make clinical decisions for their patients. It is the cornerstone of our program and the key to our clinically based, patient-focused program for those

10 Adams, Mike. Forbes.com. May 15, 2018. https://www.forbes.com/sites/mikeadams/2018/05/15/pennsylvania-to-lead-nation-in-medical-marijuana-research/#3bc5fb6c1ff2. Accessed 7/12/2018.

suffering with cancer, PTSD and other serious medical conditions."

The first three clinical registrants are PA Options for Wellness Inc., affiliated with Penn State College of Medicine, Hershey; Agronomed Biologics LLC, affiliated with Drexel University College of Medicine, Philadelphia; and MLH Explorations LLC, affiliated with Sidney Kimmel Medical College at Thomas Jefferson University, Philadelphia.

In July 2019, the department said it would bring together all eight academic clinical research centers and the three clinical registrants to discuss the research to be conducted and how it would help patients. Also in July, Levine approved treatment for Tourette syndrome and anxiety disorders to be part of the program.

In December 2018, Governor Wolf tweeted, "More and more states are successfully implementing marijuana legalization and we need to keep learning from their efforts. Any change would take legislation. But I think it is time for Pennsylvania to take a serious and honest look at recreational marijuana."

Chapter 8
Cannabis Medicine: Who Has Access?

More than half of US states have approved the use of medical cannabis, but only California's program lets doctors recommend cannabis for any reason. The thirty-four states with comprehensive public medical cannabis programs have lists of medical conditions that can officially be treated, and those with other conditions (or no health problems at all) mostly can't access legal medical cannabis. Yes, healthy people also benefit from medical cannabis.

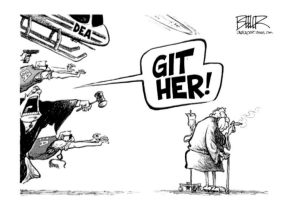

Medical cannabis legal constraints cartoon. (By Nate Beeler, courtesy Cagle Cartoons)

A Big Problem for Public Health

Given the continuing lack of education about the endocannabinoid system and cannabinoid science, it's no big leap to think that many of the 19,254 medical students who graduated as doctors in 2016–2017,[1] and at any time before that, know zip about the endocannabinoid system or medical cannabis and its value to patients.

It's a big problem for public health and for cannabis research, medical cannabis, and medical cannabis dispensaries and patients, and its root cause is the nearly fifty-year criminalization of

cannabis by the Comprehensive Drug Abuse Prevention and Control Act of 1970. This legislation put cannabis on Schedule I of the act along with heroin, LSD, peyote and all the other drugs the DEA thought, and still thinks, have high abuse potential, no medical value, and are too dangerous to study.

Now, even in the fourteen states and territories where anyone over twenty-one can buy and use certain amounts of cannabis for any reason, federal drug laws and the fledgling nature of the medical cannabis enterprise can make getting proper treatment difficult for patients.

---

1 Association of American Medical Colleges. https://www.aamc.org/data/facts/enrollmentgradu ate/148670/total-grads-by-school-gender.html Accessed 4/18/2018.

And in the states and territories that have what are called "comprehensive" public medical cannabis programs, only California, as mentioned, doesn't restrict the use of medical cannabis to specific conditions.[2]

This means that unless you have one of the specific conditions, unless the state you're in allows exceptions to these constraints, or unless you're in one of the legal cannabis states, you probably have no legal access at all to medical cannabis, even if you live in a medical cannabis state.

For patients, lack of knowledge about the endocannabinoid system and medical cannabis means that too few doctors know enough to treat the range of disorders cannabinoids can positively affect. Even in states like California where cannabis is legal and there are no constraints on medical cannabis, it can fall to dispensary staff to guide patients' searches for the right varieties or doses to treat their illnesses.

"Dispensaries are the only places you can get legal marijuana here, above ground," Martin A. Lee said during a July 27, 2017, interview. Lee is cofounder and director of the California-based Project CBD, and an author and activist.

Even before voters made recreational cannabis legal in California in January 2018 and available only from licensed dispensaries, Lee said lots of people visited the state as medical cannabis tourists. Before legalization it was necessary only to have a doctor's recommendation letter to buy medical cannabis at a dispensary. And patients can only get recommendations, not prescriptions, because cannabis is illegal under federal law, even in states where it's legal, and doctors aren't allowed to write them for medical cannabis.

Thanks to the 2018 Farm Bill, though, nearly anyone in any state can buy CBD.

The Doctor is Out

"It used to be very easy to get a [recommendation] letter from a doctor if you're in California," Martin Lee said. "You'd probably have to wait about an hour [and] you can do it all over the phone. I'm not enamored of the model," he added, "but you can call and get a letter. So if you're traveling from out of the [state or] country and you're inside a dispensary and are willing to wait an hour, you can get everything you need. That would happen on a regular basis, as far as I can tell."

Now, in post-legalization California, anyone over twenty-one can walk into a dispensary and buy up to an ounce of cannabis. And if you're seeking help for a medical condition and don't have a doctor who understands medical cannabis, you can ask dispensary staff for advice.

---

2 NORML.org.

"The burden tends to fall on the people in dispensaries and staff to guide the patients, which is not the best situation," Lee said, adding that dispensary workers get a lot of feedback from patients, and if they're conscientious they can help those seeking advice.

In a 2018 *Surgical Neurology International* paper,[3] neurosurgeons Joseph Maroon and Jeff Bost of the University of Pittsburgh Medical Center in Pennsylvania discussed the need for education among health-care providers.

"Because of the rapid legalization of medical marijuana by the majority of state legislatures in the US, physicians are faced with a lack of formal education and basic knowledge as to the possible indications, side effects, interactions, and dosing when prescribing medical marijuana," they wrote, adding, "Because of federal restrictions on human research in the US, we lack the number and quality of human trials typically used when prescribing a medication."

Despite the relatively few doctors who understand medical cannabis, books by doctors who do treat cannabis patients are increasingly available. The books discuss how they treat patients, conditions that respond to medical cannabis, and

things like treatment options and dosing for specific illnesses. And some doctors are writing books and articles that help make up for the lack of knowledge about medical cannabis among other physicians.

One of these is a 2018 *European Journal of Internal Medicine* paper[4] by Dr. Caroline MacCallum of the University of British Columbia, Canada, and Dr. Ethan Russo, founder and CEO of credo-science.com.

The paper is a guide for physicians and other health-care providers who are being called on to use cannabis as a medical treatment for patients and who need basic information about how to use it in their practice. It acquaints readers with cannabis pharmacology, modes of administration, therapeutic uses, dosing strategies, and clinical pearls ("The general approach to cannabis initiation is 'start low, go slow . . . and stay low'"), titration tactics, contraindications, adverse events, drug interactions, and monitoring.[5]

The authors also add information on what they call special cases. These include epilepsy, cancer, pain, the elderly ("THC has been used to advantage to treat agitation in dementia, and the neuroprotective effects of it and

3 Maroon, J., and J. Bost. "Review of the neurological benefits of phytocannabinoids." *Surg Neurol Int* 9:91 Published online April 26, 2018 (doi: 10.4103/sni.sni_45_18).
4 MacCallum, C. A., and E. B. Russo. "Practical considerations in medical cannabis administration and dosing." *Eur J Intern Med* 49: 12–19 (doi: https://doi.org/10.1016/j.ejim.2018.01.004).
5 Ibid.

CBD portend to offer possible advantages in this and related pathologies"), Parkinson's disease, pediatrics, opioid and other addictions, and driving and safety-sensitive occupations.[6]

"As cannabis-based medicines return to mainstream usage," MacCallum and Russo concluded, "it is essential that clinicians gain a greater understanding of their pharmacology, dosing, and administration to maximize therapeutic potential and minimize associated problems. With standardized modern products and educated caregivers, these are worthy and attainable goals."

MacCallum and Russo wrote the paper for physicians and other healthcare providers, but there's no reason you shouldn't have a read if you're interested in medical cannabis, whether or not you have access to medical cannabis doctors. Some of the words are long and hard to pronounce, but the internet is handy and it knows everything.

Lots of organizations have grown up around medical cannabis and offer manuals and other guidance for those who want more information or who want or need to treat their own illnesses with cannabis or hemp products. An explosion of expert medical cannabis websites (some better than others) and podcasts (some short-lived) tackle everything from

advocating cannabis law reform and guides to the best cannabis accessories and tech, cannabis horticulture, cannabis therapy, cannabis culture, and cooking and baking with cannabis for people and pets. You'll find a guide to reliable sites in this book's resources section.

Getting Around Barriers to Medical Cannabis

If you're like me and you live in a state where cannabis or medical cannabis aren't yet legal, you still have options. Using cannabis medically is different than using it recreationally.

As the Project CBD Cannabis Dosing section[7] notes, "Cannabis therapeutics is personalized medicine. There is no single CBD:THC ratio or dose that's optimal for everyone. As little as 2.5 mg of CBD combined with a small amount of THC can have a therapeutic effect. If they're necessary, much higher doses of good quality CBD-rich formulations are safe and well tolerated," although drug interactions can be an issue, particularly with high doses of CBD isolates.

For those of us who don't have access to legal or medical cannabis, and if we don't want to hit the streets looking for nonlegal cannabis, the internet is the best place to look for alternatives. Nowadays, all over the net, companies are selling

---

6   Ibid.
7   Project CBD, CBD and Cannabis Dosage Guide, https://www.projectcbd.org/how-to/cbd-dosage. Accessed 4/21/19.

what they claim is "legal in all 50 states" CBD oil, capsules, edibles, and all kinds of isolates and concentrates. You'll see what I mean if you google "CBD oil." I just did that and got 124 million results in 0.89 seconds. It's pretty hard to decide on CBD products with nothing to go on but 124 million results and everyone saying their product is the greatest.

The reason sellers feel like they can say their products are legal in all fifty states is because lots of the products are made not from cannabis but from hemp, also called industrial hemp (less than 0.3 percent THC, at least theoretically), which is legal, but CBD products from hemp that aren't approved by the FDA are in legal limbo.

In a 2016 article, "Sourcing CBD: Marijuana, Industrial Hemp and the Vagaries of Federal Law,"[8] Project CBD Director Martin A. Lee clarified a key difference between cannabis hemp plants and cannabis drug plants, which is resin content. Resin from cannabis flowers is where the plant makes cannabinoids, terpenes, and other important constituents, and hemp plants don't have as many resin-producing trichomes.

Lee said that a number of "high-CBD/low-THC cannabis strains are being grown in Colorado under the guise of that state's industrial hemp program . . . [but] instead of growing hemp for research purposes as part of a federally sanctioned pilot initiative, Colorado leapfrogged official protocol and went straight to large-scale commercial cultivation . . . [and] several Colorado start-ups (and others) [are] marketing CBD-rich 'hemp' oil to all 50 states and beyond."[9]

This is good for those of us who can't access medical cannabis; this way we can get broad-spectrum CBD, meaning the hemp that has CBD also may have small amounts of THC (they work best together) and for sure have other cannabinoids and terpenes. When you're online, maybe look for CBD that comes from a cannabis-legal state, our best bet for the broadest-spectrum CBD health products.

Whether the ACDC cannabis strain "or any other high-resin, non-euphoric [you won't get high], CBD-rich cannabis strain measures very slightly above or slightly below the 0.3 percent THC limit [which makes it legally qualify as industrial hemp] won't make any appreciable difference in terms of the quality of the CBD-rich oil extract or its therapeutic impact," Lee says.[10]

---

8 Lee, M. A. "Sourcing CBD: Marijuana, Industrial Hemp and the Vagaries of Federal Law." March 28, 2016. Project CBD, https://www.projectcbd.org/about/cannabis-facts/sourcing-cbd-marijuana -industrial-hemp-vagaries-federal-law. Accessed 7/17/2018.
9 Ibid.
10 Ibid.

But having small amounts of THC along with the CBD makes it better for your health, and that doesn't mean you have to get high to use medical cannabis. Along with ACDC (20:1 CBD/THC), for those who have access, other CBD-rich varieties of cannabis, according to Leafly.com,[11] include Ringo's Gift (24:1 CBD/THC), Sweet and Sour Widow (1:1 CBD/THC), Stephen Hawking Kush (no ratio given), Cannatonic (ranges from 5:1 to 1:1 CBD/THC), Harle-Tsu (no ratio given), Canna-Tsu (no ratio given), Sour Tsunami (no ratio given), and Pennywise (1:1 CBD/THC). Also according to Leafly, Harlequin, with a standard CBD/THC ratio of 5:2, is "renowned for its reliable expression of CBD" and is one of the most effective for treating pain and anxiety.

Just so you understand the real situation, here is Lee's blunt assessment of the 0.3 percent THC legal limit for industrial hemp: "When it comes to CBD-rich oil production, the 0.3 percent THC legal limit is an absurd, impractical, resin-phobic relic of reefer madness. It has become the linchpin of cannabis prohibition, a venal, dishonest policy that impedes medical research and blocks patient access to valuable therapeutic options, including herbal extracts with various CBD:THC ratios. For patients struggling with a wide range of conditions, CBD and THC work best together, enhancing each other's beneficial effects."[12]

During a March 2018 episode of the podcast *Anslinger: The Untold Cannabis Conspiracy*,[13] Annie Rouse interviewed David Spalding, a former US Department of Agriculture economist, horticulturist, and hemp expert. Rouse is cofounder of online retailer Anavii Market (anaviimarket.com), which uses a third-party verification system to analyze the quality of the CBD and other products it sells. She's also a producer, activist, and environmentalist.

Spalding discussed the difference between hemp and cannabis: "The technical difference is that hemp is cannabis that is 0.3 percent THC or less (by law). Technically, anything that's over 0.3 percent THC is marijuana." The reality, he added, "is that hemp is really anything that's less than about 3 percent THC. It takes 3 percent to 5 percent THC for anybody even to notice that [cannabis] has any buzz to it at all."

(Good news for us broad-spectrum and THC-microdosing fans.)

---

11 Leafly.com, "The 10 Best CBD Cannabis Strains According to Leafly Users," https://www.leafly.com/news/strains-products/10-best-cbd-cannabis-strains-according-to-leafly-users. Accessed 4/20/19 (really!).

12 Lee, M. A.

13 Rouse A. *Think Hempy Thoughts*, podcast episode "Murderous Marihuana," S1E6, David Spalding. https://www.thinkhempythoughts.com/murderous-marihuana/. Accessed 4/21/19.

Spalding added, "Most marijuana these days is in the 12 percent to 15 percent THC category. There are some nowadays that are as high as 30 percent, but the bulk of it is in probably in the 12 percent to 15 percent range."

Better than Nothing and Maybe Better than That

When looking for products online, oils, capsules and other products that contain all the elements—mainly cannabinoids, terpenes, and flavonoids—of the whole plant are called full-spectrum products, and that's an important thing to remember and to look for.

Before shopping, it's best to get recommendations from friends or from organizations like Colorado-based nonprofit Realm of Caring: Providing Support to Medical Cannabis Patients at theroc.us. They've partnered with three companies that sell high-quality CBD online: Colorado-based CW Botanicals (cwhemp.com), Colorado-based Mary's Nutritionals (marysnutritionals.com), and Colorado-based Elixinol (elixinol.com). Realm of Caring gives clients discounted prices on some products.

I've been buying CBD online since about 2014 and I've seen the marketplace explode. Prices have gone down (but good CBD still is pricey) and quality has gone way up. In the beginning I was looking for gel caps (capsules with CBD oil in them), which I figured were better

products than capsules that held dried and ground-up plant material. Really, though, I'd been using the dried and ground-up plant capsules when I realized that CBD made me feel better.

When I first started looking, it was hard to find gel caps (easier to dose but less bioavailable than smoking or vaping), and those I could find were $300 or more for ten or fifteen capsules that each contained five or ten milligrams (mg) of CBD, and most sellers didn't even pretend their products were full- or broad-spectrum. Also, the websites had almost no specific information about what else was in the caps, like the carrier oil for the CBD or the cannabinoid and terpene profiles. But every few months I'd go back online looking for new CBD products, and each time I'd find more websites and companies carrying more products at better prices, and offering more information about the products.

Today, for those who don't live in legal states or who have health problems that don't rise to those required by medical cannabis states, you can find absolutely full-spectrum organic hemp oil or even cannabis oil and other products online, and the best sites have testing documents and product assays. Prices are lower—still not exactly what I'd call affordable, but they still seem to be coming down.

I don't mind sharing the brands I use, at least those whose companies gave me permission to name them. These are products that have worked for me and that I'm sure are broad spectrum. I haven't tried everything on the market, though, so look around and do some homework, taking your own health needs into consideration. Remember, start low and go slow to find an effective dose and the best way, based on your needs, to use CBD—smoke, vaporize, capsules, or others. All have benefits and limitations.

My reasons for trying CBD were pretty nonserious—arthritis in knees and thumb joints—so I was worried about inflammation, which underlies lots of chronic diseases. One of the first products I tried looked like that dried stuff I mentioned. I had no idea about the quality, but I bought some. After I'd been taking the CBD capsules for about a week, one day in the middle of some project I stopped what I was doing and thought, "I feel better."

Looking back, it must have been reduced everyday stress or anxiety that made the difference. Sometime after that I noticed the pain in my hands was gone. I still had knee pain, but I was excited that what I'd been reading about CBD was true, at least at my level of medical need. I continued to look for gel caps with higher doses of CBD to see what really worked best. As mentioned, quality has gone up and prices have gone down. The prices I cite here are from 2019 and will change over time. Here are some of the CBD brands I've used (and I'm not being paid to say so).

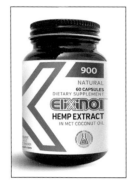

Elixinol CBD capsules (Courtesy Elixinol)

- Elixinol (elixinol.com) already mentioned. These organic hemp oil caps (CBD 900 mg total in the bottle)—full spectrum, the Colorado-based company says—each have 15 mg of CBD, 375 mg of hemp extract, and there are 60 caps in a bottle for $79.99. The company, which has other CBD products, publishes certificates of analysis per product. I think this is a good product at a really good price.

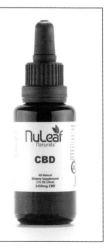

NuLeaf Naturals CBD oil (Courtesy NuLeaf Naturals)

- Organic CBD oil by Colorado-based NuLeaf Naturals (nuleafnaturals.com). I've used their 1,450 mg-per-ounce CBD bottle (there are others with less and more CBD), and each serving size (10 drops) has 450 mg of organic hemp oil and 24 mg of CBD, $179 per bottle. All are broad spectrum. NuLeaf charges less if you buy two bottles at a time (you'd save $74) and has assistance programs for retired military members and vets; police, EMT, and firefighters; low-income and long-term disability customers; and others.

• Endoca (endoca.com), a European company that grows and manufactures its organic CBD products in Denmark. They have a range of oils, capsules, crystals, edibles, and lotions, and their prices, like those of many CBD companies, have come down since the products were first available online. What's different about Endoca, at least for those of us in nonlegal states, is that they offer CBD products that contain cannabidiolic acid (CBDA), the raw form of CBD, which has its own health properties (see chapter 4). The company also has a pretty high-dose capsule. For example, I use their 50 mg raw hemp oil CBD+CBDA capsule (1500 mg total for 30 caps), $129, and their 10 mg CBD+CBDA capsules start at $31. The company also has regular sales and promotions.

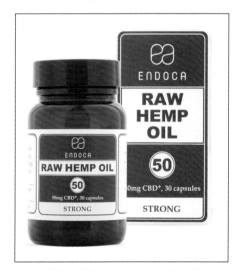

Endoca raw CBD-CBDA 50 mg capsules (Courtesy Endoca)

I use others, too, like the broad-spectrum CBDPure 25 mg caps, and I'm sure other great products are sold online, and especially in legal-state dispensaries, but it takes time to figure out medical cannabis products and how they work best for each person, no matter where you live. Good luck and do your homework. The range of broad-spectrum CBD products is growing, and its legal status won't be up in the air forever.

"If This Were Any Other Drug . . ."

According to Dr. Ethan Russo, the study of medicinal plants has historically helped people better understand their own body chemistry. One example is aspirin, a semisynthetic derivative of

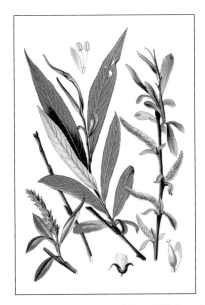

Salix alba, the white willow. (From Wikimedia with permission granted to use under GNU Free Documentation License by Kurt Stueber. Original book source: Prof. Dr. Otto Wilhelm Thomé Flora von Deutschland, Österreich und der Schweiz 1885, Gera, Germany.)

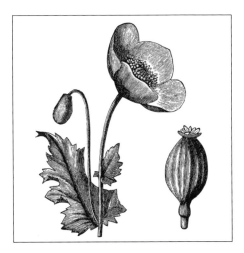

Vintage engraved illustration of a poppy flower by Jules Trousset, 1891, Paris, from the *Dictionnaire encyclopedique universel illustre*. (From Shutterstock by lynea)

salicylic acid from willow bark. This was available for a century before the basis of its ability to treat pain and inflammation led to the discovery of prostaglandins (lipids involved in recovery at sites of tissue damage or infection).[14]

Opium was also used for thousands of years before scientists identified endogenous (made in the body) opioids called endorphins and enkephalins.[15] It wasn't until 1973 that Dr. Candace Pert, at the Johns Hopkins School of Medicine in Baltimore, Maryland, biochemically proved the existence of an opiate receptor.[16]

Even LSD, the psychedelic drug that Swiss scientist Albert Hofmann discovered in 1943, led to the discovery in 1953 of serotonin in the mammalian brain and later to the finding that LSD contained a tryptamine functional group that researchers quickly saw as a scaffold for the chemical structure of serotonin.[17]

14 Russo, E. B., white paper, January 2015.
15 Russo, E. B.
16 Pert, C. B., and S. H. Snyder. "Opiate receptor: demonstration in nervous tissue." *Science* 179(4077):1011–4. http://candacepert.com/library. Accessed 11/26/2017.
17 Nichols, D. E. "Psychedelics." *Pharmacol Rev* 68(2):264–355 (doi: 10.1124/pr.115.011478).

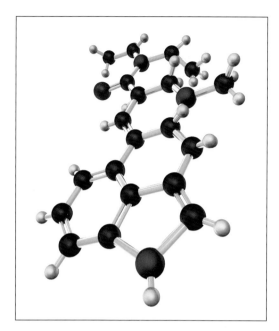

LSD molecule (From Shutterstock by Alexander Limbach)

"One could reasonably argue," author and medicinal chemist Dr. David E. Nichols wrote in his 2016 *Pharmacological Reviews* paper, "that the whole field of serotonin neuroscience, and especially the role of serotonin in brain function, was catalyzed by the discovery of LSD."[18]

In a similar way, cannabis research created a trail that eventually led to discovery of the endocannabinoid system, Russo said, "and the future of therapeutics appears much brighter as a result, since an understanding of the endocannabinoid system portends to offer many more effective and safer remedies for

disorders that have previously proven intractable to conventional treatment."[19]

What's needed, Russo says, "are better and safer treatments that address the larger problems of disease pathophysiology (changes that happen in disease) and degeneration. Botanicals, or plant-based medications, often fit this profile in contrast to the single-chemical model that is most prevalent in contemporary Western medicine."[20]

On the involvement of endocannabinoids and cannabinoids in a range of health effects, Dr. Greg Gerdeman said in a 2017 interview: "The endocannabinoid system as a protective system in the body and brain against non-protein insults really speaks to things like inflammation and free-radical oxidative stress, which is part of the normal wear and tear on cells. Endocannabinoids prevent against that in a variety of ways."

And for cannabinoids, "their targets are much more than just the brain. They're protecting against oxidative stress in the vasculature [the body's blood vessel system] and that's huge."

Years ago, a study showed that repeated microdosing of THC (regularly taking in amounts of THC way below the intoxicating dose) in mice made them less likely to develop atherosclerosis (when fatty deposits clog arteries),

18 Ibid.
19 Russo, E. B., white paper, January 2015.
20 Ibid.

even on high-cholesterol diets and with a genetic background of animals that were prone to atherosclerosis, Gerdeman said, adding, "Low-dose frequent THC diminished that outcome." Now, he said, "you're talking about the leading killer in the United States when you talk about atherosclerosis and the subsequent cardiovascular disease that comes from it."

About cannabinoids as dietary supplements, Gerdeman said, "I fully anticipate that we are very close to the time, especially in people who are fully grown and looking toward the second half of their lives, when people are going to say, 'You're not on some sort of cannabis supplement? Why not?'"

The scientific evidence for medical cannabis is so compelling, Gerdeman added, "that if this were any other drug, if this was something that was not associated with cannabis, it would have been in clinical development decades ago."

Chapter 9
Cannabinoids for Inflammation, Stress, and PTSD

Before we get into the second part of the book, this chapter is about clinical trials, because after each disorder I list some of the studies that have investigated or are ongoing for cannabis and cannabinoids in mid-2019. I'd also like to explain why there aren't more cannabis clinical studies, even though cannabis is allowed in some states for adults and in dozens of states as medical cannabis.

After decades as an illegal plant, and now, in the early years of a time when medical cannabis could become a safe and effective treatment or add-on treatment for illnesses ranging from minor to fatal, there isn't enough clinical evidence (based on human trials) to prove the scope of cannabis's worth to organizations like the National Academies of Sciences, Engineering, and Medicine, the Food and Drug Administration, and the Drug Enforcement Administration.

Why isn't the evidence there? Because getting approval to do human research with a plant/drug that's on Schedule I of the Controlled Substances Act of 1970 requires meeting many requirements of the FDA (to approve a research protocol),

the US Department of Health and Human Services (to approve a revised protocol), the DEA (to review the protocol), and the National Institute on Drug Abuse (for approved drugs to use in the clinical trial, but only if the study is about drug safety or abuse). At the very least.

So there aren't enough of what scientists call "gold standard" clinical trials for cannabinoids in different disorders, and a lot of the research described in the next few chapters is based on preclinical (in culture dishes/test tubes or in animal models) work, or clinical studies of synthetic or purified single-molecule cannabinoids like dronabinol (synthetic THC, brand names Marinol, Syndros) or nabilone (synthetic THC, brand name Cesamet). This gives researchers some information, at least about THC as a single molecule in people, but not about how botanical cannabis and its many cannabinoids, terpenes, flavonoids, and other components work, and not how safe and effective full- and broad-spectrum products are in healthy people and in those with specific disorders.

A growing number of clinical trials of botanical cannabis and of combinations of THC and CBD are in progress, though. And the removal of hemp and its constituents (including CBD), at least, from the Controlled Substances Act Schedule 1 for "dangerous" drugs and from DEA oversight should make it much easier for scientists to study it in people. I accessed the clinical trials described in the following chapters at clinicaltrials .gov, a web-based resource maintained by the National Library of Medicine at the National Institutes of Health.[1]

A clinical trial is a research study in which human volunteers are assigned to interventions (a medical product, behavior, or procedure) based on a protocol (plan). At the end of the study, the results are evaluated for effects on biomedical or health outcomes. Clinicaltrials.gov also has records describing observational studies and programs that offer access to investigational drugs outside of clinical trials (expanded access).

Studies listed in the database are conducted in all fifty states and in 204 countries, but it doesn't list every clinical study conducted in the United States because not all studies are required by law to be registered (observational studies, for example, and trials that don't study a drug, biologic [manufactured in a living system, like some vaccines], or device). But some sponsors and investigators voluntarily register their studies.[2]

In the clinical trials listed after specific disorders, I haven't included studies that use nabilone or dronabinol unless they're the only ones available, and I don't list every trial, just the latest ones and those I hope will be most useful. You can search for clinical trials yourself at the website—and should, because there will be more and more—and if you'd like more information about the studies themselves or the language used to describe them, clinicaltrials.gov has an info page at clinicaltrials.gov/ct2/about-studies/learn.

Inflammation: An Immune Response

Inflammation is the immune system's response to a stimulus like bacteria, a virus, or another kind of insult to the body, according to PubMed Health, a service of the National Center for Biotechnology Information at the US Library of Medicine.[3]

When a wound swells, turns red, and hurts, this can signal the presence

---

1 National Institutes of Health, National Library of Medicine clinical trials, https://clinicaltrials .gov/. Accessed 9/7/18.
2 Ibid.
3 PubMed Health. https://www.ncbi.nlm.nih.gov/pubmedhealth/PMH0072482/. Accessed 7/21/2018.

of inflammation. Inflammation doesn't start with the wound itself, but arises as the body starts fighting the stimulus. Some inflammation happens silently and causes no immediate symptoms, like the chronic inflammation that researchers and physicians are starting to think is at the root of most major diseases, including neurodegenerative diseases, heart disease, and some aspects of aging.[4]

So inflammation starts out as a natural response to threats and seeks to protect the body, but as a chronic condition it can end up doing the worst kind of damage. Inflammation does one more thing, according to Dr. Matthew Hill at Canada's University of Calgary Hotchkiss Brain Institute: "it profoundly stresses the body."

People generally think of stress as arising from things in their environment that psychologically stress them out, like relationship troubles, financial troubles, and work troubles, Hill said in a September 2017 interview.

"These and other variables we see as being adverse and stressful to us, and that makes us feel like crap and we get stressed out and anxious and depressed from it," he added, noting that stress at a biological level is really anything that challenges the body or makes the body move out of its standard state. People get stressed because of relationships, for example, but evolutionarily that stress response was built into the body to deal with predators and to mobilize energy to get away from dangerous or threatening situations.

"Inflammation in the body is also a stressor, it's just a different kind," Hill said. "We refer to psychological stressors as top-down because we have to process them cortically [in the brain] and understand that they're a threat to us. Once we recognize that, we mount a stress response."

Inflammation is more of a bottom-up stressor, "because it's a challenge, it's a disturbance in the body that requires the physiology of the body to change, and one of the ways it does this is by mounting a stress response." Inflammation drives the same hormonal stress response—elevating cortisol, sometimes called the stress hormone—as psychological stress.

"In the context of chronic psychological stress," Hill said, "cortisol is a big

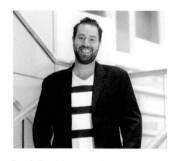

Assistant Prof. Dr. Matthew Hill, University of Calgary (Canada) Hotchkiss Brain Institute. (Photo by James May, Hotchkiss Brain Institute, used with permission)

---

4   Ibid.

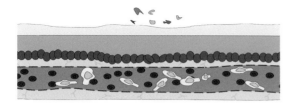

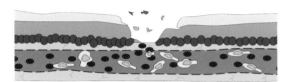

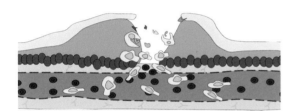

In inflammation the body's white blood cells and substances they produce protect the body and brain from infection by foreign organisms like bacteria and viruses. White blood cells called phagocytes are a nonspecific immune response, meaning they attack any foreign body. In some diseases, like rheumatoid arthritis, the immune system triggers an inflammatory response when there are no foreign invaders. In these autoimmune diseases, the body's immune system mistakenly damages its own tissues. (From Wikimedia Commons by Nason Vassiliev. This file is licensed under the Creative Commons Attribution-Share Alike 4.0 International license.)

stress because both of them [recruit] the same hormonal systems."

Clinical Trials: Cannabinoids for Stress
Anxiety, Inflammation and Stress
A Colorado observational study is investigating whether anxiety-relieving and anti-inflammatory cannabis effects vary with CBD:THC ratio to shed light on mixed data linking cannabis use and anxiety. The study start date was April 2018 and the estimated completion date will be June 2022. Estimated enrollment will be 210 adults. Study details are available at clinicaltrials.gov/ct2/show/NCT03491384

Keep checking clinicaltrials.gov for new studies. Start by searching for the disease name and the terms cannabis and cannabinoids.

mediator of a lot of the adverse effects on the brain and body that are related to chronic stress. So our reasoning is essentially that, if inflammation is just a different flavor of stressor, it's probably mediating its effects on anxiety and depression in a similar manner as psychological

ECS Signaling Collapse: Chronic Stress

Several years ago, Dr. Hill and colleagues established that chronic psychological stress could modulate anxiety related to changes in endocannabinoid function.

"Chronic stress seems to cause a collapse of the endocannabinoid system . . . so you have fewer receptors and fewer endocannabinoid molecules in the brain.

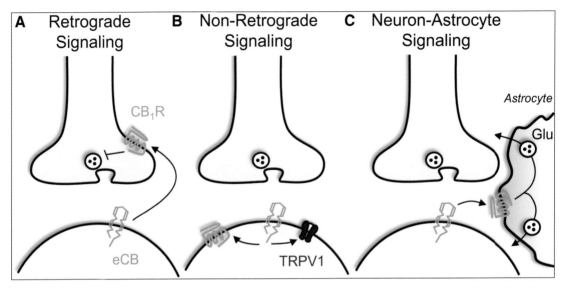

Three kinds of endocannabinoid signaling at the synapse, including retrograde signaling (From Castillo PE, Younts TJ, Chávez AE, Hashimotodani Y. *Endocannabinoid Signaling and Synaptic Function. Neuron* 2010;76(1):70-81, used with permission)

. . . The things that [the ECS] normally does to buffer against the effects of stress on anxiety and other aspects of the brain, that doesn't work so good anymore under conditions of chronic stress." Hill added, "In the brain, what endocannabinoids do is kind of temper neurotransmitter release."

Neurons "talk to each other by releasing chemicals that often excite other neurons, so while it's an electrical current that goes down one neuron, it's a chemical signal that drives communications between neurons. This is how neurons talk to each other, and basically endocannabinoids limit the amount of transmitter chemical that gets released. Therefore, they can act to quiet down parts of the brain that become hyperactive."

According to Hill's website at the Hotchkiss Brain Institute, research from his and other labs shows that endocannabinoid signaling tends to relax stress responses.

"Deficits in endocannabinoid signaling in rodents can increase neuroendocrine [cells that help nerve cell signals release hormones into the bloodstream] and behavioral responses to stress, and in people disruption of endocannabinoid signaling can produce symptoms of depression and anxiety," he wrote. Hill and colleagues have shown that stress can mobilize endocannabinoid signaling, and that this increase is needed for normal recovery from acute (short-duration) stress and the larger adaptive processes created by repeated exposure to stress.

Such chronic stress—experiencing stressors over an extended period of time—can be a long-term drain on the body, according to the American Psychological Association,[5] affecting the musculoskeletal system, respiration, the heart and blood vessels, the adrenal glands, the liver, and the gastrointestinal system.

Hill and colleagues also have found that, under conditions of chronic stress, endocannabinoid signaling breaks down. The loss of this buffer system may be one of the ways chronic stress increases the risk of mood disorders like depression and anxiety.

"This hypothesis," he wrote on his website, "has been supported by translational clinical studies we have performed demonstrating that circulating levels of endocannabinoids are reduced in individuals afflicted with major depression."

ECS Signaling Collapse: Chronic Inflammation

In their research, Hill and colleagues found that, just as chronic stress seemed to cause a collapse of the endocannabinoid system, chronic inflammation pretty much did the same thing.

Chronic inflammation "seemed to compromise the way the endocannabinoid system functioned, and that seems

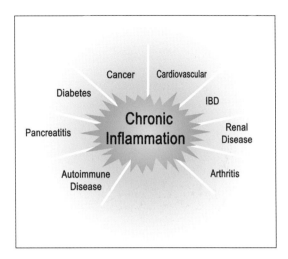

Health consequences of chronic inflammation (From Shutterstock by arka38)

to contribute to the elevations in anxiety. So one of the thoughts is that, in some of these disease states where the endocannabinoid system isn't functioning properly, people may have a propensity to self-medicate with cannabis."

Mentioning a severe form of stress, Hill said that with posttraumatic stress disorder (PTSD), the endocannabinoid system may not be functioning properly. By supplementing with something like THC, people are normalizing a deficit in the system, and that may help improve some of their symptoms.

"This, of course, is still a theory [and] we're trying to conceptualize why there's so much consistency in the reports of people who self-medicate with cannabis," he

---

5 American Psychological Association, http://www.apa.org/helpcenter/stress-body.aspx. Accessed 7/23/2018.

said, adding the problem is that reports of self-medication are anecdotal so it's hard to capture the information scientifically. But Hill said he and colleagues use the reports to generate hypotheses about how things might work.

"That's kind of where we are," Hill said of his inflammation studies. "We think that maybe these comorbid behavioral psychiatric changes associated with inflammatory diseases like anxiety and depression may relate to a dysfunctional endocannabinoid system that's driven by the chronic inflammation itself." Hill says he thinks this is true for most stress-related psychiatric illnesses: If the system isn't working properly, some things may become apparent.

"You might be more sensitive to developing anxiety after stress or you might not recover as quickly from stressful experiences in your life. We know the endocannabinoid system is very important for processing rewarding stimuli," he added, "so if it's not working properly you might become more anhedonic," meaning unable to find joy in life.

All these systems engage the same biological processes in the body, and the hypothesis is that, if the ECS isn't working properly, someone with this problem may be more vulnerable to developing a psychiatric illness like depression or PTSD.

Cannabinoids, Inflammation, and Mood

In earlier work with colleagues in Calgary's Department of Physiology and Pharmacology, Dr. Hill examined early-life inflammation and how that influences the endocannabinoid system. More recently they've explored the idea that psychiatric behavioral comorbidities (two or more disorders occurring at once) are present in people who have chronic inflammatory diseases like inflammatory bowel disease, arthritis, multiple sclerosis, and even things like asthma, Hill said during the interview.

"You often see high incidences of anxiety and depression in these populations," he added, "and it's always been hard to understand if this is just a consequence of having a chronic disease and [the accompanying] emotional burden." But, he said, it's becoming more apparent that a biological underpinning related to chronic inflammation seems to modify how the brain works in a way that makes some people more prone to anxiety and depression. Anxiety disorders affect about 40 million people in the United States alone, according to the National Institute of Mental Health, and antianxiety medications are among the top prescription drugs.[6]

"What's interesting," Hill said, "is that a lot of the chronic inflammatory diseases like arthritis, multiple sclerosis, and inflammatory bowel [disease]

---

6 National Institute of Mental Health anxiety disorders, https://www.nimh.nih.gov/health/topics/anxiety-disorders/index.shtml. Accessed 7/23/2018.

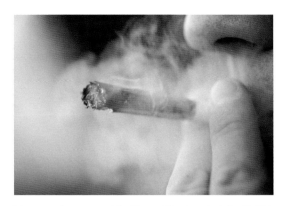
Man smokes cannabis (From Shutterstock by Pe3k)

have the largest patient populations who self-medicate with cannabis." He said there's evidence from animal testing that cannabinoids are anti-inflammatory, but the data from clinical (with people) studies involving inflammatory diseases hasn't been very impressive.

"That's not surprising," he said, "just because there's a lot of heterogeneity [diversity] in the clinical inflammatory conditions and they probably have a lot of different causes. But there is certainly a subset of people who seem to respond to [cannabinoids] positively—it's just a matter of whether it's a genuine effect or not."

Hill said a recent review paper by a colleague—Dr. David Finn, professor of pharmacology and therapeutics at the National University of

Ireland–Galway—said that in all the studies he reviewed,[7] comorbid changes in anxiety and depression often improved in people who used cannabis or cannabinoid therapy in some way, even if it didn't cure the disease. Hill said this finding suggests the disease somewhat induces the emotional comorbidities, but the comorbidities might be unrelated to the disease biology.

"There may be some changes going on in the brain," Hill said, "so we've started investigating this."

Clinical Trials: Cannabinoids, Inflammation and Mood
Cannabis Observational Study on Mood, Inflammation and Cognition (COSMIC)
A Colorado observational study examines cannabis effects on cognition and inflammation, inflammatory response, and mood, and whether the effects depend on the product's CBD:THC ratio. The study began in July 2016 and the estimated end date is April 2021. The study will have 280 adult participants. Study details are available at clinicaltrials.gov/ct2/show/NCT03522103.

---

7   Fitzgibbon, M., D. P. Finn, and M. Roche. "High Times for Painful Blues: The Endocannabinoid System in Pain-Depression Comorbidity." *Int J Neuropsychopharmacol* 19(3) (https://doi.org/10.1093/ijnp/pyv095).

Posttraumatic Stress Disorder

PTSD is a mental health problem that some people develop after experiencing or witnessing life-threatening events like combat, natural disasters, car accidents, or sexual assaults, according to the Department of Veterans Affairs' National PTSD Center.[8]

After these events it's normal to have upsetting memories, feel on edge, or have trouble sleeping. At first, it may be hard to do normal daily activities like going to work or school, or spending time with family and friends. But most people start feeling better after a few weeks or

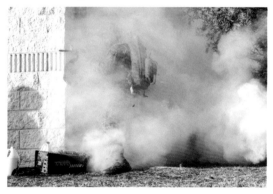

A corpsman with 2nd Medical Battalion, 2nd Marine Logistics Group, provides security during a Tactical Combat Casualty Care training exercise at Camp Lejeune designed to help corpsmen practice medical techniques in stressful environments. (U.S. Marine Corps photo by Pfc. Nicholas Guevara)

months. If symptoms continue for more than a few months, it could be PTSD.[9]

For some people, PTSD symptoms may start later, or come and go over time. In the case of service members, some may carry psychological and physical wounds of their military service back into civilian life. In one study, according to the National PTSD Center, one in four veterans returning from Iraq and Afghanistan reported symptoms of a mental or cognitive disorder; one in six reported PTSD.[10]

The *Diagnostic and Statistical Manual of Mental Disorders*, fifth edition, lists PTSD in the trauma- and stressor-related disorders category, according to N. Korem and colleagues in their 2015 *Journal of Basic and Clinical Physiology and Pharmacology* paper,[11] "Targeting the endocannabinoid system to treat anxiety-related disorders." The paper lists four diagnostic clusters of behavioral symptoms:

- Reexperiencing symptoms involves spontaneous, uncontrollable intrusions of the traumatic memory that manifest themselves as nightmares or memory flashbacks

8   US Department of Veterans Affairs, National Center for PTSD, https://www.ptsd.va.gov/index.asp. Accessed 1/12/2018.
9   Ibid.
10 Ibid.
11 Korem, N., T. M. Zer Aviv, E. Ganon-Elazar, H. Abush, I. Akirav "Targeting the endocannabinoid system to treat anxiety-related disorders." *J Basic Clin Physiol Pharmacol* 27(3):193–202 (doi: 10.1515/jbcpp-2015-0058).

- Avoidance symptoms or an individual's efforts to distance himself or herself from trauma-related stimuli. These can include emotional and social withdrawal
- Negative changes in cognition and mood
- Hyperarousal symptoms that include physiological reactions like irritability, hypervigilance, and an exaggerated startle response

Korem and colleagues described the ECS as a potential target for preventing and treating anxiety-related disorders, especially PTSD.

"Preclinical and clinical data strongly suggest that anxiety is associated with decreased endocannabinoid tone," they wrote, "and that CB1 receptors in the fear circuit in the brain are crucially involved in the [anxiety-reducing] effects of cannabinoids." The authors also called for extensive clinical research on the effects of cannabinoids in PTSD patients.[12]

A Natural Response to Extreme Circumstances

Networks of stress in the brain are interconnected with networks broadly attributed to emotional processing in the brain, so there are well-studied, discrete brain networks responsible for emotional well-being, emotional affect, and how people integrate fear and stress, Dr. Greg Gerdeman said in a 2017 interview.

"The neurobiology of emotion is highly dependent on the network called the limbic system or the corticolimbic-midbrain system, but these cortico-limbic [cor-tih-co-lim-bick] networks of emotion, affect [expression of emotion], and stress are highly regulated by the endocannabinoids," he said.

These areas have dense expressions of CB1 receptors, Gerdeman added, "and it's possible that every single neuron in these networks that are so important for emotion and personality and our responses to the world either releases endocannabinoids in certain circumstances or responds to them or both." So the endocannabinoid system can be fully expected to regulate the neuroscience of emotion, and therefore disorders of emotional processing like PTSD.

"This is what matters to us in life, right? Our sense of joy, our sense of resilience, our sense of fear and vulnerability," Gerdeman said, "these involve the senses in so many different disorders, whether it's posttraumatic stress or general anxiety or major depression or part of the suite of symptoms in schizophrenia."

Gerdeman thinks posttraumatic stress shouldn't be called a disorder

12 Ibid.

because it's "a natural defensive extreme response to extreme circumstances that human beings are exposed to." It's an adaptive response to shut down and become hypervigilant when someone is exposed to things that are inescapable, and such narrow adaptations result in the dysfunction called posttraumatic stress.

Anandamide as a Stress Buffer

In animal models of stress, Gerdeman explained, some research focuses on homotypic stress—the same stress over and over again, like an animal being restrained in a little tube repeatedly against its will. The repeated homotypic stress that the animal has no control over causes changes in the endocannabinoid system.

"It upregulates the FAAH enzyme [which breaks down the endocannabinoid anandamide] in numerous brain areas, including limbic system areas like the amygdala that control fear and stress. FAAH levels go up and that means anandamide levels go down," he said during the interview.

"In the cortical limbic system and particularly the amygdala, anandamide acts like a buffer to stress. And when anandamide levels drop, it's more likely that stress-evoking stimuli are going to activate your physiological stress response—the whole hypothalamic-pituitary-adrenal axis," Gerdeman explained. "But when your anandamide levels are high

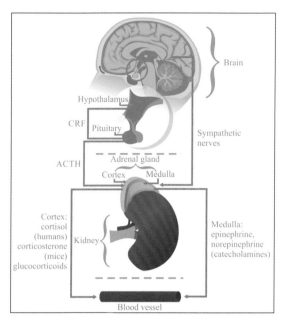

In response to stress, the hypothalamus releases corticotrophin releasing factor into the anterior pituitary, causing adrenocorticotropic hormone release into the blood flow. ACTH stimulates glucocorticoid generation in the adrenal gland cortex, and glucocorticoids then are released into the blood. (By Campos-Rodríguez R, et al. Stress modulates intestinal secretory immunoglobulin A. Front *Integr Neurosci.* 2013;7:86. This file is licensed under the Creative Commons Attribution 3.0 Unported license.)

in the amygdala, you're more resilient to potential stressors actually stressing you out."

Part of what goes on with posttraumatic stress "is that the buffer system has gotten shocked, we believe. There's a really good body of evidence that supports this from many different lines of work . . . and it's coming into a pretty coherent picture.

"In the neurobiology of stress, anandamide is a buffer, and 2-AG, the other endocannabinoid, is used in other important ways that are relevant to how you turn off the stress response. Both of the endocannabinoids are," Gerdeman said.

He recalled a 2002 *Nature* paper in which G. Marsicano and colleagues, writing about the endocannabinoid system, showed that the ECS is critical when extinguishing learned fear in animals.[13]

"Part of the study of this limbic system of fear and emotion includes the biology of learned fear, and classical associative conditioning is how you study this in rodents, and humans, really. You get them to associate a neutral stimulus with a so-called unconditioned aversive stimulus," Gerdeman said.

"The animal gets in a room, a light comes on, and it hears a tone and gets a shock in the foot. In short order, after a few of those sessions, when the animal hears the tone in the context with which the shock could occur, it freezes up. It's scared. It's learned to anticipate and be afraid.

"That's learned fear," he added, noting that the neural circuitry of the amygdala is highly involved in the process. So the animal learns fear, Gerdeman says, "but then there's a process called extinction where, if the animal is exposed to that conditioned cue over time and does not receive the shock, then the memory is, as we say, extinguished. The animal stops being afraid of the cue. The tone is now neutral again. And it's not just a matter of forgetting, it's active relearning . . . or maybe call it unlearning."

Gerdeman said the Marsicano paper showed that when an animal is undergoing the extinction training, anandamide—the stress buffer—is being actively released in the amygdala.

Supplementing the ECS for Resilience

Since that time, more sophisticated studies have shown in animal models that during fear extinction, if anandamide levels are high, the animal—or the human, Gerdeman says—moves past the fearful memory more rapidly. If CB1 receptors

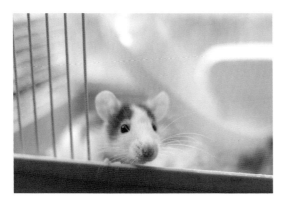

Rodent in a cage (From Shutterstock by sakavichanka)

13 Marsicano, G., C. T. Wotjak, S. C. Azad, T. Bisogno, G. Rammes, M. G. Cascio, H. Hermann, J. Tang, C. Hofmann, W. Zieglgänsberger, V. Di Marzo, and B. Lutz. "The endogenous cannabinoid system controls extinction of aversive memories." *Nature* 418(6897):530–4.

are blocked, either with a drug or with genetic techniques, fear extinction is harder—animals hold on longer to that fearful stimulus and reactivity. The same sort of thing is shown in studies with animals that are made to have the same kind of genetic variant as a substantial number of Western Europeans have.

"This variant in the human population, the FAAH enzyme, has a single nucleotide difference that leads to lower levels of activity, and lower levels of the FAAH enzyme mean that anandamide is not broken down as effectively," Gerdeman said. "So we believe that in these variants in human beings you will have a greater level of anandamide signaling" and a faster fear-extinction process.

With people this is tested using virtual reality, he said, "where you've got a VR headset and you're walking through a building and you subconsciously detect cues before something jumps out and scares you. Then later in the behavioral testing those cues are popped up and you can measure autonomic responses like sweat production and that kind of thing."

Gerdeman says the paradigm of learned helplessness—which psychologist Martin Seligman discovered in 1965 in experiments with dogs—also stems from studies where a pair of rats got foot shocks on an electric grid delivered at exactly the same time. One rat has a lever in the cage and if he presses it, the shocking will stop. He has to learn this, but they do, Gerdeman said. The other rat is called a yoked control, and his shocks depend on what the other rat does, but he's completely unaware of it. The magnitude of shocks delivered between the two animals is precisely the same, but

A traumatic brain injury patient walks through a virtual reality scenario at the Computer Assisted Rehabilitation Environment Laboratory at the National Intrepid Center of Excellence in Bethesda, MD. Cameras track patient movements and supply data to physical therapists. (U.S. Air Force photo by J. M. Eddins Jr.)

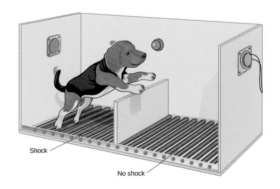

Dr. Martin Seligman's learned helplessness experiments with dogs used an apparatus that documented when the animals moved from a floor that delivered shocks to one that didn't. (From Wikimedia Commons by Rose M. Spielman PhD. This file is licensed under the Creative Commons Attribution 4.0 International license.)

only one animal can learn that it has the power to turn the shocks off.

The animal that learns it has no control over the stressor goes through a whole constellation of gene changes, physiological changes associated with the chronic stress. These don't happen in the animal that learns it can control the stress. Later on in the animals' lives, Gerdeman says, "the animal that had control over its early life stress in that experiment is much more likely to be resilient to future stressors and not go into a locked-down, fearful animal model of PTSD."

Part of what may go on in the war theater, or in abuse by a spouse or in a troubled childhood, "is if someone grows up in a situation where as a child they learned helplessness, they may be more vulnerable to being triggered into what we call PTSD."

Gerdeman said this information is "hugely relevant" to the idea that using cannabinoid supplements to balance the endocannabinoid system is therapeutic. Doing so "makes all the sense in the world," he said.

A Consistent Kind of Neural Signature

Dr. Matthew Hill, through his research in determining the endocannabinoid system's role in the effects of stress on neuroendocrine function, emotional behavior, and other conditions, said in a 2017 interview that researchers don't totally understand what's different in the brain of someone who's been exposed to trauma and develops PTSD, versus someone who's been exposed to trauma and doesn't.

"But one of the things that reliably pops up from study to study in humans," Hill said, "is that people with PTSD have what appears to be hyperactivity of neurons in an area of the brain called the amygdala," the part of the brain "involved

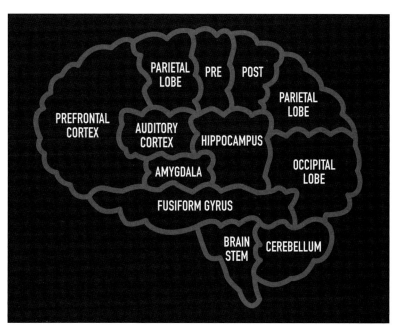

A brain with sections named, including the amygdala. (From iStock by Jobalou)

in understanding the emotional salience [weight] of, let's say, stimuli in your environment."

He explained, "If you put your hand on a hot oven and burn your hand and it's a very aversive experience, your amygdala is important for recognizing that it was bad and learning the association between the stovetop and the burning pain. And you don't want to do that again." The amygdala is important in understanding cues in the environment related to emotional responses and threatening outcomes, and it's important for scanning the environment almost unconsciously to determine if there's a threat that could cause harm.

"In PTSD it's thought that individuals start generalizing. A trauma can be a very specific thing, like a car accident, for example," Hill said. "But someone who got PTSD after the accident starts to generalize to all cars and to traffic in general, and may start to exhibit anxiety and panic responses when they see any stimulus that's similar to what was associated with their initial trauma." Depending on how common or familiar the stimulus is, Hill said, generalizing can cause a huge amount of distress. But cannabinoids seem to be very efficient at calming down neural activity in the amygdala, at least in animal studies.

"This is probably not the only way [cannabinoids] influence aspects of PTSD," Hill added, "because there's a huge sleep component as well in PTSD, but hyperactivity of the amygdala seems to be a relatively consistent kind of an abnormality that's present in PTSD." This has been a lot of the focus, for example in looking at drugs that may have benefit in PTSD, he said, "by looking at whether the drugs have the ability to blunt amygdala reactivity to the threat cues in your environment."

PTSD: Acquired Endocannabinoid Deficiency

The concept of endocannabinoid deficiency, which neurologist and psychopharmacology researcher Dr. Ethan Russo proposed in 2001, is based on the concept of endocannabinoid tone.

Endocannabinoid tone reflects a person's levels of the endocannabinoids anandamide and 2-AG and their production and metabolism, and the relative abundance and states of the cannabinoid receptors, among them CB1 and CB2. If endocannabinoid levels drop, this tone

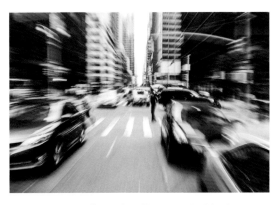

Camera zoom effect of traffic scene in Manhattan NYC (From Shutterstock by Christian Mueller)

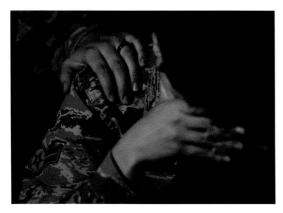

September is Suicide Prevention Month in the United States, when organizations show how to identify warning signs of suicide, increase understanding of what leads to suicide and offer resources. (Illustrative photo by U.S. Air Force Airman 1st Class Kathryn R. C. Reaves, in the public domain.)

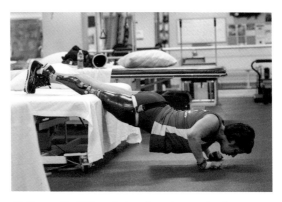

Air Force Staff Sgt. Sebastiana Lopez Arellano, a patient at Walter Reed National Military Medical Center, does push-ups during her therapy session at the center's Military Advanced Training Center in Bethesda, Maryland, April 13, 2016. (U.S. Air Force photo by Sean Kimmons)

declines and illness results, Russo said, adding that PTSD could be one of those illnesses.

When he proposed the concept, Russo named migraine, fibromyalgia, and irritable bowel syndrome, all of which are common subjective pain syndromes, as indicative of clinical endocannabinoid deficiency. But PTSD is an example of an acquired endocannabinoid deficiency, Russo said in a 2017 interview.

"Some of these things are genetic, but here you've got a situation of, say, a young soldier, well-adjusted before, has this terrible experience and comes back with this florid syndrome that subsequently is ruining their life. The Department of Defense needs to be interested in this explanation because the areas of application are legion."

For victims of PTSD, Russo added, "and those who get blown up and have traumatic brain injuries, and people who have lost limbs and have phantom limb pain, absolutely the best thing is cannabis."

For example, when people have an amputation they're at risk for developing phantom-limb pain. "This is not just a phenomenon in which the patient says, 'I still feel my leg even though it's not there any longer.' Rather, it is a severe and chronic form of neuropathic pain—a burning, relentless, difficult-to-treat pain originating from the severed nerves," Russo said. "The conventional drugs to treat this are pretty ineffective, so often the cases are intractable to treatment."

Russo says such patients may not be taken care of properly and doctors find themselves using chronic narcotics in efforts to control the pain. Opioids don't work in this context and eventually create problems of their own, he said, including exacerbating neuropathic pain, developing tolerance requiring ever-higher dosages, and risking addiction and overdose. This process of neuropathic pain seems to be driven by an excess of the excitatory neurotransmitter glutamate.

"When present in excess, [glutamate] spills over and drives the neuropathic pain. Similarly, in the brain after head injury, there's so much glutamate that it actually produces what's called excitotoxicity—an overreaction that kills the cells." The initial injury may kill certain brain cells, but in the next few days the cells that are only damaged become so driven by this release of glutamate that they also succumb, even though they may have been salvageable with the right treatment, he said.

"Cannabinoids, and especially CBD, turn off this process and can save the damaged-but-not-yet-dead cells from the head injury," Russo said. "THC specifically and CBD probably, when used chronically, also turn down this glutamate excitability and can reduce, and eventually in some cases extinguish, neuropathic pain."

Preventing PTSD?

Russo says that when a patient has an established PTSD syndrome they need

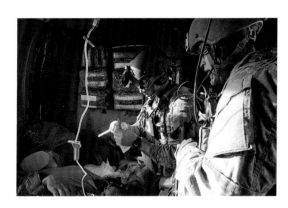

Special operations combat medics from the 10th Special Forces Group (Airborne) render in-flight medical attention to a mock casualty during MedEvac training Nov. 8, 2016. (Defense Department photo by Air Force Staff Sgt. Jorden M. Weir, in the public domain)

to be treated on an ongoing basis, but he also advocates prevention.

"If we had the option to jump in at the beginning of a traumatic event with opiates and cannabinoids in combination, maybe PTSD doesn't eventuate, or at least not with the terrible frequency that it now occurs in warfare," he said.

If battlefield medics had opiates and cannabinoids to administer acutely in the field, Russo added, "you could

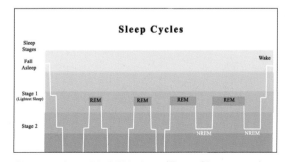

Sleep cycles with REM sleep (From Shutterstock by arca38)

probably substantially eliminate PTSD if you treated them [with cannabinoids] at the time you controlled their pain [with opioids]. You may allow them to sleep. The multifaceted therapeutic effects of cannabis on these biochemical mechanisms may prevent the development of the PTSD cycle in the brain that doesn't allow you to forget and that is producing intrusive dreams and making it impossible to function in society."

One of the things THC does is suppress rapid-eye movement (REM) sleep—dreaming sleep. "If REM sleep is suppressed, you can't have nightmares. What's one of the cardinal side effects of THC? Forgetfulness. In PTSD you can't forget. So with THC you're reinforcing the ability to forget, and that's what patients with PTSD need so they can once again look forward in their lives," he said.

If society really wants an approach that's cost effective, Russo added, "it is, treat in the field and follow up with those people while they're recovering physically with counseling so they can process what they've been through, and I think you can prevent almost all of this. But this is a crazy idea in the estimation of most people."

The alternative is the status quo, "a huge population of victims who suffer endlessly along with their families, and who end up as suicide victims with horrible frequency." Russo added, "If you've actually got the chance to intervene on behalf of injured soldiers at risk for PTSD, you can treat them acutely, prevent it, and they can return to a normal life. That's good for him or her, for the family, and for society." For treating PTSD if it can't be prevented, Russo said, researchers and physicians don't yet know what treatment is optimal.

"My suspicion is that, like with a lot of things, you'd need a little THC to work on the memory and intrusive dream aspect, and a larger amount of CBD to increase endocannabinoid tone and help with any pain and other damage. It's a formula that has a lot of applicability broadly because there are so many things that it would help."

Mired in PTSD Symptoms

The federal classification of cannabis as essentially too dangerous to study is a barrier to research and keeps patients whose illnesses don't respond well to traditional medicines—opioids, for example—mired in pain, anxiety, insomnia, and other symptoms. Severe PTSD is one of those illnesses.

Because of the federal restriction on cannabis, even the US Department of Veterans Affairs can't prescribe, and until recently couldn't even discuss, medical cannabis for veterans with PTSD, pain, anxiety, or any other illness that cannabis could help treat. The same restriction has created a research environment in which most studies of cannabinoids and PTSD are done with animal models of PTSD, and only a few small studies have examined PTSD and cannabinoids in people.

One small 2014 study[14] in Israel by P. Roitman and colleagues, for example, explored using THC as an add-on to traditional treatments. The researchers knew that many PTSD patients got only partial relief with current treatments and that patients with uninterrupted PTSD showed high rates of substance abuse.

The open-label study (investigators don't disguise the THC or use a placebo) evaluated the tolerance and safety of orally absorbable THC for chronic PTSD. The ten patients, who already were on stable medication for PTSD, received 5 mg of THC (a low dose, also called a microdose, that wouldn't necessarily be intoxicating) twice a day as an add-on treatment.[15]

The researchers reported that three patients had mild adverse effects but didn't drop out of the study, and the THC intervention improved the severity of all symptoms—sleep quality, nightmare frequency, and PTSD hyperarousal (increase in anxiety and irritability, among others) symptoms. They concluded that THC was safe and well tolerated by patients with chronic PTSD.[16]

PTSD: A Handful of Small Studies

Dr. Hill said there isn't a lot of well-executed clinical work in the realm of looking at cannabinoids for PTSD, but there are a handful of small studies.

"These . . . usually don't have enough subjects in them to make strong conclusions or to generalize at all, but what I find interesting . . . is that three or four of them have been done now and only one of them has been done properly, with a placebo-controlled double-blind trial," he said. That study was done by the

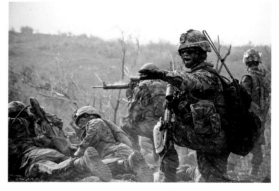

Royal Canadian Army Warrant Officer Robby Fraser, with Princess Patricia's Canadian Light Infantry, directs machine gun fire at a support-by-fire position during a live-fire assault July 22, 2012. (Defense Department photo by Lance Cpl. Robert Bush, U.S. Marine Corps, in the public domain)

---

14 Roitman, P., R. Mechoulam, R. Cooper-Kazaz, and A. Shalev. "Preliminary, open-label, pilot study of add-on oral Δ9-tetrahydrocannabinol in chronic post-traumatic stress disorder." *Clin Drug Investig* 34(8):587–91 (doi: 10.1007/s40261-014-0212-3).

15 Ibid.

16 Ibid.

Canadian military with ten patients. This kind of study uses a placebo—a harmless substance with no drug effect—and makes sure that no one among the participants or investigators knows which substance is the study drug and which is the placebo (blinded), eliminating the possibility of some kind of bias. Double-blind means that no information about test results is released until after the test.

The 2015 *Psychoneuroendocrinology* study[17] by R. Jetly and colleagues that Hill discussed used a synthetic cannabinoid called nabilone. Nabilone (trade name Cesamet) mimics THC but has more predictable side effects and few or no intoxicating effects, both important for studying other kinds of effects. The researchers wanted to see if nabilone capsules would reduce the frequency and intensity of nightmares in Canadian male military members with PTSD who were already on standard treatment (psychotherapy, antidepressants).

During the study, which was registered with Health Canada, the Canadian public health department, subjects received 3 mg of nabilone before bed each night for seven weeks. Afterward, the researchers said nabilone had "provided significant relief for military personnel with PTSD, indicating that it shows promise as a clinically relevant treatment for patients with nightmares and a history of non-response to traditional therapies." The findings, they wrote, should be replicated in a larger group of subjects and more research should explore the effect of nabilone on other PTSD symptoms, like reexperiencing hypervigilance and insomnia.[18]

"What the people who had PTSD found from taking [nabilone]," Hill said, "was that it dramatically reduced their frequency of nightmares and it improved their quality of sleep, and in PTSD sleep disturbances are a massive problem." PTSD sufferers "have a lot of vivid, lucid nightmares. They wake up a lot so their sleep is fragmented through the night. The thought is, these memories that come back in the form of nightmares are almost hyper-consolidating (hyper-stabilizing) the memory . . . and the lucid nightmares during REM sleep are thought to be one of the things that sensitizes the disease."

Because this was a double-blind placebo-controlled trial, the research staff could switch subjects over to the placebo without anyone involved in the study knowing who was on the drug and who was on the placebo at what time. Almost

---

17 Jetly, R., A. Heber, G. Fraser, and D. Boisvert. "The efficacy of nabilone, a synthetic cannabinoid, in the treatment of PTSD-associated nightmares: A preliminary randomized, double-blind, placebo-controlled cross-over design study." *Psychoneuroendocrinology* 51:585–8 (doi: 10.1016/j.psyneuen.2014.11.002).

18 Ibid.

immediately, when the subjects who had been on the drug went on the placebo, all the nightmares came back within a day or two.

"It seemed to be a pretty robust effect," Hill said, "but again, it's a very small sample size." Still, he hopes the Canadian government, especially in light of cannabis legalization across that country, will put more money into cannabinoid research, which would help produce more well-rounded and broader clinical trials.

The First Placebo-Controlled, Triple-Blind, Randomized PTSD Trial

After seven years of submitting applications and working with multiple federal agencies, the Multidisciplinary Association for Psychedelic Studies (MAPS) received permission in 2014 to conduct the very first clinical trial of smoked cannabis for PTSD. MAPS, whose mission since 1986 has included collecting objective information about the efficacy of cannabis-based treatments for PTSD and other disorders, sponsored the study.

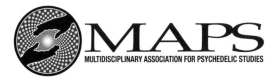

Multidisciplinary Association for Psychedelic Studies logo (Courtesy MAPS)

The Colorado Department of Public Health and Environment awarded a $2.1 million grant for the study. Its official title was "Placebo-controlled, triple-blind, randomized crossover pilot study of the safety and efficacy of four different potencies of smoked marijuana in 76 veterans with chronic, treatment-resistant posttraumatic stress disorder (PTSD)." So this clinical trial, also called the WeCan Study, covered a lot of research-standards bases.

Sue Sisley, MD, is a physician and was the study's principal investigator at Scottsdale Research Institute in Phoenix, Arizona. The study enrolled its first participant in 2017 and in October 2018 enrolled its seventy-sixth and final participant to explore whether smoked cannabis could help reduce PTSD symptoms in US military veterans with chronic, treatment-resistant PTSD.

Participants had to be military veterans, men or women eighteen or older, with a diagnosis of PTSD that hadn't improved with medication or psychotherapy. According to the study website, "Results from the WeCan Study will help advance the standard of care for PTSD in veterans, potentially providing avenues for new research and treatment, as well as providing clear, scientifically sound data on the efficacy of cannabis for PTSD."

Clinical Trials: Cannabinoids for PTSD

Study of Four Different Potencies of Smoked Marijuana in 76 Veterans With PTSD
Here's the listing for the WeCan Study mentioned above. The sponsor is MAPS. The start date was January 2017, the end date January 2019. During the study, each participant smoked two of four types of cannabis, up to 1.8 grams per day, for three weeks. After each three-week cannabis-use period, they stopped smoking cannabis for two weeks and no cannabis use was allowed. Study details are available at clinicaltrials.gov/ct2/show/NCT02759185.

Evaluating Safety and Efficacy of Cannabis in Participants with Chronic PTSD
The triple-blind placebo-controlled crossover study seeks to evaluate the safety and efficacy of vaporized cannabis in forty-two adults with chronic, treatment-resistant PTSD. The study—of cannabis with high THC/low CBD, high THC/high CBD, and low THC/low CBD—began in September 2016 and ends in June 2020. Study details are available at clinicaltrials.gov/ct2/show/NCT02517424.

Chapter 10
Cannabinoids for Brain Trauma and Neurodegeneration

Endocannabinoids and phytocannabinoids have a range of protective actions in the body and brain, and one of them is to regulate brain cell balance and survival.[1]

They can do this because the endocannabinoid system (ECS) produces protective effects that include preserving, rescuing, repairing, and replacing neurons and glial cells against multiple insults that could damage the cells. Because CB1 and CB2 receptors, endocannabinoid-related enzymes, and non-endocannabinoid targets all are located on nearby neurons, glial cells, and neural progenitor cells (cells that can differentiate into new brain and glial cells[2]), endocannabinoid protective effects can begin taking place as soon as damage occurs at those sites.[3]

The ECS also has modulatory effects on important functions like neurotransmission, glial activation, oxidative stress, and protein homeostasis. Dysregulation in these cellular processes is a hallmark of aging and of central nervous system neurodegenerative diseases. The broad spectrum of endocannabinoids and cannabinoids lets them target different aspects of these multifactorial diseases, Aymerich and colleagues wrote in a 2018 *Biochemical Pharmacology* paper.[4]

Cannabinoids for Stroke and Brain Trauma

Stroke is the second most common cause of death and the third most common cause of disability worldwide. About 80 percent of strokes happen because a blood vessel is blocked; these are called ischemic (iss-keem-ick) strokes. The rest are mainly associated with a blood vessel rupture, called hemorrhagic

---

1 Fernández-Ruiz, J., M. A. Moro, and J. Martinez-Orgado. "Cannabinoids in neurodegenerative disorders and stroke/brain trauma: From preclinical models to clinical applications." *Neurotherapeutics* 12:793–806 (doi: 10.1007/s13311-015-0381-7).

2 Nature.com, https://www.nature.com/subjects/neural-progenitors. Accessed 8/10/2018.

3 Fernández-Ruiz, J, M. A. Moro, and J. Martinez-Orgado.

4 Aymerich, M. S., E. Aso, M. A. Abellanas, R. M. Tolon, J. A. Ramos, I. Ferrer, J. Romero, and J. Fernández-Ruiz.

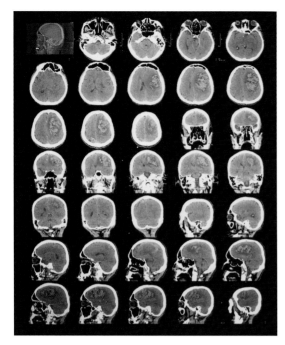

Computerized tomographic scan a brain with hemorrhagic stroke. Red identifies the lesion focus. (From iStock by sudok1)

(hem-or-ah-jick) strokes, according to a 2015 *Neurotherapeutics* paper by J. Fernández-Ruiz and colleagues.[5]

When a blood vessel that supplies blood to brain tissue is blocked, a large release of the excitatory neurotransmitter glutamate triggers ischemic brain damage. This reverses glutamate uptake by glutamate transporters and related effects promote cell death, disrupt mitochondrial function, and irreversibly injure or kill cells, and the injury from ischemic stroke is made worse by a vigorous inflammatory response.[6]

A treatment used very soon after the stroke occurs is a clearing of the blocked blood vessel using a tissue plasminogen activator, a protein that helps break down blood clots. This narrow window means that less than 5 percent of stroke patients can benefit from the treatment.[7]

Traumatic brain injury (TBI) is an acquired focal (located in one brain area) injury that happens when sudden trauma damages the brain. These injuries often happen because of car or firearm accidents or falls. TBI disease processes have many of the same mechanisms as stroke.[8]

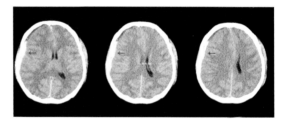

An axial computerized tomography scan of a patient with traumatic injury shows right subdural hemorrhage and edema with shifting of the brain to the left. Intra-cerebral bleeding and blood clots are from a car accident. (From Shutterstock by Tomatheart)

Promising Treatments

Cannabinoids have been proposed as promising neuroprotective compounds for treating stroke and TBI, but, because

5 Fernández-Ruiz, J., M. A. Moro, and J. Martinez-Orgado.
6 Ibid.
7 Ibid.
8 Ibid.

whole-plant cannabis is federally illegal, they've been studied mainly in experimental or genetic models of both disorders using animal models of the injuries and synthetic cannabinoids and phytocannabinoids. And because it's illegal, no standardized whole-plant cannabis products yet have been developed that could be used in human studies, except the plant-derived—and very expensive—CBD product Epidiolex.

Still, according to Fernández-Ruiz and colleagues, over time and based on lab and animal studies, the cannabinoid-related compounds improved neurological performance; reduced infarct size (localized dead tissue caused by failed blood supply), edema (swelling caused by accumulating fluid), blood-brain barrier disruption, inflammation, and gliosis (reactive change of glial cells caused by CNS damage); and increased control of immunomodulatory (regulatory adjustment) responses.[9]

Similar findings were shown in experiments using mice that were genetically altered to lack or have deficient CB1 cannabinoid receptors and, to a lesser extent, CB2 receptors. The researchers said that CB2 was a good target for TBI and stroke candidate drugs because cannabinoid-related compounds that activate CB2 receptors aren't intoxicating.

The psychoactive phytocannabinoid THC activates the CB1 receptor[10] and binds less strongly to CB2.

The research on cannabinoid treatments for TBI and stroke has mainly taken place in culture dishes/test tubes or in animal models of the disorders, but Fernández-Ruiz and colleagues say several clinical studies also have taken place. The most relevant was a multicenter, placebo-controlled phase 3 trial (comparing the effectiveness of an experimental drug with a standard drug) conducted in 2005 that was held to determine the safety and effectiveness of dexanabinol (dex-ah-nab-in-all, HU-211) in TBI patients. Dexanabinol is a synthetic compound that has the chemical structure of a classic cannabinoid but no activity at cannabinoid receptors (although it was active at a glutamate receptor called NMDA, for N-methyl-D-aspartate.[11] This will not be on the test).

The trial showed that HU-211 was safe but didn't effectively treat TBI. The researchers said that because it's a synthetic cannabinoid and has no activity at the CB1 or CB2 receptors, clinical studies should be repeated with compounds that do act at the cannabinoid receptors.[12]

---

9 Ibid.
10 Ibid.
11 Ibid.
12 Ibid.

Or, Fernández-Ruiz said during a 2017 interview, the lack of effective TBI treatment may have been a timing issue.

"Brain trauma is very similar to a stroke in terms of the neurotoxic processes, so the problem with brain trauma, like stroke, is that they are very fast disorders. Nobody knows when someone riding on a motorcycle is going to have an accident. So the damage is very fast, it's a question of an hour and treatments would be initiated and would have an opportunity for neuroprotection very early." But in clinical trials, he said, people "are recruited for the clinical trials one to two days after they have the trauma. Possibly it was too late."

In a 2014 *Frontiers in Pharmacology* paper, cannabinoid researchers Aso and Ferrer wrote that "interest in the role the endocannabinoid system may play in neurodegenerative processes is based on findings revealing that the augmentation of cannabinoid tone contributes to brain homeostasis and neuron survival, suggesting that [augmenting endocannabinoid tone] may offer protection against the deleterious consequences of pathogenic molecules."[13]

So, as other researchers have mentioned, boosting endocannabinoid tone may act as a preventive measure against brain trauma.

Cannabinoids and Other Brain Injuries

In his 2018 *Frontiers in Integrated Neuroscience* paper,[14] Dr. Ethan Russo wrote that cannabinoids' neuroprotective antioxidant effects are particularly relevant in their ability to counteract the neurotransmitter glutamate's excitotoxicity (excessive stimulation), which leads to neuronal death after traumatic brain injury.

Anecdotally, he added, cannabis, particularly chemovars (chemical varieties) combining THC and CBD, has been very helpful in treating chronic traumatic encephalopathy (CTE) symptoms: headache, nausea, insomnia, dizziness, agitation, substance abuse, and psychotic symptoms.

"CTE, previously known as *dementia pugilistica* or 'punchdrunk syndrome,'" Russo wrote, "has garnered a great deal of attention due to its apparent frequency among long-term players of American football but including victims of repetitive head injury from causes as diverse as other contact sports, warfare, and even 'heading' in soccer."[15]

---

13 Aso, E., and I. Ferrer. "Cannabinoids for treatment of Alzheimer's disease: moving toward the clinic." *Front Pharmacol* 5(37):1–11 (doi: 10.3389/fphar.2014.00037).
14 Russo, E. B. "Cannabis therapeutics and the future of neurology." *Front Integr Neurosci* 12:51 (doi: 10.3389/fnint.2018.00051).
15 Ibid.

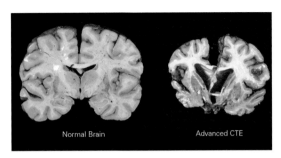

Normal brain and brain with advanced chronic traumatic encephalopathy (From the Boston University Center for the Study of Traumatic Encephalopathy. This file is licensed under the Creative Commons Attribution-Share Alike 4.0 International license.)

A 2017 study showed that 87 percent of autopsied American football players showed CTE with tau aggregates in neurons and astrocytes, neurofibrillary tangles in superficial cortical layers and hippocampus, and beta-amyloid deposition, among others, Russo wrote. Microglia were present early in the course, whose premonitory (predictive warning) symptoms include dementia, personality change, rage, and attention problems. Ninety-six percent showed a degenerative course.

Physicians and others have long considered CTE a postmortem pathological diagnosis, Russo wrote, but two current studies support the ability to identify symptoms while a patient is alive (pre-mortem). Also, he added, positron emission tomography (PET) imaging binding levels in a living CTE patient correlated with the patient's postmortem

tau deposition. The greatest tau concentration was seen in cortical and brainstem areas, allowing pre-mortem diagnosis and distinction from Alzheimer's.[16]

Cannabinoids and Contact Sports

During a February 20, 2019, webinar hosted by Dr. Dustin Sulak's medical cannabis Healer Training and Certification Program at healer.com,[17] Dr. Greg Gerdeman, a neuroscientist chief scientific officer with Colorado-based United Cannabis Corporation, was a guest speaker.

During the webinar's question and answer segment, one attendee asked about using cannabinoids to treat people who already have injuries like post-concussive syndrome or TBI and who have recently started using cannabis, and about the prophylactic use of CBD for people who play contact sports.

"I'm not a clinician," Gerdeman said, "but I certainly have been around a number of clinical success stories of people taking CBD and getting at least some rapid recovery from brain injury that was better than their initial prognosis. I don't know that we know enough to say one thing or another, but CBD and THC are both neuroprotective for brain injury in many different ways. It's a pleiotropic [having multiple effects] kind of mechanism and all these receptor targets protect against ischemic damage and glial

16 Ibid.
17 Sulak, D.

infiltration and so many other aspects that lead to TBI."

There are no clinical studies to discuss, Sulak said, "but as I say in these webinars and in the [healer.com] training material, 'treat the patient, not the diagnosis.' What's the patient having trouble with? Is it sleep, cognition, focus, awareness? And we could tailor the treatment using THC and CBD and possibly acidic cannabinoids [for example like the nonintoxicating THCA and CDBA], so I wouldn't think there's a one-size-fits-all answer for that." To the next part of the question—can CBD be used preventively in contact sports?—Sulak said, "I hear that a lot of NFL players use CBD before practices and games, and I think there's very little downside to that."

"I think they should all do it," Gerdeman added. "I think CBD should be on the sidelines of all of those football and contact sports." He said he was recently part of a panel discussion about sports and cannabis at the Emerald Cup (an annual organic cannabis competition in Santa Rosa, California), and he'd spoken with a National Football League player and with a former National Basketball Association player.

"It was a really illuminating conversation," Gerdeman said. "The NFL player . . . was telling me it's not football players using CBD alone. He's like, you wouldn't believe the number of playmaker NFL players who are on the field and they're hitting vape pens at halftime. And not just CBD—a lot of guys are using THC before games in the NFL."

Look at people like Junior Seau, Gerdeman added, "who had such a tragic story from chronic head injury." Seau was a gifted NFL linebacker (1990–2009) who killed himself in 2012 and whose family, after a postmortem of his brain, learned that he'd had chronic traumatic encephalopathy—concussion-related brain damage—that may have contributed to his suicide.

Gerdeman added, "If he'd been taking CBD before and after games, would that have happened to him? We can't really say we know, but it would not have hurt one bit to try, and I think all those athletes should be taking CBD and low-dose THC."

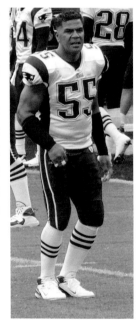

New England Patriots linebacker Junior Seau during a 2008 game against the Oakland Raiders (From Wikimedia Commons by J. J. Hall. This file is licensed under the Creative Commons Attribution 2.0 Generic license.)

Cannabinoids and Neurodegeneration

Aging is a natural process that in the brain leads to changes and adaptations in molecules, cells, and tissues. The changes—less predominant for healthy people, more for those who aren't so healthy[18]—can include the following range of results:

- Reduced glucose metabolism; glucose, critically, is the brain's main source of energy[19]
- Oxidative stress, created when antioxidants fail to control cellular waste products called free radicals that damage energy-producing mitochondria and disrupt cell signaling
- Impaired cellular calcium signaling; calcium underlies the brain's ability to control synaptic activity and form memories and maintains neuronal integrity and long-term cell survival[20]
- Slower protein synthesis and degradation, which may slow new neuron production and

reduce glial reactivity and lets damaged proteins clump together and neurons to atrophy[21]

Aging and the Endocannabinoid System

Results from animal models and human studies over twenty years has increased researchers' understanding of how the endocannabinoid system, THC, and synthetic THC work at the molecular level to influence cannabinoid receptors, Di Marzo and colleagues wrote in a 2015 *Nature Reviews Neuroscience* paper.[22] Studies discussed in the paper also lent "scientific support for targeting the endocannabinoid signaling system to treat several devastating diseases, including neurodegenerative and chronic inflammatory diseases." Their review focused on "recent evidence that added a new layer of complexity to the idea of targeting the endocannabinoid signaling system for therapeutic benefit," because it's now clear that expression levels of endocannabinoid system receptors, and enzymes that make or break down

---

18 Fernández-Ruiz, J. "The biomedical challenge of neurodegenerative disorders: An opportunity for cannabinoid-based therapies to improve on the poor current therapeutic outcomes." *Br J Pharmacol* (doi: 10.1111/bph.14382).

19 Mosconi, L. "Glucose metabolism in normal aging and Alzheimer's disease: Methodological and physiological considerations for PET studies." *Clin Transl Imaging* 1(4) (doi: 10.1007/s40336-013-0026-y).

20 Marambaud, P., U. Dreses-Werringloer, V. Vingtdeux. "Calcium signaling in neurodegeneration." *Mol Neurodegen* 4:20 (doi: 10.1186/1750-1326-4-20).

21 Fernández-Ruiz, J.

22 Di Marzo, V., N. Stella, and A. Zimmer.

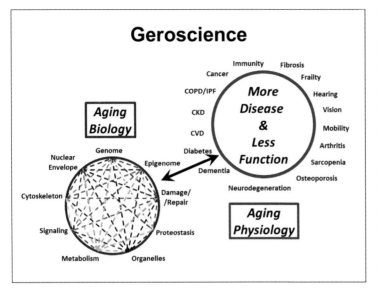

Geroscience

Immunity   Fibrosis
Cancer   Frailty
COPD/IPF   Hearing

**More
Disease
&
Less
Function**

CKD   Vision
CVD   Mobility
Diabetes   Arthritis
Dementia   Sarcopenia
                                  Osteoporosis
Neurodegeneration

**Aging
Biology**

Genome
Nuclear
Envelope   Epigenome

Cytoskeleton   Damage/
                          /Repair

Signaling   Proteostasis

Metabolism   Organelles

**Aging
Physiology**

Geroscience, a National Institutes of Health-wide initiative, accelerates research into the basic biological mechanisms driving aging and that could lead to improved clinical interventions for diseases and conditions experienced by many older people. (Courtesy NIH National Institute on Aging)

endocannabinoids, change substantially in the brain and in other organs as people age.

"This suggests that the bioactivity of endocannabinoid-based therapeutics is likely to vary depending on the age of the patient, the disease type and the stage of disease at the time of treatment," Di Marzo and colleagues wrote, and "such treatments may have to be tailored for different subsets of patients."

The researchers also wrote that expression levels of cannabinoid and endocannabinoid-related receptors in neurons and glial cells can change with

normal aging, or earlier in life in response to a neurological disease. In neurological disease, they added, chronic changes in endocannabinoid signaling often come with chronic activation of the immune system. Some of the immune cells that invade the brain parenchyma (functional tissue) also express cannabinoid receptors, and this increases the number of cells that respond to endocannabinoids and cannabinoids.[23]

"This dynamic change in brain neuroinflammation in endocannabinoid signaling in neurons, glia, and immune cells has been mapped in detail in mice undergoing experimental allergic encephalomyelitis (EAE), a model of multiple sclerosis," Di Marzo and colleagues wrote, adding that they don't yet know whether the ability to control neuroinflammation changes as people age, or how aging might predispose people with multiple sclerosis or other neuroinflammatory disorders to cannabinoid-based treatments.

Some of the studies reviewed in the paper, and evidence suggesting that changes in endocannabinoid levels might have a role in amyotrophic lateral

23 Ibid.

sclerosis and Parkinson's disease, "outline a molecular framework that connects [cannabinoid signaling outside and inside cells] to an age- and cell-metabolism-dependent deterioration of neural cells that might contribute to some neurodegenerative diseases."[24]

Common Mechanisms

Because people live longer than they used to, often reaching eighty, ninety, or beyond, regular changes and adaptations in some aging brains could aggravate and drive processes that lead to the increasingly common neurodegenerative condition Alzheimer's disease (AD), and to

Clinical Trials: Cannabinoids and Aging

Acute Effects of Cannabis on Cognition and Mobility in Older HIV-infected and HIV-Uninfected Women This randomized crossover study of sixty women sought to understand why HIV-infected and uninfected women who use cannabis now or have in the past had higher risk of experiencing a fall in the earlier Women's Interagency HIV Study. The present study compared cannabis with placebo on the women's measures of mobility, balance, and cognition. The study began in November 2018 and ended in August 2019. Study details are available at clinicaltrials.gov/ct2/show/NCT03633721.

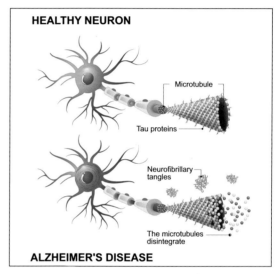

In Alzheimer's disease, the change in tau protein results in the breakdown of microtubules in neurons. Shown are tau proteins, neurofibrillary tangles and microtubule breakdown. (From iStock by ttsz)

Parkinson's disease (PD), Huntington's disease (HD), amyotrophic lateral sclerosis (ALS), and multiple sclerosis (MS).

Each disorder has a different cause and disease progression, but common mechanisms underlie their

---

24 Ibid.

neurodegenerative components, including neuroinflammation, excitotoxicity, mitochondrial dysfunction, and reduced neuronal maintenance support.[25] The number of people worldwide who have the most common neurodegenerative diseases is increasing.

In age ranges 60–64 and 85–89, the number of people with Alzheimer's increases fifteen-fold, those with Parkinson's increases seven-fold, and those with Huntington's increases five-fold, according to Dr. Javier Fernández-Ruiz, head of the Department of Biochemistry and Molecular Biology (Faculty of Medicine) at Complutense University of Madrid in Spain. He and his lab study cannabinoids and their effects

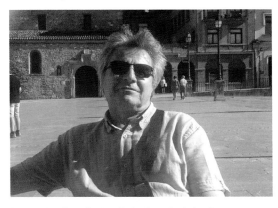

Dr. Javier Fernández-Ruiz, head of the Department of Molecular Biology (Faculty of Medicine) at Complutense University-Madrid in Spain. (From Dr. Javier Fernández-Ruiz. Used with permission.)

on neurodegenerative diseases, and here he was speaking in 2017 at the eighth European Workshop on Cannabinoid Research held in Roehampton, London.[26]

The increase in these degenerative diseases is grim, and the drugs developed to treat them are few and don't work well. But there's better news that involves cannabinoids.

"Despite the large number of therapeutic agents investigated to combat AD . . . only four agents with modest efficacy [effectiveness] have been approved to date," Fernández-Ruiz said, noting that the failure rate also has been high for drugs at preclinical and clinical evaluation stages, and the same situation exists for PD, HD, and ALS.[27]

The problem may be that each drug targets only one aspect of a neurodegenerative disease that was created by many neurotoxic events that combine to damage and disable neurons and glia. But a potentially viable option is emerging to treat neurodegeneration—the endocannabinoid system—and researchers have found endocannabinoid signaling to be altered in many neurodegenerative disorders.[28]

"These types of disorders with poor therapeutic outcomes represent a great opportunity for cannabinoids,"

25 Fagan, S. G., and V. A. Campbell. "The influence of cannabinoids on generic traits of neurodegeneration." *Br J Pharmacol* 171: 1347–60.
26 Fernández-Ruiz, J.
27 Ibid.
28 Fagan, S. G., and V. A. Campbell.

Fernández-Ruiz said in an interview (September 8, 2017), "which have particular neuroprotective properties that it's important to explore in order to develop novel disease-modifying medicines for these disorders. This is something cannabinoids can provide, so it's an opportunity for their therapeutic progress."

A second reason that cannabinoids should be studied for their use as medicines for treating acute (stroke, brain trauma) and chronic (AD, PD, HD, ALS) neurodegenerative disorders, he added, is the broad-spectrum profile of cannabis. Current therapies try to treat ALS, for example, with antioxidants that control only oxidative stress. For Alzheimer's, a therapy may control only excitotoxicity using agents that address a problem with homeostasis (balance) in the body's excitatory neurotransmitter, glutamate.

"This means we tried to control the disorder treating only one aspect of the mechanism that kills the neurons," Fernández-Ruiz said. "And we know that the enemies of neuronal integrity work together, they cooperate to kill neurons. So when neurons die, it's not only from one factor, it's the result of synergies [interactions] of different factors—oxidative stress, inflammation, excitotoxicity, aggregation of proteins [misfolded proteins clumped together]—that produce the apoptosis [programmed death] of neurons," he explained.

"If we want to control the progression of the disease by protecting neurons against these insults," he added, "we'll need to find or combine neuroprotective components that can also cooperate to control the different cytotoxic [toxic to cells] mechanisms." This is what cannabinoids, especially CBD, already do naturally.

"They cooperate to reduce excitotoxicity, oxidative stress, glia-driven inflammation, and protein aggregation," Fernández-Ruiz said, "and they do it through the endocannabinoids anandamide and AG-2, and through CB1, CB2, and other receptors, and their properties are active against most pathological events."

Ultimately, he said at the conference in London, "therapeutic events driven by endocannabinoid signaling reflect the activity of an endogenous system that regulates the preservation, rescue, repair and replacement of neurons and glia."[29]

Recent studies even have shown that CB1- and CB2-mediated signaling helps preserve the integrity and function of the blood-brain barrier, which is essential in neuroprotection and whose high-density cells protect the brain from harmful ions, molecules, and cells in the bloodstream. Fernández-Ruiz said CB1 and CB2

---

29 Fernández-Ruiz, J.

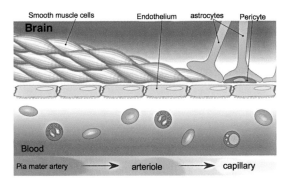

The blood-brain barrier is essential in neuroprotection; its high-density cells protect the brain from harmful ions, molecules, and cells in the bloodstream. (From Wikimedia Commons by Armin Kubelbeck. This file is licensed under the Creative Commons Attribution 1.0 Generic license.)

receptors are located in specific cells in the blood-brain barrier, where they contribute to its integrity and function.[30]

Given the broad spectrum of cannabis effects for neurodegenerative disorders, Fernández-Ruiz said during the interview, "some people considered that cannabis medicine or a combination would work the same way independent of the type of disorder—so the same for Parkinson's, the same for ALS, etc. But this is not true. We need to go to a selection, a particular choice of the best combination, the best components, depending on the disease."

Yes, it's complicated, he acknowledged. "Science is always complicated, but this is very important so it's worthy, and we're interested in exploring these very complicated things."

Cannabinoids and Alzheimer's Disease

Alzheimer's disease is an age-dependent neurodegenerative disorder in which brain changes begin years before people show signs of the disease, and progressive declines over time affect memory, attention, and language. The three stages, according to the Alzheimer's Association,[31] are early (mild disease), middle (moderate), and late (severe).

In a 2015 *Neurotherapeutics* paper,[32] Fernández-Ruiz and colleagues discussed the major Alzheimer's tissue-damaging events in the brain:

- Formation outside the cells of accumulations of beta-amyloid proteins called senile plaques
- Development inside the cell of (neurofibrillary or tau) tangles among the network of protein filaments caused by an uptick in the activity of enzymes called tau kinases

30 Ibid.
31 Alzheimer's Association, Alzheimer's and Dementia, https://www.alz.org/alzheimer_s_dementia. Accessed 8/11/2018.
32 Fernández-Ruiz, J., M. A. Moro, and J. Martinez-Orgado.

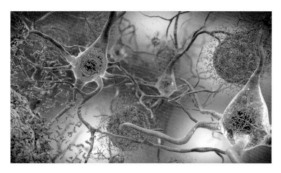

In the Alzheimer's affected brain, abnormal levels of the beta-amyloid protein clump together to form plaques (brown) that collect between neurons and disrupt cell function. Abnormal collections of the tau protein accumulate and form tangles (blue) within neurons, harming synaptic communication between nerve cells. (Courtesy National Institutes of Health)

- A high degree of wasting away of axons and dendrites that project out from the neuron, and neuronal death[33]

Cannabinoid Pharmacology and Alzheimer's Disease

In a 2018 *Frontiers in Integrated Neuroscience* paper,[34] Dr. Ethan Russo discussed Alzheimer's as a neurodegenerative disease with senile plaques formed of fibrillar beta-amyloid, identified by the presence of neurofibrillary tangles composed of tau protein. Every now and then tau tangles precede beta-amyloid deposition, but once the process begins, deterioration is inexorable.

Other pathology includes functional mitochondrial defects, increased reactive oxygen species (ROS, free radicals whose buildup can damage DNA, RNA, and proteins, and can cause cell death) and reactive nitrogen species (antimicrobial molecules that act with ROS to damage cells), and a failure of enzymes involved in energy production that leads to nerve cell exhaustion.[35]

"Eventually," Russo wrote, "synapses and dendritic branching fail, with consequent progressive neuronal wastage. Dementia and cognitive decline develop and no treatment arrests the process. Intervention must begin at an early preclinical stage to have any hope of success."[36]

Endocannabinoids modulate the primary pathological processes of Alzheimer's during the silent phase of neurodegeneration: protein misfolding, neuroinflammation, excitotoxicity, mitochondrial dysfunction, and oxidative stress. CB2 levels increase in Alzheimer's, especially in microglia around senile plaques, and CB2 stimulates macrophages to remove beta-amyloid. Head trauma increases beta-amyloid deposition and neuronal tau expression, and diabetes, obesity, trans fats, and head trauma all increase Alzheimer's risk; the

---

33 Ibid.
34 Russo, E. B. "Cannabis therapeutics and the future of neurology."
35 Ibid.
36 Ibid.

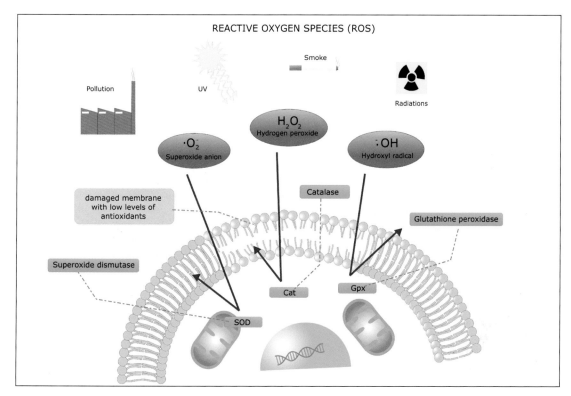

REACTIVE OXYGEN SPECIES (ROS)

Smoke

Pollution

UV

Radiations

H_2O_2
Hydrogen peroxide

$\cdot O_2^-$
Superoxide anion

$\cdot OH$
Hydroxyl radical

Catalase

damaged membrane with low levels of antioxidants

Glutathione peroxidase

Superoxide dismutase

Cat

Gpx

SOD

Main reactive oxygen species (ROS) and inhibition by antioxidants (From Shutterstock by ellepigrafica)

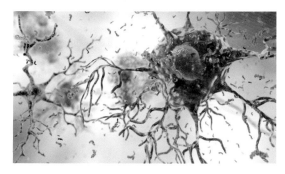

Neuroinflammation in Alzheimer's disease (Courtesy National Institutes of Health image gallery)

Mediterranean diet, education, and physical activity reduce it, Russo wrote.[37]

No current pharmacotherapy is approved for agitation in Alzheimer's. Commonly used antipsychotics, antidepressants, anxiolytics (anxiety-reducing drugs), and hypnotics (sleeping pills) often are associated with increased mortality in demented patients.[38]

Current drugs to treat memory and disease progression have been ineffective or toxic. But treatment with cannabinoids seems to be more promising and benign,

37 Ibid.
38 Ibid.

Russo wrote, noting, "As demonstrated in 1998 . . . and the subject of USA patent US09674028, CBD is a neuroprotective antioxidant, more potent than ascorbate [a mineral salt of vitamin C] or tocopherol [a form of vitamin E], that works on the same NMDA target [N-methyl-D-aspartate receptor agonists are used to treat Alzheimer's] without attendant toxicity."[39]

Later research showed that CBD inhibited beta-amyloid plaque formation, prevented reactive oxygen species production, limited neuronal apoptosis (programmed cell death), and had other positive effects related to beta-amyloid. CBD was anti-inflammatory in an animal model of Alzheimer's, and it inhibited tau protein hyperphosphorylation (transformation of normal tau into neurofibrillary tangles).[40]

Also, the endocannabinoid anandamide and CBD promoted neurogenesis after beta-amyloid exposure. THC, along with its neuroprotective antioxidant effects, inhibited acetylcholinesterase (increasing levels and the span of action of the neurotransmitter acetylcholine) and prevented beta-amyloid aggregation into plaques by binding in a critical brain region to the enzyme that affects amyloid production.[41]

On the clinical side, Russo wrote, various trials of THC in Alzheimer's have produced positive results. In 1997, in fifteen institutionalized dementia patients refusing nutrition, a randomized placebo-controlled six-week crossover trial of synthetic THC (Marinol), 2.5 mg twice daily, led to increased body-mass index with decreased agitation scores, improved negative affect (negative emotional expression) scores, and a notable carryover effect during the placebo period when THC was administered first.[42]

In 2006, an open-label two-week study of five Alzheimer's patients and one vascular dementia patient taking THC 2.5 mg at 7:00 p.m. showed benefit for nighttime motor activity, agitation, appetite, and irritability with no adverse effects.[43]

Russo wrote that initial trials of herbal cannabis for Alzheimer's have begun sporadically, with a more focused effort undertaken in 2017 by Jeffrey Hergenrather, MD—a cannabis consultant in Sebastopol, California, and a founding member of the Society of Cannabis Clinicians—in a California nursing home.[44]

---

39 Ibid.
40 Ibid.
41 Ibid.
42 Ibid.
43 Ibid.
44 Ibid.

Patients were given tinctures and edibles treated with various preparations: THC-predominant (2.5–30 mg/dose), CBD predominant, and the nonintoxicating acidic THC version THCA, which has its own positive health effects, including being anti-inflammatory and neuroprotective. Marked benefit was reported on neuroleptic drug sparing (able to use lower doses), decreased agitation, increased appetite, aggression, sleep quality, objective mood, nursing care demands, self-mutilation, and pain control.[45]

Based on their pharmacology, Russo wrote, cannabis components (like the terpenes named below) may provide benefits in target symptoms in this complex disorder:

- Agitation: THC, CBD, linalool
- Anxiety: CBD, THC (low dose), linalool
- Psychosis: CBD
- Insomnia/restlessness: THC, linalool
- Anorexia: THC
- Aggression: THC, CBD, linalool
- Depression: THC, limonene, CBD
- Pain: THC, CBD
- Memory: alpha-pinene and THC

- Neuroprotection: CBD, THC
- Reduced beta-amyloid plaque formation: THC, CBD, THCA[46]

"Thus," Russo wrote, "an extract of a Type II chemovar [has a THC-CBD balance] of cannabis with a sufficient pinene fraction would seem to be an excellent candidate for clinical trials."[47]

Cannabinoids Reduce Classic Neurotoxic Events

Few drugs are available today for Alzheimer's disease, especially therapies that might delay disease progression. But cannabinoids and their ability to reduce classic neurotoxic events have attracted research interest.

In a 2014 *Frontiers in Pharmacology* paper,[48] researchers Aso and Ferrer wrote that endocannabinoid signaling has been shown to modulate the main pathological processes that occur during the silent period (early disease stages) of the neurodegenerative process, including protein misfolding, neuroinflammation, excitotoxicity, mitochondrial dysfunction, and oxidative stress.

Several findings indicate that activating CB1 and CB2 receptors with natural or synthetic agonists, at nonintoxicating doses, have beneficial effects in

---

45 Ibid.
46 Ibid.
47 Ibid.
48 Aso, E., and I. Ferrer.

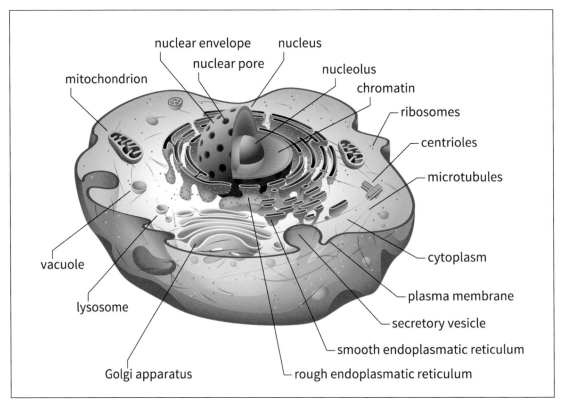

Eukaryotic cell diagram with mitochondrion. (From iStock by jackOm)

experimental models of Alzheimer's by reducing beta-amyloid peptide action and tau phosphorylation, and by promoting the brain's own repair mechanisms, the researchers wrote. Endocannabinoid signaling also has been shown to modulate several co-occurring pathological processes, including neuroinflammation, excitotoxicity, mitochondrial dysfunction, and oxidative stress.[49]

Aso and Ferrer noted that most evidence indicating the potential therapeutic use of cannabinoids in Alzheimer's has come from cell and animal models of the range of AD-related changes. But at the time of their paper, a few clinical trials and a case report were available, the trials all using synthetic THC (dronabinol or nabilone, both of which are THC alone with no CBD or other cannabinoids or terpenes).[50]

One six-week clinical trial of fifteen Alzheimer's patients with dronabinol decreased the severity of altered behavior and increased body weight in AD patients who previously refused to eat, the researchers wrote, and two pilot

49 Ibid.
50 Ibid.

studies with dronabinol that included eight dementia patients showed reduced nighttime agitation and behavioral disturbances with no adverse effects.[51]

In line with these observations, Aso and Ferrer wrote, using the cannabinoid receptor agonist (activator) nabilone correlated with prompt and dramatic improvements in severe agitation and aggression shown by an advanced AD patient for whom antipsychotic and anxiolytic (anxiety-reducing) medications were ineffective.[52]

Below is a summary of the main findings showing beneficial effects of cannabinoid compounds in Alzheimer's disease models. The researchers said that despite the low number of patients in the trials, and that none of the trials evaluated cognitive or neurodegenerative markers, the positive behavioral results represent limited but valuable information, especially considering that no remarkable side effects were reported.[53]

Aso and Ferrer also reported protective roles for cannabinoids and synthetic cannabinoids on the following Alzheimer's-related conditions: cannabinoids and beta-amyloid plaques outside the neuron, cannabinoids and aggregated

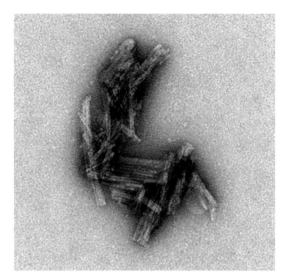

Electron micrograph of tau clusters. (Courtesy National Institutes of Allergy and Infectious Diseases)

tau filaments (neurofibrillary tangles) inside the neuron, neuroinflammation, and mitochondrial dysfunction and oxidative stress.[54]

They also cited the 2013 *Journal of Alzheimer's Disease* study by M. J. Casarejos and colleagues[55] that reported a marked reduction in neurofibrillary tangles in a mouse model of frontotemporal dementia, parkinsonism, and lower motor neuron disease after prolonged exposure to Sativex (prepared by combining cannabis extracts, one high in THC

---

51 Ibid.
52 Ibid.
53 Ibid.
54 Ibid.
55 Casarejos, M. J., J. Perucho, A. Gomez, M. P. Muñoz, M/ Fernandez-Estevez, O. Sagredo, J. Fernández-Ruiz, M. Guzman, J. G. de Yebenes, and M. A. Mena. "Natural cannabinoids improve dopamine neurotransmission and tau and amyloid pathology in a mouse model of tauopathy." *J Alzheimers Dis* 35(3):525–39 (doi: 10.3233/JAD-130050).

and the other high in CBD, with a ratio of about 1:1), and a reduction in free radicals and mitochondrial activity in a mouse model of tau protein pathology that was chronically treated with Sativex.

"In light of the polyvalent properties for the treatment of AD and the limited side effects exhibited by these compounds," Aso and Ferrer wrote, "progress toward a clinical trial to test the capacity of cannabinoids to curb this neurodegenerative disease seems to be fully justified."[56]

Positive Results in Preclinical Models of Alzheimer's Disease

At the time of the 2015 *Handbook of Experimental Pharmacology* paper[57] by Fernández-Ruiz and colleagues, many beneficial effects of cannabinoids reported in preclinical studies involved CB1 and CB2 receptors. Activating the receptors improved cognitive impairment, preserved neuronal cells, prevented beta-amyloid-induced microglia activation and generation of pro-inflammatory mediators, and removed pathological deposits in different lab and animal models of Alzheimer's.

In the case of antioxidant phytocannabinoids, Fernández-Ruiz and colleagues wrote in a 2015 *Neurotherapeutics* paper, cannabinoids may exert more specific effects on AD pathogenesis, for example preventing beta-amyloid aggregation and, by doing so, hindering plaque formation and reducing the density of plaques affecting axons and dendrites. Antioxidant phytocannabinoids also inhibit beta-amyloid-induced tau protein tangling.[58] Amyloid plaques (also called senile plaques) are microscopic masses of fragmented, decaying nerve terminals surrounding an amyloid core.[59]

Despite positive results with cannabinoids in preclinical models of Alzheimer's disease, "the clinical development of cannabinoids for patients with AD is still very poor and will be a complicated task given that these preclinical models only partially reproduce the disease."[60]

The few clinical studies conducted so far have concentrated on specific symptoms like dementia-induced appetite loss, but studies have not investigated disease-modifying effects, the researchers said, noting that Sativex, used with multiple sclerosis patients and others, should be investigated at the clinical level. Based on the activity of Sativex, Fernández-Ruiz and colleagues wrote, its CBD and THC components at complementary targets

---

56 Aso, E., and I. Ferrer.
57 Fernández-Ruiz, J., J. Romero, and J. A. Ramos.
58 Fernández-Ruiz, J., M. A. Moro, and J. Martinez-Orgado.
59 *Journal of Alzheimer's and Dementia.*
60 Fernández-Ruiz, J., M. A. Moro, and J. Martinez-Orgado.

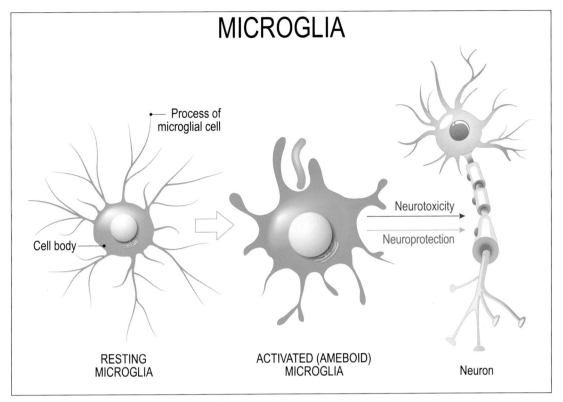

MICROGLIA

Process of microglial cell

Cell body

Neurotoxicity

Neuroprotection

RESTING MICROGLIA

ACTIVATED (AMEBOID) MICROGLIA

Neuron

Microglial activation (From iStock by ttsz)

(CB1, CB2, and other receptors), identified as neuroprotective in Alzheimer's disease, "could become a promising novel disease-modifying therapy for patients with AD, as has been recently demonstrated in a mouse model of the AD-related disorder, frontotemporal dementia."[61]

THC Removes Beta-Amyloid and other Clumping Proteins

In a 2016 *npj Aging and Mechanisms of Disease* paper, A. Currais and colleagues showed in a preclinical study that cannabinoids like THC help remove beta-amyloid and other aggregating (clumping) proteins from inside neurons.[62] This finding was important because beta-amyloid and other misfolded proteins in the brain increase with age and often are found

---

61 Ibid.

62 Currais, A., O. Quehenberger, A. M. Armando, D. Daugherty, P. Maher, and D. Schubert. "Amyloid proteotoxicity initiates an inflammatory response blocked by cannabinoids." *npj Aging Mech Dis* 2:16012 (doi: 10.1038/npjamd.2016.12).

inside neurons, and nerve-cell death from accumulating, clumping amyloid-like proteins is common in most age-dependent neurodegenerative diseases.

The accumulation of intracellular beta-amyloid is an early event in Alzheimer's disease, and in people and rodents beta-amyloid accumulation is seen inside the cell well before it's seen outside the cell. Currais and colleagues said central nervous system (CNS) inflammation also increases with age and in disease. Because Alzheimer's is associated with neuron dysfunction, the researchers hypothesized that proteotoxicity (cell function impairment caused by misfolding proteins) in nerve cells themselves may initiate an inflammatory response that can lead directly to their deaths and contribute to overall CNS inflammation.[63]

The researchers used a human CNS nerve-cell line that expresses beta-amyloid to show, among other things, that there's a complex and inflammatory response inside nerve cells caused by the accumulation of intracellular beta-amyloid, and that this early form of cell-function impairment can be blocked by activating cannabinoid receptors. If the result were to hold up eventually in human testing, Currais and colleagues

wrote, it could mean that endocannabinoids and cannabinoid receptor activation may help slow or halt Alzheimer's and other neurodegenerative diseases in their early stages.[64]

Advances in Evaluating CBD for Alzheimer's Treatment

In a 2017 *Frontiers in Pharmacology* paper,[65] G. Watt and T. Karl reviewed the broad utility of CBD and CBD/THC for the disease mechanisms and the neurodegenerative cascade that results in Alzheimer's disease. They also discussed recent advances in evaluating therapeutic CBD properties in AD rodent models.

CBD has been found in vitro (test tube, culture dish) to be neuroprotective, to prevent neurodegeneration in the brain's hippocampus (center of emotion, memory and the autonomic nervous system) and cortex (outer layer of the cerebrum—folded gray matter with an important role in consciousness), to fight inflammation and oxidative stress, to reduce the tau protein hyperphosphorylation (a signaling mechanism the cell uses to regulate a kind of cell division called mitosis) that creates tangles, and to regulate microglial cell migration,[66] which is essential for many pathophysiological

---

63 Ibid.
64 Ibid.
65 Watt, G., and T. Karl. "In vivo evidence for therapeutic properties of cannabidiol (CBD) for Alzheimer's disease." *Front Pharmacol* 8:20 (doi: 10.3389/fphar.2017.00020).
66 Ibid.

processes, including immune defense and wound healing.[67]

Watt and Karl summarized the status of in vivo effects of CBD in two animal models of Alzheimer's disease—pharmacological and transgenic. One model is created using drugs and the other by injecting human genes into the mouse genome. For pharmacological models of AD in mice, the researchers said several studies have reported the effects of CBD as anti-inflammatory and neuroprotective. The in vivo anti-inflammatory effects of CBD were confirmed in a mouse model of AD.[68]

In one study, the results implied that CBD is able to reduce beta-amyloid-induced reactive gliosis (a reactive change of glial cells in response to central nervous system damage). Glial cells include astrocytes, microglia, and others.[69] Reactive gliosis and scar formation after brain injury can interfere with the recovery process.[70] Another study of AD-related neuroinflammation in adult male rats showed, among other things, that CBD could restore certain pyramidal neurons nearly to the integrity of those in control rats.[71]

Pyramidal neurons are excitatory cells found in the cerebral cortex, hippocampus, amygdala, and elsewhere in the brain.[72] In the hippocampus, pyramidal cells process sensory and motor cues to form a cognitive map that encodes spatial, contextual, and emotional information, and the cells transmit this throughout the brain.[73]

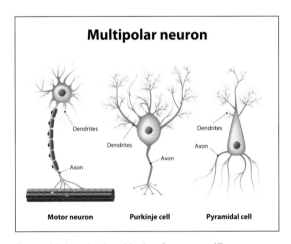

Pyramidal and other kinds of neurons (From Shutterstock by Designua)

---

67 Network Glia (Berlin), http://www.networkglia.eu/en/microglia. Accessed 8/24/18.

68 Watt, G., and T. Karl.

69 Ibid.

70 Andersson, H. C., M. F. Anderson, M. J. Porritt, C. Nodin, F. Blomstrand, and M. Nilsson. "Trauma-induced reactive gliosis is reduced after treatment with octanol and carbenoxolone." *Neurol Res* 33(6):614–24 (doi: 10.1179/1743132810Y.0000000020).

71 Watt, G., and T. Karl.

72 Ibid.

73 Graves, A. R., S. J. Moore, E. B. Bloss, B. D. Mensh, W. L. Kath, and N. Spruston. "Hippocampal pyramidal neurons comprise two distinct cell types that are countermodulated by metabotropic receptors." *Neuron* 76(4):776–789 (doi:10.1016/j.neuron.2012.09.036).

Also in the study, CBD reduced gliosis and repaired neurogenesis (when neural stem cells produce new neurons) in the dentate gyrus,[74] which is part of the hippocampus and helps form new memories, among other things.

Watt and Karl said one study to date in a pharmacological AD model has investigated CBD effects on cognition, and CBD treatment reversed cognitive deficits in beta-amyloid-treated mice. With AD transgenic mice, studies were conducted in the Watt and Karl labs to examine chronic CBD treatment's curative and preventive potential. For the curative study, adult male transgenic mice were treated for three weeks with CBD after the onset of cognitive deficits and AD pathology. CBD treatment reversed cognitive deficits in object recognition memory and social recognition memory.[75]

"This suggests," Watt and Karl wrote, "that when CBD and THC are combined there may be either a summative effect or an interaction effect between the compounds which potentiates their therapeutic-like effects." The studies in their paper "provide 'proof of principle' that CBD and possibly CBD-THC combinations are valid candidates for novel Alzheimer's disease therapies."[76]

In a 2013 *Annual Review of Psychology* paper,[77] Mechoulam and Parker wrote that the action of the endocannabinoid system may work to protect memory decline in aging. They noted, "Mice lacking CB1 receptors showed accelerated age-dependent deficits in spatial learning [and] a loss of principal neurons in the hippocampus, which was accomplished by neuroinflammation."

"These exciting findings suggest that CB1 receptors on hippocampal GABAergic neurons [gamma-aminobutyric acid is one of the central nervous system's inhibitory neurotransmitters] protect against age-dependent cognitive declines," Mechoulam and Parker added.[78]

They also noted that "interesting recent work suggests that cannabidiol [CBD] reduces [harmful] microglial activity after beta-amyloid administration in mice and prevents subsequent spatial learning impairment, suggesting that this nonintoxicating compound in marijuana may be useful in treating Alzheimer's disease."[79]

---

74 Watt, G., and T. Karl.

75 Ibid.

76 Ibid.

77 Mechoulam, R., and L. A. Parker.

78 Ibid.

79 Ibid.

Clinical Trials: Cannabinoids and Alzheimer's Disease

Safety and Efficacy of Nabilone in Alzheimer's Disease

An ongoing phase 2 and phase 3 pilot trial studied synthetic THC's safety and efficacy in Alzheimer's disease. Participating were forty adults in moderate-to-severe disease stages. The study start date was January 2015 and the estimated completion date was March 2019. The objective was to provide pilot data on whether the THC analogue nabilone is a pharmacological option for managing agitation, and to gather double-blind information on tolerability and safety. Study details are available at clinicaltrials.gov/ct2/show/NCT02351882.

Trial of Dronabinol Adjunctive Treatment of Agitation in Alzheimer's Disease

A phase 2 clinical study of Alzheimer's disease for 160 older adults was a pilot trial of dronabinol (synthetic THC) to be used with a primary agitation treatment in Alzheimer's. The start date was March 2017 and the estimated completion date is December 2020. The investigators wrote that this pilot trial could open the door to repurposing dronabinol (Marinol) as a novel, safe treatment for Alzheimer's agitation, with significant public health impact. Study details are available at clinicaltrials.gov/ct2/show/NCT02792257.

The Effect of Cannabis on Dementia Related Agitation and Aggression

Sixty adults aged sixty and older will participate in this study of agitated behavior in dementia, some receiving placebo and others receiving study medication (cannabis oil 20:1 CBD:THC). Medical cannabis patients have reported that cannabis aids in pain relief, increased appetite, and a sense of calm. Elderly patients suffering from dementia who experience this syndrome could benefit from other quality-of-life aspects of cannabis treatment like reduced medication, weight gain and sleep improvement. The study began in December 2017 and the estimated completion date is May 2020. Study details are available at clinicaltrials.gov/ct2/show/NCT03328676.

Cannabinoids and Parkinson's and Huntington's Diseases

Parkinson's disease (PD) is a progressive neurodegenerative disease, the second most common disorder of this kind after Alzheimer's. PD is associated with the gradual loss of dopamine-producing neurons in the midbrain and the accumulation of intracellular Lewy bodies—clumps of protein that arise inside neurons and contribute to Parkinson's and other dementias.[80]

Parkinson's Disease

Parkinson's disease progresses slowly with the deaths of small clusters of dopamine-producing neurons in the midbrain, creating a gradual loss of dopamine, a

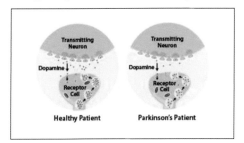

Parkinson's patients have less dopamine in their brains than healthy people do. (Courtesy NIH National Institute of Environmental Health Sciences)

critical neurotransmitter that transmits messages to parts of the brain that coordinate muscle movement. Studies have shown that Parkinson's symptoms usually appear when 50 percent or more of the dopamine neurons in midbrain are lost. Symptoms begin gradually and typically worsen over time, according to the Parkinson's disease page of the National Institutes of Health National Institute of Environmental Health Sciences.[81]

According to the Parkinson's Foundation, more than 10 million people worldwide live with PD, and nearly a million Americans will have the disease by 2020.

Common Parkinson's motor (movement) symptoms include tremors of shaking in hands, arms, legs, jaw, and face; stiffness of limbs and trunk; slow movement; and difficulties with balance, speech, and coordination. Non-motor symptoms that may develop years before movement problems begin may include poor sense of smell, constipation, depression, cognitive impairment, and fatigue.[82]

In the disease, according to the National Institutes of Health National Institute on Aging,[83] nerve cells are

---

80 Catlow, B., and J. Sanchez-Ramos. "Cannabinoids for the treatment of movement disorders." *Curr Treat Options Neurol* 17:39 (doi: 10.1007/s11940-015-0370-5).

81 National Institute of Environmental Health Sciences (National Institutes of Health) Parkinson's disease, https://www.niehs.nih.gov/health/topics/conditions/parkinson/index.cfm. Accessed 8/27/18.

82 Ibid.

83 National Institute on Aging (National Institutes of Health) Parkinson's disease. https://www.nia.nih.gov/health/parkinsons-disease. Accessed 8/26/2018.

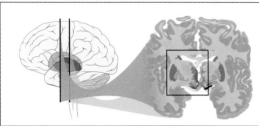

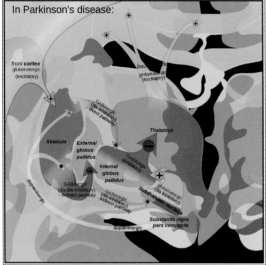

In Parkinson's disease:

Showing circuits of the basal ganglia in Parkinson's disease: Picture shows 2 coronal slices that have been superimposed to include the basal ganglia. Green arrows refer to excitatory glutamatergic pathways, red arrows to inhibitory GABAergic pathways, and turquoise arrows to dopaminergic pathways that are excitatory on the direct pathway and inhibitory on the indirect pathway. (From Wikimedia Commons by Mikael Häggström, based on an image by Andrew Gillies/User:Anaru. This file is licensed under the Creative Commons Attribution-Share Alike 3.0 Unported license.)

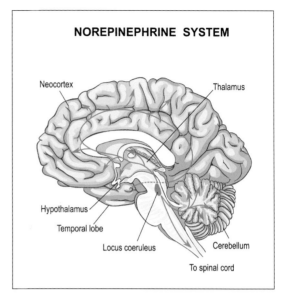

Norepinephrine system deficiency has been associated with Parkinson's disease postural instability and gait disorder, and with depression, apathy, attention problems, and sleep disturbance. (From Shutterstock by Vasilisa Tsoy)

damaged or die in part of the brain called the basal ganglia that's responsible for motor control, executive function, and behavior, among other things. Neurons produce the neurotransmitter dopamine, and when the cells are damaged or die they produce less dopamine, causing the movement problems of Parkinson's.

But, according to A. J. Espay and colleagues, growing evidence supports an earlier deficiency of norepinephrine caused by the degeneration of neurons of the locus coeruleus and sympathetic ganglia. This results in "some of the motor, behavioral, cognitive, and auto-nomic impairments that are directly or indirectly associated with the marked deficiency of norepinephrine in the brain and elsewhere."[84]

Huntington's Disease

Huntington's disease (HD) is a fatal genetic disorder that causes the progressive breakdown of nerve cells in the brain. It deteriorates a person's physical and mental abilities during their prime working years and has no cure. Every child of a parent with HD has a 50/50 chance of carrying the faulty gene, and today about 30,000 Americans have symptoms and

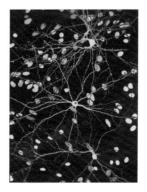

A montage of three images of single striatal neurons transfected with a disease-associated version of huntingtin, the protein that causes Huntington's disease. (From Wikimedia Commons by Dr. Steven Finkbeiner, Gladstone Institute of Neurological Disease, Taube-Koret Center for Huntington's Disease Research, and the University of California-San Francisco. This file is licensed under the Creative Commons Attribution 3.0 Unported license.)

more than 200,000 are at risk of inheriting the disease, according to the Huntington's Disease Society of America.[85]

HD symptoms include personality changes, mood swings, and depression; forgetfulness and impaired judgment; unsteady gait and involuntary movements called chorea (from the Latin word for dance); and slurred speech, difficulty swallowing, and significant weight loss. Symptoms usually appear between ages thirty to fifty, and worsen over ten to twenty-five years. Ultimately, a weakened HD patient dies of pneumonia, heart failure, or other complications.[86]

Huntington's disease is caused by changes (mutations) in the HTT gene, which carries instructions for making a protein called huntingtin, according to the NIH National Library of Medicine's Genetics Home Reference website.[87]

The exact function of huntingtin isn't yet known, but it seems to have an important role in neurons, and it's essential for normal development before birth. Huntingtin is in many body tissues but its highest activity levels are in the brain. Inside cells, the protein may be involved in chemical signaling, transporting materials, binding to proteins and other

84 Espay, A. J., P. A. LeWitt, and H. Kaufmann. "Norepinephrine deficiency in Parkinson's disease: The case for noradrenergic enhancement." *Mov Disord* 29(14) (doi: 10.1002/mds.26048).

85 Huntington's Disease Society of America, http://hdsa.org/what-is-hd/. Accessed 8/27/18.

86 Ibid.

87 National Institutes of Health, National Library of Medicine Genetics Home Reference, https://ghr.nlm.nih.gov/gene/HTT. Accessed 8/27/18.

structures, and protecting the cell from apoptosis (programmed self-destruction). One region of the HTT gene has a DNA segment called a CAG trinucleotide repeat (nucleotides form the basic structure of nucleic acids like DNA), meaning it's made up of a series of three DNA building blocks (cytosine, adenine, and guanine) that appear multiple times in a row.[88]

Normally, the CAG segment is repeated ten to thirty-five times in the gene. The inherited mutation that causes Huntington's disease is called a CAG trinucleotide repeat expansion, and this mutation increases the size of the CAG

segment in the HTT gene. People with Huntington's usually have 36 to more than 120 CAG repeats. People with 36 to 39 CAG repeats may or may not develop the signs and symptoms of Huntington's disease. Those who have 40 or more repeats almost always develop the disorder.[89]

The expanded CAG segment helps produce an abnormally long version of the huntingtin protein, and this is cut into smaller toxic fragments that bind together and accumulate in neurons, disrupting the cells' normal functions.[90]

This process especially affects brain regions (striatum and cerebral cortex) that help coordinate movement and control thinking and emotions. The dysfunction and eventual death of neurons in these brain areas underlie the signs and symptoms of Huntington's. Everyone has the gene that causes HD, but only those who inherit the gene expansion will develop HD and perhaps pass it on to their children. Every person who inherits the expanded HD gene eventually will develop the disease.[91]

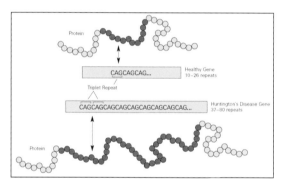

Graphic showing excessive repetitions of the cytosine-adenine-guanine (CAG) nucleotide sequence in a gene from a Huntington's disease patient (bottom) compared to a gene from a person without the neurodegenerative disorder (top). (Courtesy NIH National Institute of General Medical Sciences)

88 Ibid.
89 Ibid.
90 Ibid.
91 Ibid.

Cannabinoids for Both Diseases

In a 2015 *Current Treatment Options in Neurology* paper,[92] B. Catlow and J. Sanchez-Ramos reviewed the rationale for using cannabinoid drugs to treat a range of movement disorders. The CB1 receptor is heavily distributed in the basal ganglia of rodent and human brains, and Parkinson's and Huntington's diseases both are considered disorders of the basal ganglia.

The basal ganglia is a set of interconnected deep gray structures in the brain (substantia nigra, subthalamic nucleus, putamen, caudate, globus pallidus) responsible for the automatic execution of learned motor behaviors. Dysfunction among the components, or disruption of neural circuitry in the basal ganglia, leads to diseases characterized by involuntary movements, or difficulty starting or halting movement.[93]

Parkinson's is a prototype of a basal ganglia disorder, characterized clinically by slow movement, rigid muscles, tremors, and loss of balance. Huntington's disease is another example, a hereditary (genetic) neurodegenerative disease known for its involuntary movements. In both diseases, the endocannabinoid system changes as the diseases progress.[94]

Early presymptomatic phases in both disorders are associated with downregulating CB1 receptors, Catlow and Sanchez-Ramos wrote. And because activating CB1 receptors inhibits release of the excitatory neurotransmitter glutamate, CB1 downregulation, seen in both disorders, leads to higher glutamate levels and excitotoxicity, so decreased expression of CB1 receptors likely has an important role in disease progression. In intermediate and advanced disease stages, when neurons are dying, CB1 changes are characterized by opposite changes in both disorders.[95]

In the case of Huntington's, CB1 receptor loss is associated with the death of striatal neurons (the striatum is a critical part of the motor and reward system) that express those receptors. These changes correlate with the choreic (involuntary twitching) movements typical of HD. In HD patients, this loss of CB1 receptors has been documented by in vivo (in the body) imaging of CB1-related activity. But in Parkinson's there is significant upregulation of CB1 receptors, consistent with the bradykinetic (slowed ability to start and keep moving) feature of the disease.[96]

---

92 Catlow, B., and J. Sanchez-Ramos. "Cannabinoids for the treatment of movement disorders." *Curr Treat Options Neurol* 17:39 (doi: 10.1007/s11940-015-0370-5).

93 Ibid.

94 Ibid.

95 Ibid.

96 Ibid.

CB2 receptors, typically abundant in the immune tissues outside the central nervous system, in what's called the periphery, have been found in a few neuronal subpopulations, Catlow and Sanchez-Ramos wrote, but most of the brain's CB2 receptors are expressed in glial cells. Because activated astrocytes and microglia in HD and PD are associated with upregulatory CB2 receptor responses, these receptors are a potential target for cannabinoid agents to confer neuroprotection by reducing microglia-dependent toxic influences and promoting beneficial effects of activated astrocytes.[97]

"Both CB1 and CB2 receptors and other elements of the endogenous cannabinoid signaling system provide attractive targets for novel pharmacotherapies useful in PD and HD and other basal ganglia disorders," the researchers wrote. "Patients may benefit from symptom-alleviating actions of cannabinoid medications but perhaps more importantly cannabinoids can serve as neuroprotective agents to mitigate progression of disease."[98]

Clinical Trials: Cannabinoids and Huntington's Disease

Neuroprotection by Cannabinoids in Huntington's Disease

In a 2016 *Journal of Neurology* paper, López-Sendón Moreno and colleagues reported on the results of their 2011 double-blind, randomized, crossover, placebo-controlled pilot trial with Sativex in Huntington's disease.[99] The trial was based on the endocannabinoid system's involvement in the pathogenesis of HD mouse models and therapeutic effects in HD of stimulating specific ECS targets. The main objective was safety, assessed by the absence of more severe adverse events, and no greater deterioration of motor, cognitive, behavioral or functional scales during active treatment. During the twelve-week trial, Sativex was shown to be safe and well tolerated in HD patients, but the researchers found no clinical improvement or worsening for any motor, cognitive or psychiatric measures. Study details are available at clinicaltrials.gov/ct2/show/NCT01502046.

---

97 Ibid.
98 Ibid.
99 López-Sendón Moreno, J. L., J. García-Caldentey, P. Trigo-Cubillo, C. Ruiz-Romero, G. García-Ribas, M. A. Alonso-Arias, M. J. García de Yébenes, R. M. Tolón, I. Galve-Roperh, O. Sagredo, S. Valdeolivas, E. Resel, S. Ortega-Gutierrez, M. L. García-Bermejo, J. Fernández-Ruiz, M. Guzmán, J. García de Yébenes, J. Prous. "A double-blind randomized, cross-over, placebo-controlled, pilot trial with Sativex in Huntington's disease." *J Neurol* 263(7):1390–400 (doi: 10.1007/s00415-016-8145-9).

The Complex Reality of Neurodegenerative Disease Treatment

In an October 2017 interview, Dr. Javier Fernández-Ruiz, head of the Department of Biochemistry and Molecular Biology (Faculty of Medicine) at Complutense University of Madrid in Spain, discussed the complex reality of using cannabinoids in Huntington's disease, or any degenerative disease that progresses in stages.

In the 2011 clinical trial in Madrid described above, Fernández-Ruiz said researchers, he among them, used Sativex in a twelve-week double-blind, randomized, crossover, placebo-controlled pilot trial of twenty-four patients with HD. At the end of the trial, the researchers reported no differences in motor, cognitive, behavioral or functional scores during Sativex treatment compared to placebo, and no significant molecular effects. To be effective, Fernández-Ruiz explained, the Sativex 1:1 THC/CBD combination would need to be varied along the disease progression for each different neurodegenerative disorder.

"Using THC is good in the first stage of Huntington's but it's not very good when the disease progresses because CB1 receptors [where THC binds] are lost early in the disease," he said. "If you're trying to activate CB1 receptors with THC later in the disease progression, you have no target for controlling the disease, so it may be better to increase the CBD [which protects against HD neuroinflammation and

excitotoxicity] in Sativex as soon as the disease progresses to advanced stages."

Working in the Right Direction

By the time Parkinson's is diagnosed, Dr. Fernández-Ruiz said, when a patient shows the first symptoms—slow walking, tremor when resting, postural instability—"these are related to great damage already produced in the brain. So when these symptoms are visible they facilitate the clinical diagnosis, but the disease started probably ten years before, remaining silent and not being visible."

He added, "This is really a problem because if you try to develop treatments, if they are initiated at the clinical diagnosis, they will not be enough to arrest the disease, to limit the progression of the disease. [Treatments] need to be initiated during the silent period. By contrast, when the disease is diagnosed, what we need are ways to repair the tissue that was damaged, to replace the neurons that were lost in the prodromal [period between initial symptoms and the disease's full development] phase of the disease."

Happily, he said, "the cannabinoid system can stimulate neurogenesis, the production of new neurons, the production of new glial cells, and this is important. We need not only neuroprotection, we need also neurorepair, neuroreplacement—so neuroprotective and neurorepair medicines to control the disorder.

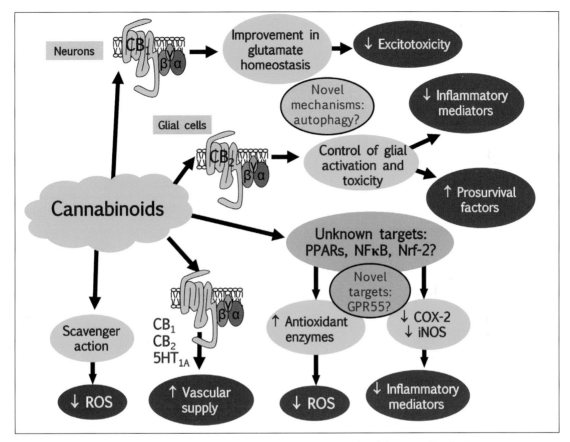

Cannabinoids that are being explored for treating neurodegeneration (Courtesy Dr. Javier Fernández-Ruiz)

Cannabinoids are an opportunity because they have this kind of broad-spectrum profile, so they can work against all the different events that kill neurons and they can restore those neurons lost in the silent phase of the disease." Fernández-Ruiz said his research team is working in that direction.

"We work with Parkinson's disease, we work with mouse models, basically we work with neurotoxin-based or transgenic models, and also for Huntington's chorea, for amyotrophic lateral sclerosis, for ataxias, etcetera. This is our area of work."

The work includes testing cannabinoid components for the effects they produce in the diseases and attempting to understand the progression of each specific disease.

"In Parkinson's, for example, in one animal model, the endocannabinoid system is altered along the progression of the disease. What happens when we are in the asymptomatic period or in early phases of the disease with mild symptoms? What happens in the middle of the disease, and what is happening when the disease is in advanced stages? The disease progresses significantly," Fernández-Ruiz added, "so change in this moment can be different compared with changes in the initial stages. It's important to follow this because we need to align pharmacological treatment to the specific moment of the disease."

An Area of Active Research

Parkinson's has been an area of active research because of the density of cannabinoid receptors in basal ganglia, but therapeutic results have been mixed, Dr. Ethan Russo wrote in a 2018 paper about cannabinoids and neurology.[100]

In a 2004 study, an oral THC:CBD extract showed no significant benefits on dyskinesia (movement that is uncontrolled and involuntary) or other signs in seventeen patients, but in other studies CBD was helpful in five Parkinson's patients with psychosis, in twenty-one patients with more general symptoms, and on REM sleep disorder in four patients, Russo wrote.[101]

An observational study showed that twenty-two of twenty-eight patients tolerated smoked cannabis, presumably THC-predominant, and showed acute benefits for tremor, rigidity, and bradykinesia (slow movement). Five of nine patients using cannabis reported great improvement, particularly on mood and sleep. And a carefully crafted survey of 339 Czech patients using oral (raw) cannabis leaves reported significant effects on multiple symptoms, particularly patients who used the treatment for three or more months, with improvement in general function, resting tremor, bradykinesia, and rigidity with few side effects, suggesting that THCA may have an important role to play in treatment of Parkinson's.[102]

"Whereas PD is commonly attributed to cell loss in the substantia nigra, with chronicity [long duration] widespread pathology is the norm," Russo wrote.[103]

"In common with Alzheimer disease," he added, "tau proteins that regulate microtubule assembly, cytoskeletal integrity [filaments and tubules give cells shape], and axonal transport in neurons develop neurofibrillary tangles. Interestingly, nabiximols [Sativex] reduced such tangles in [mouse models of PD], with improvement in dopamine metabolism, glial function, oxidative stress, anxiety, and self-injury."[104]

---

100 Russo, E. B. "Cannabis therapeutics and the future of neurology."
101 Ibid.
102 Ibid.
103 Ibid.
104 Ibid.

A Thousand Years to Progress

The medical use of cannabinoids has a long history, but cannabis's prohibition is a major barrier to studying them in a systematic way, including as treatments for symptoms of Parkinson's and other movement disorders, according to researchers Catlow and Sanchez-Ramos in their 2015 *Current Treatment Options in Neurology* paper.[105]

"The first description of cannabis to specifically treat muscle spasms was in the writings of Al-Kindi [an Islamic philosopher] in the 9th century AD. Almost 1,000 years later, cannabis extracts were used to increase survival from tetanus in India, and the use of cannabis preparations as muscle relaxants and antispasmodics became prevalent in Britain and North America."[106]

A British physician brought a supply of cannabis herbal material (in the form of "Squire's Extract," a tincture [a concentrated liquid form of herbs] of Indian hemp) from Calcutta, India, to England. The physician also gave it to other practitioners in the British Isles.[107]

"The use of tincture of Indian hemp to treat the tremor of Parkinson's disease was first described by Sir William Gowers in his landmark textbook of neurology published in the late 19th century.

'In one case tremor had commenced in the right arm and leg an hour after a railway accident and extended, three months later, into the left arm,' Gowers wrote. 'Two years subsequently there was a constant lateral movement at the wrist joints, but no tremor in the fingers. A great improvement occurred on Indian hemp and, a year later, the tremor had almost ceased, being occasional only.'"[108]

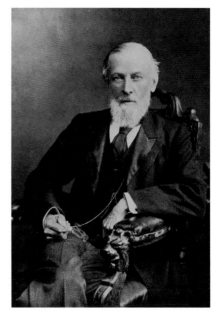

Sir William Richard Gowers, a British neurologist (1845–1915) and author of the two-volume *Manual of Diseases of the Nervous System* (1886 and 1888), in which he documented Parkinson's disease. (Photogravure after Maull & Fox, courtesy Wellcome Collection under the Creative Commons Attribution license)

---

105 Catlow, B., and J. Sanchez-Ramos.
106 Ibid.
107 Ibid.
108 Ibid.

Clinical Trials: Cannabinoids and Parkinson's Disease

A Study of Tolerability and Efficacy of Cannabidiol on Tremor in Parkinson's Disease

In this clinical trial, researchers were studying CBD tolerability and effectiveness on tremor in Parkinson's disease. About sixty adults participated. The study began in October 2016 and the estimated completion date was June 2019. The investigators hypothesized that CBD would be well tolerated and would reduce tremor, anxiety, and psychosis, and would stabilize cognitive decline in PD. Study results and details are available at clinicaltrials.gov/ct2/show/record/NCT02818777.

A Study of Tolerability and Efficacy of CBD on Motor Symptoms in Parkinson's Disease

A clinical trial was developed to assess the effectiveness of CBD on PD motor symptoms, and to study the safety and tolerability of CBD and other effectiveness, particularly for tremor in PD. The start date was August 2018 and the estimated completion date was June 2019. This is a 1:1 parallel, double-blind, randomized controlled trial with sixty adult participants. Study results and details are available at clinicaltrials.gov/ct2/show/NCT03582137.

Cannabis Oil for Pain in Parkinson's Disease

A phase 2, randomized, open-label, double-blind, two-center study seeks to evaluate the tolerability, safety, and dose finding of an oil cannabis preparation for pain in Parkinson's disease. The study recruited fifteen adults with Parkinson's disease and pain but without cognitive impairment. The start date was December 2018 and the estimated completion date is July 2020. Study details are available at clinicaltrials.gov/ct2/show/NCT03639064.

Cannabinoids and Amyotrophic Lateral Sclerosis

Amyotrophic lateral sclerosis (ALS) is part of a group of rare neurological diseases that mainly involve nerve cells (neurons) that control voluntary muscle movements like chewing, walking, and talking. ALS is progressive, so symptoms quickly get worse over time, and so far there's no cure or effective treatment to halt or reverse disease progression, according to the ALS website[109] at the National Institute of Neurological Disorders and Stroke, part of the National Institutes of Health.

ALS belongs to a group of disorders called motor neuron diseases, caused by gradual deterioration and death of motor neurons, Aymerich and colleagues wrote in a 2018 *Biochemical Pharmacology* review paper.[110] These nerve cells—extending from the brain to the spinal cord and to muscles throughout the body—initiate and act as communication links between the brain and voluntary muscles.

Messages from motor neurons in the brain (upper motor neurons) are transmitted to motor neurons in the spinal cord and motor nuclei (lower motor neurons) and from the spinal cord and motor nuclei of the brain to a particular muscle or muscles.[111] A characteristic feature of ALS disease development is the extreme vulnerability of the axonal transport of proteins or cell organelles because motor neurons have short dendrites and long axons.[112]

In ALS, upper and lower motor neurons degenerate or die and stop sending messages to muscles, which gradually weaken, start to twitch, and waste away (atrophy). Eventually, the brain loses the ability to initiate and control voluntary movements. Early symptoms include muscle weakness or stiffness. Gradually, all muscles under voluntary control are affected and ALS patients lose strength

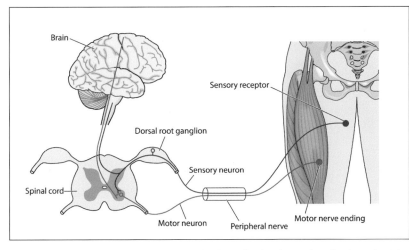

Control of muscle showing nerve paths from brain through spinal cord and peripheral nerves (From Shutterstock by Blamb)

109 National Institutes of Health, National Institute of Neurological Disorders and Stroke, ALS, https://www.ninds.nih.gov/Disorders/Patient-Caregiver-Education/Fact-Sheets/Amyotrophic-Lateral-Sclerosis-ALS-Fact-Sheet. Accessed 9/1/18.
110 Aymerich, M. S., E. Aso, M. A. Abellanas, R. M. Tolon, J. A. Ramos, I. Ferrer, J. Romero, and J. Fernández-Ruiz.
111 National Institutes of Health, National Institute of Neurological Disorders and Stroke, ALS.
112 Aymerich, M. S., E. Aso, M. A. Abellanas, R. M. Tolon, J. A. Ramos, I. Ferrer, J. Romero, and J. Fernández-Ruiz.

and the ability to speak, eat, move, and even breathe, the researchers wrote. Most ALS patients die from respiratory failure within three to five years from the time symptoms appear, but about 10 percent live for ten or more years. Most ALS cases occur seemingly at random and 5 percent to 10 percent are familial,[113] but familial and sporadic forms of ALS are indistinguishable, sharing pathogenic events and therapeutic intervention.[114]

Aymerich and colleagues said solid evidence from studies describing changes in specific elements of the endocannabinoid system in the spinal cord, brainstem, and motor cortex—the central nervous system areas more affected in patients with ALS and in ALS animal models—have "placed cannabinoids as a possible and potential disease-modifying therapy in ALS."[115]

In ALS, the endocannabinoid system is affected in specific ways. For one thing, the researchers wrote, the endocannabinoid 2-AG is elevated in the spinal cords of the classic ALS mouse model based on a mutation in the SOD-1 gene (discovered in 1993), and this "was interpreted as an endogenous protective response, fueling the idea that inhibiting endocannabinoid inactivating enzymes [and therefore

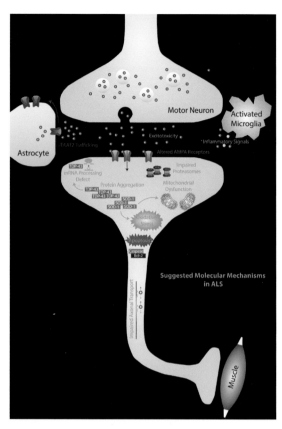

Suggested molecular mechanisms in amyotrophic lateral sclerosis at the synapse (From Wikimedia Commons by User:Rcchang16. This file is licensed under the Creative Commons Attribution-Share Alike 4.0 International license.)

increasing 2-AG levels] may be neuroprotective in ALS." Also in ALS, CB2 receptors were upregulated (activated), mainly in astrocytes, in ALS mouse models, in dogs with degenerative myelopathy

---

113 National Institutes of Health, National Institute of Neurological Disorders and Stroke, ALS.

114 Aymerich, M. S., E. Aso, M. A. Abellanas, R. M. Tolon, J. A. Ramos, I. Ferrer, J. Romero, and J. Fernández-Ruiz.

115 Ibid.

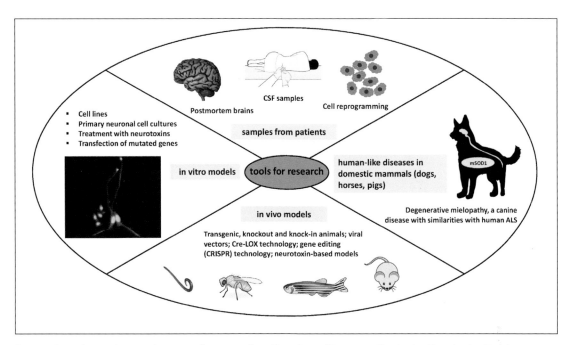

Research tools used to study neurodegenerative disorders. (Courtesy Dr. Javier Fernández-Ruiz)

(the canine version of ALS), and in ALS patients.[116]

CB2 receptor expression also was upregulated in the spinal cords and brains of transgenic ALS mice and in postmortem spinal cord samples from ALS patients.[117]

These observations suggested to the researchers that beneficial effects might come from targeting the CB2 receptor to control astrocyte support or microglial toxicity for motor neurons. Changes in the expression of CB1 receptors in animal models were inconclusive, Aymerich and colleagues wrote, and in ALS patient spinal cords CB1 receptors seemed to be reduced.[118]

Most pharmacological studies on the use of cannabinoids in experimental ALS were conducted with the classic transgenic mouse model, developed in the 1990s and used to investigate the neuroprotective effects of THC, cannabinol, and CB1 and CB2 receptor agonists (activators), in all cases with beneficial effects, the researchers said, noting that similar findings came from other genetic ALS mouse models.[119]

116 Ibid.
117 Ibid.
118 Ibid.
119 Ibid.

In recent studies involving a new transgenic mouse model that's based on a new ALS-related gene (TARBD gene), activating CB2 receptors improved motor behavior, preserved spinal motor neurons, and reduced the effect of glial reactivity. CB1 receptor activation decreased glial reactivity to a lesser extent. But clinical evidence for using cannabinoids in ALS is scarce, they wrote.[120]

The first studies were observational, based on subjective impressions of ALS patients who self-medicated with cannabis, and the results suggested a mild improvement of different symptoms. A randomized double-blind crossover trial conducted with oral Sativex showed that patients tolerated the drug well but it didn't reduce cramp frequency or intensity (details in the clinical trials section below).[121]

"No clinical studies have been attempted to investigate the potential of cannabinoids as disease-modifying therapies," Aymerich and colleagues wrote, adding, "There is an urgent need for additional clinical investigations in ALS,

and cannabinoids might represent an interesting therapeutic approach."[122]

An International DM-ALS Research Collaboration

In 2009, the *Proceedings of the National Academy of Sciences* published a research paper[123] whose topic was good news for dogs and for people with ALS. One of the researchers was Dr. Joan R. Coates, a veterinary neurologist and associate professor of veterinary medicine and surgery at the University of Missouri College of Veterinary Medicine.

"We uncovered the genetic mutation of degenerative myelopathy [DM], which has been unknown for 30 years, and linked it to ALS, a human disease that has no cure," she said in a university press release at the time. "Dogs with DM are likely to provide scientists with a more reliable animal model for ALS, [and] this discovery will pave the way for DNA tests that will aid dog breeders in avoiding DM in the future."[124]

The study was a collaborative project with Missouri researchers and Kerstin Lindblad-Toh and Claire Wade, who

---

120 Ibid.
121 Ibid.
122 Ibid.
123 Awano, T., G. S. Johnson, C. M. Wade, M. L. Katz, G. C. Johnson, J. F. Taylor, M. Perloski, T. Biagi, I. Baranowska, S. Long, P. A. March, J. Natasha, N. J. Olby, G. D. Shelton, S. Khan, D. P. O'Brien, K. Lindblad-Toh, J. R. Coates. "Genome-wide association analysis reveals a SOD1 mutation in canine degenerative myelopathy that resembles amyotrophic lateral sclerosis." *Proc Natl Acad Sci* 106(8):2794–99 (doi: 10.1073/pnas.0812297106).
124 Ibid.

are researchers at the Broad Institute of Harvard and the Massachusetts Institute of Technology. The American Kennel Club Canine Health Foundation and participating breed clubs funded the study.[125]

The researchers found that the genetic mutation responsible for DM in dogs is the same mutation that causes ALS. Because of the discovery, researchers now can use dogs with DM as animal models to help identify therapeutic interventions for treating ALS and simi-

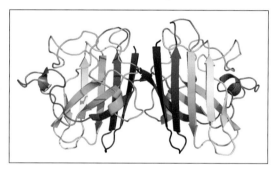

Structure of the SOD1 protein (From Wikimedia Commons by User:Emw. This file is licensed under the Creative Commons Attribution-Share Alike 3.0 Unported license.)

lar disorders.[126]

For years, ALS research has relied heavily on transgenic mice that expressed the mutant human gene called SOD1, which causes ALS. Coates and colleagues

found that dogs with DM also had SOD1 gene mutations. Lots of mouse models have high levels of SOD1 that produce pathologic processes different from those of ALS patients. Because the SOD1 mutation is spontaneous in dogs, the clinical spectrum in dogs may more accurately represent that of human ALS.[127]

DM is reported most commonly in German shepherds but also exists in Cardigan and Pembroke Welsh corgis, Rhodesian Ridgebacks, Chesapeake Bay retrievers, and boxers. There are no treatments yet for ALS or DM that clearly slow or stop disease progression.[128]

Canine Degenerative Myelopathy

M. Fernández-Trapero and colleagues, among them Coates and Fernández-Ruiz, wrote in the May 2017 *Disease Models and Mechanisms* about CB2 upregulation in reactive astrocytes (abnormal increase in astrocytes after nearby neurons are destroyed by CNS disease or trauma) in canine degenerative myelopathy.[129]

Researchers already had seen CB2-generated neuroprotection in transgenic (SOD1) ALS mice, and Fernández-Trapero and colleagues now wanted

---

125 Ibid.
126 Ibid.
127 Ibid.
128 Ibid.
129 Fernández-Trapero, M., F. Espejo-Porras, C. Rodríguez-Cueto, J. R. Coates, C. Pérez-Díaz, E. de Lago, and J. Fernández-Ruiz. "Upregulation of CB receptors in reactive astrocytes in canine degenerative myelopathy, a disease model of amyotrophic lateral sclerosis." *Dis Model Mech* 10(5):551–8 (doi: 10.1242/dmm.028373).

to know if they would see similar CB2 receptor upregulation, and changes in other endocannabinoid elements, in spinal cords of DM dogs with SOD1 mutations. The study addressed changes in specific endocannabinoid elements in canine DM, the researchers wrote, noting that the endocannabinoid system had been investigated in different regions of the canine brain.[130]

"This is the first time that these elements have been investigated in the context of an important neurodegenerative disorder occurring in dogs. The benefits of such an investigation could result in the development of cannabinoid-based therapies for human ALS, but these studies may also serve as a first step in a cannabinoid-based pharmacotherapy useful for veterinary medicine." The researchers investigated six endocannabinoid elements commonly used to develop pharmacological therapies and identified the CB receptor as a promising potential target.[131]

They noted that the study showed no loss of the CB1 receptors usually found in neurons, despite the loss of motor neurons in canine DM. This suggested to the researchers that, contrary to human neurodegenerative conditions like Huntington's disease that show a profound loss of neuronal CB1 receptors, the CB1 receptor also may be a potential target in canine DM and in human ALS.[132]

The CB2 receptor is also strongly upregulated in activated glia in response to neuronal damage in transgenic ALS mouse models and in ALS patients. The same response is seen in other acute or chronic neurodegenerative disorders, including ischemia, Alzheimer's disease, Parkinson's disease, and Huntington's disease.[133]

"These findings," Fernández-Trapero and colleagues wrote, "support the idea that the rise in cannabinoid receptors in activated glial elements is an endogenous response of endocannabinoid signaling aimed at protecting neurons against cytotoxic insults [and] restoring neuronal homeostasis and integrity."[134]

In a 2017 interview, Dr. Javier Fernández-Ruiz discussed the collaboration of his research group with Coates at the University of Missouri.

"When we work with mice, we are altering the genome of the mouse to produce a mutation that produces the disease. So we artificially produce the disease in the mouse," he explained. "But in the case of the dogs, the disease

---

130 Ibid.
131 Ibid.
132 Ibid.
133 Ibid.
134 Ibid.

Clinical Trials: Cannabinoids and ALS

Safety and Efficacy on Spasticity Symptoms of a Cannabis Sativa Extract in Motor Neuron Disease (CANALS)

In 2013, researchers from San Raffaele Scientific Institute in Milan, Italy, and collaborators began a clinical study of sixty adults, eighteen to eighty years old, with spasticity caused by motor neuron disease (including ALS). Sativex was the study drug. It was a randomized, double-blind, controlled multicenter study that was completed in 2015. The results, as mentioned above by Aymerich and colleagues, were that patients tolerated the drug well but it didn't reduce cramp frequency or intensity. Study details are available at clinicaltrials.gov/ct2/show/NCT01776970.

Efficacy of Cannabinoids in Amyotrophic Lateral Sclerosis or Motor Neurone Disease

This randomized, double-blind, placebo-controlled study will examine the results of a cannabis-based medicine extract (CannTrust CBD oil), in patients with amyotrophic lateral sclerosis or motor neurone disease. Participants (thirty adults) will be randomized to receive capsulized CBD oil or placebo. Treatment duration is six months with a one-month safety follow-up. The estimated start date was December 2018 and the estimated completion date is January 2021. Study details are available at clinicaltrials.gov/ct2/show/NCT03690791.

is spontaneous and this is very good for human research because it's like this in the human." In people, he added, "the disease appears by spontaneous mutation or by another kind of process or factor, not necessarily genetic, and this has the advantage that it is spontaneous."

Canine DM is very similar to human ALS, with similar affected genes, Fernández-Ruiz said, adding that Coates and colleagues at Missouri have a collection of tissues from dogs affected by DM,

"and they are very useful for us and for other researchers around the world. They are trying to understand what's happening in the brains of the dogs and relate it to the humans to see similar mechanisms in the progression of the disease. This is very good information. Many researchers in the world are collaborating on this, something that is very important."

Now, the Missouri University Veterinary Health Center (VHC) (vhc .missouri.edu) is seeking canine patients for enrollment in clinical trials for degenerative myelopathy-affected dogs. The trials will evaluate promising new drugs as a treatment to slow DM disease progression. Depending on the research protocol, dogs will receive a drug that represses production of the mutated SOD1 gene. The drug, which has undergone preclinical testing for safety, will be injected into spinal fluid that surrounds the spinal cord. The studies will be randomized and double-blinded; neither the investigator nor the pet owner will know whether the dog receives the drug.

Researchers will monitor clinical disease progression and evaluate cerebrospinal fluid, brain MRIs, and muscle and nerve function, techniques that have been used with ALS patients to monitor and predict disease progression.

Cannabinoids and Multiple Sclerosis

In 2010, ten European countries approved the use of GW Pharmaceuticals' cannabis-based drug Sativex to treat symptoms of multiple sclerosis. It was a first for a cannabis drug, and Di Marzo and colleagues addressed this with historical perspective in their January 2015 *Nature Reviews Neuroscience* paper.[135]

"After millennia of anecdotal use (both medicinal and recreational) of cannabis plants as described in Chinese, Indian and Arab pharmacopeias, centuries of their documented medicinal use throughout the world, and nearly five decades of research on the mechanism of action of their bioactive constituents [the phytocannabinoids], the medical use of cannabis extracts was approved in June 2010 by 10 European countries," the researchers wrote.[136]

This first cannabis-based medicine—known as nabiximols in the United States (but not approved here) and marketed as Sativex in more than thirty countries worldwide—was prepared by combining botanical extracts from two varieties of cannabis sativa plants, one producing mainly THC and the other producing mainly CBD, with a ratio of about 1:1.[137]

"Thus," Di Marzo and colleagues wrote, "despite the medicinal uses of THC for the treatment of emesis [vomiting] and cachexia [wasting] in patients with cancer undergoing chemotherapy, and for promoting appetite in patients with AIDS, cannabis extracts were finally given *bona fide* therapeutic status, after a decade of clinical trials dedicated to the testing of a combination of THC and CBD on the neurodegenerative disease multiple sclerosis."[138]

---

135 Di Marzo, V., N. Stella, A. Zimmer.
136 Ibid.
137 Ibid.
138 Ibid.

An Unpredictable Disease

Multiple sclerosis is an unpredictable disease of the central nervous system and can range from being relatively benign to somewhat disabling to devastating, as communication among the brain and other parts of the body is disrupted, according to the National Institutes of Health National Institute of Neurological Disorders and Stroke (NINDS) MS Information Page.[139] About 2.3 million people around the world have MS, the most common disabling neurological condition affecting young adults, with an average onset age of thirty years.

Many researchers think MS is an autoimmune disease in which the body, through the immune system, launches a defensive attack against its own tissues, and the NINDS page says the attacks may be linked to an environmental trigger, maybe a virus.[140]

Most MS patients first experience symptoms between the ages of twenty and forty. These can include blurred or double vision, red-green color distortion, or blindness in one eye. Most MS patients have muscle weakness in arms and legs and difficulty with coordination and balance, which can be severe enough to impair walking or standing. In the worst cases, MS can produce partial or complete paralysis.[141]

Most MS patients experience paresthesias—passing abnormal sensory feelings like numbness, prickling, or pins-and-needle sensations. Some have pain. Other complaints are speech impediments, tremors and dizziness, and sometimes hearing loss. About half of MS patients develop cognitive impairments, like problems with concentration, attention, memory, and poor judgment, but these can be mild. Depression is another common complaint.[142]

In MS, nerve insulating myelin comes under attack by plaques that affect the brain's white and gray matter, which

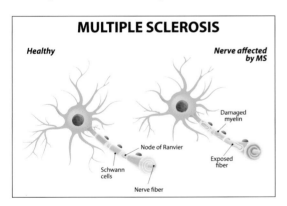

Healthy cell and nerve cell affected by multiple sclerosis (From iStock Photo by ttsz)

---

139 National Institute of Neurological Disorders and Stroke, NIH, Multiple Sclerosis Information Page, https://www.ninds.nih.gov/disorders/all-disorders/multiple-sclerosis-information-page. Accessed 9/3/18.
140 Ibid.
141 Ibid.
142 Ibid.

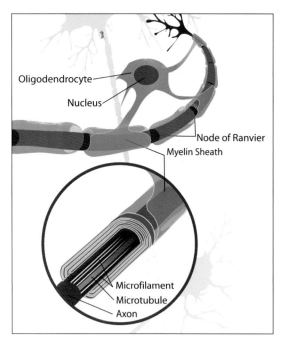

A neuron cell diagram, cropped to show an oligodendrocyte and myelin sheath (From Wikimedia Commons by User:LadyofHats, who released the work into the public domain.)

then consist of damaged myelin and oligodendrocytes (oh-lih-go-dend-roe-sites). Myelin is a mix of proteins and fatty acids that form white insulating covers, called sheaths, around nerve fibers, increasing impulse-conducting speed. Oligodendrocytes are glial cells that produce myelin in the central nervous system. Some myelin is repaired early in the disease, but later in MS there's a progressive loss of neurons, J. Rice and M. Cameron wrote in a 2018 *Current Neurology and Neuroscience Reports* paper.[143]

MS, Cannabinoids, and the American Academy of Neurology

In June 2014, conference coverage from the sixty-sixth annual meeting of the American Academy of Neurology (AAN) in Philadelphia, Pennsylvania, opened with the headline: "Medical Marijuana May Alleviate MS Symptoms." According to the report by Eric Greb, "Certain forms of medical marijuana can help treat symptoms of multiple sclerosis (MS), but they may not be helpful in treating levodopa [dopamine precursor]-induced movements in Parkinson's disease."

He wrote that the researchers didn't find enough evidence at that time to show if medical cannabis could help treat motor problems in Huntington's disease, tics in Tourette syndrome, cervical dystonia, or seizures in epilepsy. These conclusions were part of AAN's review of scientific research on the use of medical cannabis in brain diseases. The findings were published in the April 29, 2014, *Neurology Reviews*."[144]

---

143 Rice, J., and M. Cameron. "Cannabinoids for treatment of MS symptoms: State of the evidence." *Curr Neurol Neurosci Rep* 18:50 (https://doi.org/10.1007/s11910-018-0859-x).

144 *Neurology Reviews* 22(6):20–23.

Also in 2014, in March, AAN published a guideline[145] on complementary and alternative therapies, like medical cannabis, to treat MS. And in April, AAN published a systematic review[146] (1948–2013) on the efficacy and safety of medical cannabis in selected brain and nervous system disorders, like epilepsy, Parkinson's disease, MS, and Tourette syndrome.

The AAN guideline for medical cannabis and MS came to the following conclusions:

- Spasticity: Oral cannabis extract (OCE) is effective, and Sativex and THC are probably effective, for reducing patient-centered measures; it's possible oral cannabis extract and THC are effective for reducing patient-centered and objective measures at one year.

- Central pain or painful spasms (including spasticity-related pain but not neuropathic pain): OCE is effective; Sativex and THC are probably effective.

- Urinary dysfunction: Sativex is probably effective for reducing bladder voids/day; THC and OCE are probably ineffective for reducing bladder complaints.

- Tremor: THC and OCE are probably ineffective; Sativex is possibly ineffective.

- Other neurologic conditions: OCE is probably ineffective for treating levodopa-induced dyskinesias in patients with Parkinson's disease. Oral cannabinoids are of unknown efficacy in non-chorea-related symptoms of Huntington's disease, Tourette syndrome, cervical dystonia, and epilepsy. The risks and benefits of medical cannabis should be weighed carefully. Risk of serious adverse psychopathologic effects was nearly 1 percent. Comparative effectiveness of medical cannabis versus other therapies is unknown for these indications.[147]

---

145 Yadav, V., C. Bever, J. Bowen, A. Bowling, B. Weinstock-Guttman, M. Cameron, D. Bourdette, G. S. Gronseth, P. Narayanaswami. "Summary of evidence-based guideline: Complementary and alternative medicine in multiple sclerosis." *Neurology* (doi: https://doi.org/10.1212/WNL.0000000000000250).

146 Koppel, B. S., J. C. M. Brust, T. Fife, J. Bronstein, S. Youssof, G. Gronseth, D. Gloss. "Systematic review: Efficacy and safety of medical marijuana in selected neurologic disorders." *Neurology* 82(17) (doi: https://doi.org/10.1212/WNL.0000000000000363).

147 Ibid.

A Review of MS Clinical Findings

In their 2018 paper, Rice and Cameron also reported on the state of the evidence for cannabinoid treatment of MS symptoms.[148] They summarized the highest-quality evidence for cannabis use in treating MS spasticity and pain, and possible dosing regimens based on information from the studies, which included eleven randomized studies with 2,138 patients that compared cannabinoid effects with placebo on MS spasticity.

Study details varied, but most suggested that cannabinoids were associated with self-reported improvements in spasticity, even though objectively measured spasticity improvements

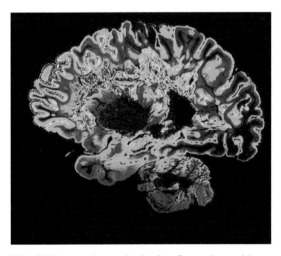

This MRI scan shows the brain of a patient with multiple sclerosis. (Courtesy the NIH Intramural Research Program)

generally didn't reach statistical significance. Overall, Rice and Cameron wrote, data supported the use of cannabinoids for reducing the severity of self-reported MS spasticity, but the study had limitations, including that it was short term and the cannabis dose varied among studies.[149]

On MS-related pain, Rice and Cameron said pain affects about two-thirds of MS patients, with headache (43 percent), neuropathic pain in arms or legs (26 percent), back pain (20 percent), painful spasms (15 percent), and trigeminal neuralgia (chronic pain affecting the nerve that carries sensation from face to brain) (3.8 percent). Central (nervous system) neuropathic pain or pain from spasms are the most common forms of pain for those with MS, the researchers wrote, and cannabinoids' role in pain relief is complex and not well understood. Some evidence suggests that CB1 receptors in brain and peripheral nerves help modulate and process pain, and cannabis also may reduce pain by reducing inflammation.[150]

A 2011 systematic review of randomized controlled trials examined studies performed before 2010 that evaluated the effects of any cannabinoid—smoked cannabis, oral extracts, nabilone (THC analogue), synthetic THC, or Sativex—on

148 Rice, J., and M. Cameron.
149 Ibid.
150 Ibid.

chronic non-cancer pain (including MS pain). In fifteen of eighteen studies, the researchers wrote, cannabinoids offered at least modest pain relief. A 2015 update by the same authors evaluated eleven more studies (2010–2014) and reported that seven of eleven studies also found cannabinoids more effective than placebo.[151]

An Early Questionnaire on MS and Cannabis Use

In the mid-1990s, Professor Roger Pertwee of the Institute of Medical Sciences at the University of Aberdeen, Scotland, was reading a newspaper when he came across an article about people with multiple sclerosis who self-medicated with cannabis.

"I eventually spoke with the writer of many of these articles, who self-medicated with cannabis herself for her MS," he said during a July 2017 interview. She was a reporter who had to give up her job because of MS but continued to write about cannabis, using a pseudonym, at a time when the plant was illegal.

Pertwee contacted her, mainly writing letters, "and eventually some colleagues and I contacted a lot of people with MS who self-medicated with cannabis in the UK or the USA. This we did both through the Alliance for Cannabis Therapeutics in the UK (ACT UK), with the help of the British reporter with MS and through Alice O'Leary of ACT USA," he said.

Pertwee and colleagues sent a lot of questions to the group of self-medicating MS patients and received many answers.

"It was clear from their answers that they all tended to have similar reasons for taking cannabis for their MS—to reduce the pain, to reduce the spasticity, and to improve sleep. And for them it appeared to work well," he said. Afterward, he and colleagues described these anecdotal claims in a 1997 *European Neurology* paper.[152] His colleagues were Drs. Paul Consroe, Whitney Tillery, and Judith Rein from the University of Arizona Health Sciences Center in Tucson, and Dr. Richard Musty of the Department of Psychology at the University of Vermont–Burlington.

In the paper, the researchers reported that fifty-three people from the United Kingdom and fifty-nine from the United States (fifty-five women, fifty-seven men) anonymously answered the thirteen-page questionnaire. From 97 percent to 30 percent of subjects reported that cannabis improved (in descending rank order)— spasticity, chronic pain of extremities, tremor, emotional dysfunction, anorexia/ weight loss, fatigue states, double vision,

---

151 Ibid.
152 Consroe, P., R. Musty, J. Rein, W. Tillery, and R. Pertwee. "The perceived effects of smoked cannabis on patients with multiple sclerosis." *Eur Neurol* 38(1):44–8.

sexual dysfunction, bowel and bladder dysfunctions, vision dimness, dysfunctions of walking and balance, and memory loss.[153]

The researchers described many study shortcomings but did say that the present study, with the content of previous reports, strongly suggested that cannabis may significantly relieve certain signs and symptoms of MS, particularly spasticity and pain, in at least some patients.[154]

"The present study also suggests that these cannabis effects occur equally across nationalities, genders and diverse clinical presentations of MS," they wrote. "We conclude from these data that there are sufficient grounds for mounting a properly controlled clinical trial that will test the most prevalent claims made about the beneficial effects of cannabis both objectively and conclusively."[155]

The paper, Pertwee said in the interview, "encouraged physicians to think about this and also I think helped to encourage someone to set up a drug company to develop a new medicine for multiple sclerosis. That company was GW Pharmaceuticals, set up by Dr. Geoffrey Guy and Dr. Brian Whittle in the late 1990s."

Pertwee said he and others testified before the Select Committee on Science and Technology of the House of Lords, which encouraged the GW effort and produced a report on cannabis in 1998 titled *Cannabis: The Scientific and Medical Evidence*. The report recommended that cannabis be looked at seriously as a source of new medicines.

Very soon, Pertwee said, "GW did develop a new medicine called Sativex, which was licensed initially in Canada in 2005 for multiple sclerosis and cancer pain, and then in the UK for multiple sclerosis."

Sativex isn't smoked, he said, "but instead sprayed into the mouth where it's absorbed. Ideally it should not all be swallowed, as you then get variable absorption from the gut, after which a lot of the drug goes straight to the liver where it gets metabolized. If you absorb it from the mouth it goes straight to the heart and from the heart to the brain and many other parts of the body, so it's a good route of administration."

Pertwee said the MS patients who self-medicated with cannabis, "were I think mainly people for whom standard medicines did not work, and so they were desperate to find something else and, for a lot of them, cannabis worked. Certainly the replies we got back to our questions from a lot of these people were very encouraging and, as I have already said, very consistent."

---

153 Ibid.
154 Ibid.
155 Ibid.

Clinical Trials: Cannabinoids, Multiple Sclerosis and Related Disorders

Neurophysiological Study of Sativex in Multiple Sclerosis Spasticity

The aim of this phase 3 randomized, double-blind, placebo-controlled crossover study was to investigate cannabinoid-induced changes in neurophysiological measures of spasticity and corticospinal excitability in forty adults with secondary or primary progressive MS. The study start date was April 2012 and the end date was November 2013. In a 2015 *Journal of Neurology* paper,[156] the investigators found the response on a scale of spasticity was significantly more frequent after Sativex than after placebo. They wrote: "Our findings confirm the clinical benefit of Sativex on MS spasticity." Study details are available at clinicaltrials.gov/ct2/show/NCT01538225.

Evaluate the Maintenance of Effect After Long-term Treatment with Sativex in Subjects with Symptoms of Spasticity Due to Multiple Sclerosis

This study was designed to evaluate how long thirty-six adults with MS spasticity maintained a beneficial effect after long-term treatment with Sativex. The study start date was November 2007 and it was completed in January 2009. In 2012 Notcutt and colleagues published their results[157] in *Multiple Sclerosis*, noting that eligible subjects with ongoing benefit from Sativex for at least twelve weeks entered the five-week placebo-controlled, parallel group, randomized withdrawal study. The main outcome was significantly in favor of Sativex, and the researchers found significant changes in two more measures in favor of Sativex. Study details are available at clinicaltrials.gov/ct2/show/NCT00702468.

A Randomized Study of Sativex on Cognitive Function and Mood: Multiple Sclerosis Patients

This safety study compared the change in cognitive performance and psychological status of 121 adults with MS spasticity when treated with Sativex or placebo, added to existing anti-spasticity therapy over fifty weeks. The start date was January 2012, end date May 2013. In 2013, Wright and colleagues

---

156 Leocani, L., A. Nuara, E. Houdayer, I. Schiavetti, U. Del Carro, S. Amadio, L. Straffi, P. Rossi, V. Martinelli, C. Vila, M. P. Sormani, and G. Comi. "Sativex(®) and clinical-neurophysiological measures of spasticity in progressive multiple sclerosis." *J Neurol* 262(11):2520–7 (doi: 10.1007/s00415-015-7878-1).

157 Notcutt, W., R. Langford, P. Davies, S. Ratcliffe, and R. Potts. "A placebo-controlled, parallel-group randomized withdrawal study of subjects with symptoms of spasticity due to multiple sclerosis who are receiving long-term Sativex® (nabiximols)." *Mult Scler* 18(2):219–28 (doi: 10.1177/1352458511419700).

published results[158] in *Multiple Sclerosis*. Antispasticity medication, taken at the same time as Sativex, included baclofen, tizanidine, benzodiazepines, and gabapentinoids; 49 percent of subjects had relapsing-remitting and 39 percent had secondary progressive MS. After twelve months, the mean change was +6.8 in both groups. Patient, physician, and caregiver global impressions of change all were significantly in favor of THC:CBD. The researchers wrote that long-term Sativex treatment wasn't associated with cognitive decline or significant mood changes. Effectiveness was maintained in long-term treatment. Study details are available at clinicaltrials.gov/ct2/show/NCT01964547.

Effects of Vaporized Marijuana on Neuropathic Pain
For this phase 1–2 study, the researchers theorized that a low dose of vaporized cannabis could alleviate nerve-injury pain. They conducted a double-blind, placebo-controlled crossover study evaluating the pain-reducing effectiveness of vaporized cannabis in thirty-nine subjects, most of whom experienced neuropathic pain despite traditional treatment. They inhaled medium-dose, low-dose, or placebo cannabis. The study began in December 2009 and ended in November 2012. In a February 2014 *Journal of Pain* paper, Wilsey and colleagues reported that cannabis has analgesic efficacy (effectively relieves pain), with the low and medium doses being about equally effective as pain relievers. The investigators concluded that "vaporized cannabis, even at low doses, may present an effective option for patients with treatment-resistant neuropathic pain." Study details are available at clinicaltrials.gov/ct2/show/NCT01037088.

Cannabinoids in the Treatment of Tics (CANNA-TICS)
This was a multicenter, randomized, double-blind, placebo-controlled, parallel-group, phase 3b trial for which ninety-six adult patients with chronic tic disorders and Tourette syndrome were recruited. The objective was to show that treatment with the cannabis extract nabiximols (Sativex, a 1:1 combination of THC and CBD) is superior to placebo in reducing tics and comorbidities in patients with Tourette syndrome and chronic tic disorders. The study start date was April 2018 and the estimated end date was May 2019. Check for study results and study details at clinicaltrials.gov/ct2/show/NCT03087201.

---

158 Wright, S., M. M. Vachova, and I. Novakova. "The effect of long-term treatment with a prescription cannabis-based THC:CBD oromucosal spray on cognitive function and mood: a 12-month double blind placebo-controlled study in people with spasticity due to multiple sclerosis." *Mult Scler* 19(11_suppl):559–73 (doi: 10.1177/1352458513502436).

Neurodegenerative Diseases: Future Perspectives

In their 2018 *Biochemical Pharmacology* paper,[159] Aymerich and colleagues wrote that cannabinoids are compounds with a broad spectrum of effects, making them suitable for targeting multiple pathological features that characterize neurodegenerative diseases.

Preclinical studies offer evidence that supports the potential of cannabinoids to treat these conditions, but each neurodegenerative disease has specific alterations of the endocannabinoid system that may offer specific targets for cannabinoid-based therapy. For example, an interesting experimental therapy for Alzheimer's disease would be a 1:1 THC:CBD combination because of synergies among each cannabinoid's mechanism of action.[160]

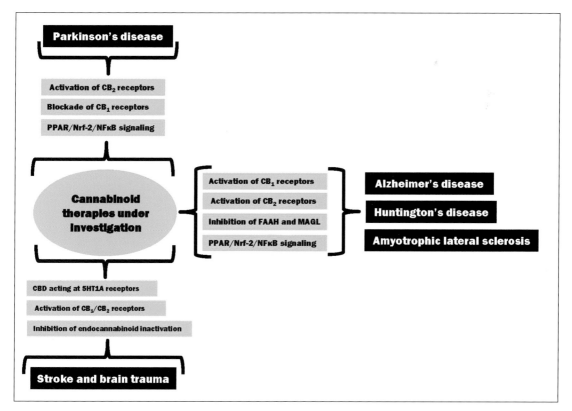

Image shows cannabinoid therapies under investigation for a range of neurodegenerative diseases. (Courtesy Dr. Javier Fernández-Ruiz)

159 Aymerich, M.S., E. Aso, M. A. Abellanas, R. M. Tolon, J. A. Ramos, I. Ferrer, J. Romero, and J. Fernández-Ruiz.

160 Ibid.

Administering both cannabinoids was more effective than each cannabinoid alone in reducing cognitive decline and some of the Alzheimer's pathological processes. Clinical data about chronic use of THC:CBD for other indications suggests it could result in a safe, well-tolerated treatment for Alzheimer patients, one that would confer virtually no THC psychoactivity because CBD reduces THC strength.[161]

For Parkinson's disease, Aymerich and colleagues said preclinical alternatives for PD treatment would be to target CB2 receptors and modulate endocannabinoid levels by inhibiting their catabolic (degrading) enzymes MAGL, which is neuroprotective, and FAAH. This would have the effect of raising CB2 activity levels The phytocannabinoid tetrahydrocannabivarin (THCV) has emerged as a valuable alternative that needs further investigation.[162]

For Huntington's disease, the researchers wrote, promising data from experimental HD models indicates that activating CB1 and CB2 receptors could be good targets for cannabinoid-based therapies, and cannabinoids that target those receptors and PPAR (works inside the cell at the nucleus) would be the best option in amyotrophic lateral sclerosis.[163]

Aymerich and colleagues noted that different strategies have been tested— directly targeting cannabinoid receptors with agonists or antagonists, or indirectly controlling endocannabinoid signaling with inhibitors of endocannabinoid degradation, or activating cannabinoid-receptor independent effects. More research is needed to investigate one of the most interesting aspects of cannabinoid pharmacology—its neuroprotective profile, which may arise from its pleiotropic (having multiple effects) activity.[164]

The nuclear receptor PPAR gamma is one of the most relevant targets for CBD and other cannabinoids and a key element for exerting anti-inflammatory and neuroprotective properties, the researchers added. The recent formulation of CBD as Epidiolex, FDA-approved for treating infantile refractory epileptic syndromes, may facilitate CBD's use in clinical trials for neurodegenerative disorders.[165]

So, Aymerich and colleagues noted, "more research is needed to identify a precise formulation for each type of pathology and each subset of patients, and for achieving a neuroprotective effect. New clinical studies involving large samples of patients, placebo groups, appropriate molecular targets, and objective

---

161 Ibid.
162 Ibid.
163 Ibid.
164 Ibid.
165 Ibid.

outcome measures are needed to clarify the effectiveness of cannabinoid-based therapies."[166]

During the 2017 United Kingdom conference that opened this chapter, Fernández-Ruiz (also a researcher in the 2018 work cited above) told conference attendees, "The intense preclinical work carried out over the past fifteen years on cannabinoid-based therapies for neuro-degenerative diseases has provided solid evidence to justify further efforts aimed at developing these molecules (or combinations) from their current preclinical state to a true clinical application."[167]

The challenge for the coming years, he added, "is to initiate clinical trials that validate in patients the promise and expectations generated by cannabinoids in cell and animal models of different neurodegenerative disorders."[168]

166 Ibid.
167 Fernández-Ruiz, J.
168 Ibid.

Chapter 11
Cannabinoids, Chronic Pain, and Other Inflammatory Disorders

Acute pain is a normal sensation triggered in the nervous system to alert the body to possible injury, but chronic pain is different, according to the National Institutes of Health National Institute of Neurological Disorders and Stroke (NINDS) Chronic Pain Information Page.[1] Chronic pain persists. Pain signals fire in the nervous system for weeks, months, or years.

The pain may have come from an initial mishap, or there's an ongoing cause of pain—arthritis, cancer, muscular dystrophy—but some have chronic pain without injury or signs of damage. Lots of chronic pain conditions affect older adults—headache, low back pain, cancer, arthritis, neurogenic pain (from damage to peripheral nerves or the central nervous system), and others. A person can have two or more chronic pain conditions at the same time, including chronic fatigue syndrome, fibromyalgia, and inflammatory bowel disease.[2]

Cannabinoids and Chronic Pain

Pain is a multidimensional disorder with sensory, emotional-affective and cognitive aspects. Chronic pain is the most commonly presented clinical complaint in the United States, affecting about 10 percent of the adult population, according to a 2017 S. G. Woodhams and colleagues *Neuropharmacology* paper.[3]

Even so, the researchers wrote, treatments for pain are an inadequate source of relief, highlighting the urgent need for effective new analgesic (pain-relieving) agents. Opioids, nonsteroidal anti-inflammatory drugs, selective COX-2 inhibitors (like Celebrex), antidepressants, anticonvulsants, and local anesthetics are all used clinically to treat pain.[4]

---

1   National Institutes of Health, National Institute of Neurological Disorders and Stroke, Chronic Pain Information web page, https://www.ninds.nih.gov/Disorders/All-Disorders/Chronic-pain-Information-Page. Accessed 9/18/18.
2   Ibid.
3   Woodhams, S. G., V. Chapman, D. P. Finn, A. G. Hohmann, and V. Neugebauer. "The cannabinoid system and pain." *Neuropharmacology* 124:105–20 (doi:10.1016/j.neuropharm.2017.06.015).
4   Ibid.

Opioids, like morphine derived from the opium poppy, have been used in pain relief for millennia, and synthetic opioids (tramadol, fentanyl, remifentanil) are routinely used to treat neuropathic and post-operative pain. But these agents have serious limitations, including constipation, tolerance, and dependence that has added to an epidemic of addiction and drug-related deaths in the United States.[5]

In the past few decades, the endocannabinoid system, its related elements, and its endogenous pain-control pathway have become a new target for pain relief, with the help of cannabinoids, terpenes, flavonoids, and more from the ancient plant and pain reliever, cannabis.[6]

"The endocannabinoid system is a major endogenous pain-control system," Woodhams and colleagues wrote, "running in parallel to the opioid system and playing crucial roles in the development and resolution of pain states, and the affective and cognitive aspects of pain." In the past two decades, a wealth of research has shown the potential efficacy of this approach to pain relief.[7]

Inhaled Cannabis for All Kinds of Pain

In a 2017 *Current Rheumatology Reports* paper, E. A. Romero-Sandoval and colleagues reviewed scientific evidence for cannabis use for chronic pain,[8] with a section on smoked or vaporized cannabis for chronic, severe, intractable, and other kinds of pain.

Cannabis is commonly used by inhalation by smoking the plant, oils, or resins, and to a lesser extent by vaporization (vaping), Romero-Sandoval and colleagues wrote.[9]

Among the thirty-four states and territories where medicinal cannabis is legal, most allow the use of inhaled (smoked or vaped) cannabis and include chronic, severe, intractable, and other types of pain in the indications they've approved for treatment with medical cannabis. Recreational cannabis legalization in a growing number of states makes it available on a broader spectrum, meaning that the whole-plant cannabis would have a broader range of cannabinoids, including THC, which is better for chronic pain.[10]

Inhaling cannabis in any of its forms has advantages and limitations, Romero-Sandoval and colleagues wrote, but the

---

5 Ibid.
6 Ibid.
7 Ibid.
8 Romero-Sandoval, E. A., A. L. Kolano, and P. A. Alvarado-Vázquez. "Cannabis and cannabinoids for chronic pain." *Curr Rheumatol Rep* 19: 67 (doi: 10.1007/s11926-017-0693-1).
9 Ibid.
10 Ibid.

pharmacokinetics of inhaled cannabis is one of its major advantages for treating pain. After inhaling (by smoke or vape), cannabis-related effects generally begin in five to fifteen minutes, peak at one hour, and stay at a steady state for three to five hours, which matches the plasma levels of THC.[11]

The pharmacokinetic profile of inhaled cannabis is similar to that of THC given intravenously, and the pharmacokinetic profile of CBD is similar to that of THC orally, intravenously, or inhaled.[12]

It's worth noting, the researchers wrote, "that the effects of cannabis could be experienced immediately after the first inhalation and these effects could increase within 1 to 10 minutes. The rapid onset, short time peak effect, and intermediate lasting effects, because they avoid first-passage metabolism [during which a drug's concentration is greatly reduced before it reaches systemic circulation], allow for self-titration [to maximize analgesic effects], reduced side effects or dysphoria, and reduced drug exposure when pain is controlled. All these advantages are virtually impossible with oral administration of cannabis or cannabinoids."[13]

The major limitation of inhaling cannabis, the researchers added, is the intake of toxic combustion by-products like carbon monoxide after smoking and its effects in the respiratory tract. But vaping is a smoke-free alternative for inhaling cannabis or cannabinoids.[14]

Cannabinoids, Pain, and the Elderly

In a 2018 *European Journal of Internal Medicine* research paper,[15] R. Abuhasira and colleagues reported that medical cannabis was safe and effective for elderly patients for indications that included pain and quality of life. Epidemiological data showed that the older population constitutes a growing segment of medical cannabis users, ranging from about 7 percent to more than a third, depending on the country.

"Despite the significant rise in use, the current evidence on the efficacy and safety of medical cannabis in the elderly is scarce. Only a small number of studies included elderly patients or analyzed them separately. The aim of this study," they wrote, "was to assess the characteristics of the older population receiving medical cannabis for a wide variety of diseases [and] evaluate the safety

---

11 Ibid.

12 Ibid.

13 Ibid.

14 Ibid.

15 Abuhasira, R., L. Bar-Lev Schleider, R. Mechoulam, and V. Novacka."Epidemiological characteristics, safety and efficacy of medical cannabis in the elderly." *Eur J Internl Med* 49:44–50 (https://doi.org/10.1016/j.ejim.2018.01.019).

Clinical Trials: Cannabinoids and Chronic Pain

Pain Research: Innovative Strategies with Marijuana (PRISM)

This observational study tested effects of cannabinoid blood levels on pain relief, inflammation, and cognitive dysfunction in chronic pain patients who used edible cannabis. Over two weeks, participants used an edible product of their choice. THC and CBD blood levels were measured before, during, and after the two weeks to see if there were associations with pain, inflammation, sleep, physical activity, anxiety/depression and cognitive dysfunction. Afterward, researchers followed participants for six months to collect self-report data on cannabis use, pain levels, sleep quality, and mental health symptoms. The estimated enrollment was about 283 adults. The estimated start date was June 2018 and the estimated completion date is March 2022. Study details are available at clinicaltrials.gov/ct2/show/NCT03522324.

MEMO—Medical Marijuana and Opioids Study

This study will examine how medical cannabis use affects opioid analgesic use over time, with attention to THC/CBD content, HIV outcomes, and severe adverse events. The study began in September 2018 and will end in June 2022. Participants are 250 adults with chronic pain who are certified for medical cannabis use in New York. Study details are available at clinicaltrials.gov/ct2/show/NCT03268551.

Cannabis Oil for Chronic Non-Cancer Pain Treatment (CONCEPT)

This randomized controlled interventional parallel-assignment study recruited 309 adults to determine whether CBD or CBD+THC reduces average pain in participants with chronic non-cancer pain. The investigators also wanted to determine whether CBD or CBD+THC is associated with reduced pain severity, pain interference, anxiety, depression, insomnia, opioids, and use of benzodiazepines, analgesics, antidepressants, anxiolytics, or hypnotics among chronic non-cancer pain patients, or with an increase in physical functioning, physical health-related role limitations, social functioning, and mental functioning. The study start date was October 2018 and it will be completed in December 2020. Study details are available at clinicaltrials.gov/ct2/show/NCT03635593.

Cannabis vs. Opioids Pain Management Objective Testing Comparisons (CVO)
This study compares cannabis and opioids to find safer, better-performing non-addictive products as an alternative for pain relief and to help alleviate the US opioid epidemic. The estimated start date was January 2019 and the estimated end date is January 2025, with 1,000 participants. The study consists of therapy of chronic pain and swelling with monochromatic infrared photo energy in combination with transcutaneous electrical nerve stimulation and cannabis or opioids to determine which treatment is most successful. Study details are available at clinicaltrials.gov/ct2/show/NCT03734731.

Treatment of Chronic Pain with Cannabidiol (CBD) and Delta-9-tetrahydrocannabinol (THC)
This study will compare the effects of THC vs. CBD vs. a placebo on chronic non-cancer pain of seventy-five participants. Participants include individuals with chronic pain who were randomized into one of three intervention conditions: high THC/low CBD, low THC/high CBD, or placebo. These measures were gathered before and after the fifth doses of CBD/THC or placebo. The study began in February 2018 and the estimated completion date was February 2019. Study details are available at clinicaltrials.gov/ct2/show/NCT03215940.

and efficacy of short- and medium-term use."[16]

Their prospective study included all patients sixty-five and older who initiated treatment with Tikun Olam Ltd.—one of Israel's largest medical cannabis suppliers—from January 2015 to October 2017 in a specialized medical cannabis clinic and were willing to answer an initial questionnaire. Outcomes were pain intensity, quality of life, and adverse events at six months.[17]

During the study period, 2,736 patients older than sixty-five began cannabis treatment and answered the initial questionnaire. The mean age was about seventy-four. For various reasons, of the total, 1,186 patients were eligible to answer the follow-up questionnaire after six months of treatment, and 901 actually responded.[18]

---

16 Ibid.
17 Ibid.
18 Ibid.

Indications for receiving a cannabis prescription were cancer-associated pain (36.6 percent), non-specific pain (30 percent), cancer-chemotherapy treatment (24.2 percent), Parkinson's disease (5.3 percent), posttraumatic stress disorder (0.8 percent), Crohn's disease (0.4 percent), amyotrophic lateral sclerosis (0.3 percent), compassion treatment (0.3 percent), ulcerative colitis (0.2 percent), Alzheimer's disease (0.1 percent), and multiple sclerosis (0.1 percent).[19]

An "others" category (1.8 percent) was made up of epilepsy, tic disorder, multiple system atrophy, essential tremor, dementia, tension headache, cluster headache, peripheral vascular disease, myelodysplastic syndrome (caused by dysfunctional blood cells), fibromyalgia, and rheumatoid arthritis.[20]

Cannabis treatment significantly reduced the intensity of reported pain, Abuhasira and colleagues wrote, from a median of 8 on a scale of 0–10 to a median of 4 after six months of treatment. Before treatment, 66.8 percent of respondents reported high pain intensity of 8 to 10, and at six months of treatment only 7.6 percent reported high pain intensity. The quality of life assessment improved with the treatment.[21]

At baseline, 79.3 percent of respondents defined their quality of life as bad or very bad, but after treatment 58.6 percent defined their quality of life as good or very good. Of the 901 patients who responded to the follow-up questionnaire (still receiving the treatment at six months), 31.7 percent reported at least one adverse event due to the treatment after six months. The most common adverse events were dizziness (9.7 percent) and dry mouth (7.1 percent). Of the 286 patients who reported adverse events, 11.5 percent rated their severity as 7 to 10 on a scale of 1 to 10.[22]

"The older population is a large and growing part of medical cannabis users," Abuhasira and colleagues wrote. "Our study finds that the therapeutic use of cannabis is safe and efficacious [effective] in this population. Cannabis use can decrease the use of other prescription medicines, including opioids. Gathering more evidence-based data, including from double-blind randomized controlled trials, in this special population is imperative."[23]

The Endocannabinoid System and Comorbid Pain-Depression

A 2016 *International Journal of Neuropsychopharmacology* paper[24] by

---

19 Ibid.
20 Ibid.
21 Ibid.
22 Ibid.
23 Ibid.
24 Fitzgibbon, M., D. P. Finn, and M. Roche.

M. Fitzgibbon and colleagues discussed some of the clinical reporting on the endocannabinoid system and its role in comorbid (present at the same time) pain-depression.

Several lines of evidence have shown changes in endocannabinoid system elements in chronic pain and in psychiatric patients. For example, genetic variations of CB1 and CB2 receptors have been seen in patients with major depression and bipolar disorder, and a single base-pair variation in a DNA sequence in the CB1 receptor was reported to enhance the risk of treatment resistance in depression and the development of anhedonic (inability to feel pleasure) depression following early-life trauma.[25]

Genetic alterations in the CB1 receptor and FAAH—the enzyme that breaks down the endocannabinoid anandamide—also have been identified in patients with pain associated with migraine, Parkinson's disease, and irritable bowel syndrome, Fitzgibbon and colleagues wrote. Endocannabinoid serum levels have been reported as reduced in depressed patients and chronic pain patients.[26]

Few clinical studies have directly investigated the role of cannabinoids in depression-pain interactions, but enhanced mood and better quality of life were reported in studies investigating the pain-relieving effectiveness of cannabinoid-based therapies.[27]

In a group of HIV patients, for example, cannabis was reported to improve muscle and nerve pain, depression, and anxiety, and improvements in anxiety and overall distress were reported in patients with advanced cancer whose pain symptoms were managed by daily adjunctive administration (added to standard treatment) of a THC analogue called Cesamet (nabilone) for thirty days. Nabilone is an FDA-approved medication available in the United States. A randomized double-blind placebo-controlled trial that examined the therapeutic benefit of nabilone for pain management and improved quality of life in fibromyalgia patients showed significant pain relief and lessened anxiety symptoms after four weeks of therapy.[28]

Another study, a retrospective evaluation investigating nabilone's effectiveness for managing concurrent disorders in seriously mentally ill prison populations, identified significantly improved symptoms related to posttraumatic stress

---

25 Ibid.
26 Ibid.
27 Ibid.
28 Ibid.

> **Clinical Trials: Cannabinoids and Comorbid Pain-Depression**
>
> *Effect of Medical Marijuana on Neurocognition and Escalation of Use (MMNE)*
>
> This study uses a randomized controlled design to test whether patients who use medical cannabis, compared to a wait-list control group, experience a change in health outcomes (relief of symptoms [pain, depression, insomnia, anxiety], or adverse health outcomes like new-onset symptoms of cannabis-use disorders or neurocognitive impairments) or brain-based changes. The trial recruited 200 adults; it began in July 2017 and ends in March 2022. Study details are available at https://clinicaltrials.gov/ct2/show/NCT03224468.

current medication, reported improved anxiety and depression after seven months of treatment.[30]

The cannabis-derived drug Sativex (1:1 ratio of THC:CBD), indicated for treatment-resistant spasticity and pain in multiple sclerosis, hasn't yet been associated directly with notable mood changes, but patients have reported a better overall quality of life after sixteen weeks of treatment. In a separate randomized controlled clinical trial evaluating Sativex's effect in patients with chronic painful diabetic neuropathy and comorbid depression, participants had significantly improved total pain scores compared with non-depressed counterparts.[31]

Collectively, Fitzgibbon and colleagues wrote, the studies suggest that when they coexist, depression/anxiety and pain respond to medical cannabinoids, but it's not yet known if the effects are coordinated by common or parallel mechanisms.[32]

disorder and a subjective improvement in chronic pain.[29]

A multicenter retrospective (looking at past records or interviewing patients about past events) survey of patients with chronic central neuropathic pain or fibromyalgia who were prescribed oral synthetic THC (dronabinol), to supplement

Cannabinoids, Pain, and Arthritis

Arthritis causes joint inflammation. Though it's a symptom rather than a diagnosis, people use the term to refer to any disorder affecting the joints, according to the National Institutes of Health's National Institute of Arthritis

---

29 Ibid.
30 Ibid.
31 Ibid.
32 Ibid.

and Musculoskeletal and Skin Diseases (NIAMS).[33]

One arthritic disorder is osteoarthritis, which damages the slippery tissue that covers the ends of bones, causing bones to rub together and producing pain, swelling, and loss of motion. Another disorder is rheumatoid arthritis, a disease that affects multiple joints, resulting in pain, swelling, and stiffness, and sometimes tiredness and fever.[34]

Osteoarthritis (OA) occurs most often in older people, and it's the most common type of arthritis. Younger people sometimes get the disease after joint injuries. No single test can diagnose osteoarthritis— doctors use several methods to diagnose the disease and rule out other problems.

Treatments for osteoarthritis include medicines, nondrug pain relief techniques, surgeries, and alternative therapies. Exercise, weight control, and other self-care activities can help. Conditions that might make getting the disorder more likely include being overweight, getting older, joint injury, joints that aren't properly formed, a genetic defect in joint cartilage, and stresses on joints from certain jobs and sports.[35]

Rheumatoid arthritis (RA) is an autoimmune inflammatory disease that causes pain, swelling, stiffness, and loss of function in the joints. It occurs when the immune system, which normally helps protect the body from infection and disease, attacks the membrane lining the joints.[36]

RA is different from other kinds of arthritis in several ways. It generally occurs in a symmetrical pattern, meaning that if one knee or hand is involved, the other one is too. RA often affects the wrist and finger joints closest to the hand. RA can affect other parts of the body—heart, lungs, blood, nerves, eyes, and skin. People with RA may have fatigue, occasional fevers, and appetite loss. Anyone can get rheumatoid arthritis, but it occurs more often in women and is most common in older people. Environmental factors and hormones may play roles in developing RA.[37]

---

33 National Institutes of Health, National Institute of Arthritis and Musculoskeletal and Skin Diseases, arthritis and rheumatic diseases, https://www.niams.nih.gov/health-topics/arthritis -and-rheumatic-diseases. Accessed 11/15/18.

34 Ibid.

35 Ibid.

36 Ibid.

37 Ibid.

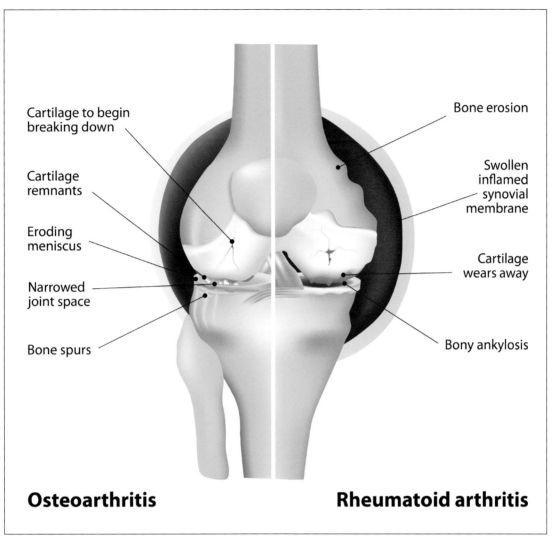

Cartilage to begin
breaking down

Cartilage
remnants

Eroding
meniscus

Narrowed
joint space

Bone spurs

Bone erosion

Swollen
inflamed
synovial
membrane

Cartilage
wears away

Bony ankylosis

Osteoarthritis

Rheumatoid arthritis

Comparing osteoarthritis and rheumatoid arthritis; RA is caused when the immune system mistakenly attacks the joints and causes inflammation. OA is a progressive degenerative joint disease. (From Shutterstock by Designua)

Cannabinoids and Osteoarthritis

In a 2018 *British Journal of Pharmacology* paper,[38] N. Malek and K. Starowicz discussed whether cannabinoids could help prevent or repair joint problems. Joints are made mainly of cartilage (flexible connective tissue), synovial fibroblasts (cells that are part of the connective

---

38 Malek, N., and K. Starowicz. "Joint problems arising from lack of repair mechanisms: can cannabinoids help?" *Br J Pharmacol*. March 25, 2018 (doi: 10.1111/bph.14204) [Epub ahead of print].

tissue [synovium] around human joints), and bone tissue.

OA was traditionally thought to be a cartilage-based disease, but scientists now know that during its development, all three components may be affected and can contribute to disease progression. OA also used to be classified as a non-inflammatory type of arthritis, but recent reports indicate that some inflammation occurs and that inflammatory cytokines (a signaling molecule excreted from immune cells that promote inflammation) are released into the joint.[39]

Ultimately, the main feature of OA is cartilage breakdown, and lots of things can contribute to it—aging, trauma, low-grade local or systemic inflammation, metabolic syndromes, obesity, and genetic predispositions. Current OA therapies mostly target pain rather than disease progression, and the researchers noted that a need to find a treatment for cartilage degeneration, bone deformation, and synovial inflammation led to research on the endocannabinoid system's involvement in how OA develops.[40]

The ECS is a protective system that switches on mainly after injury or in the presence of disease, and such activation has been shown to help control inflammation. Research has shown that ECS receptors CB1 and CB2 are expressed in chondrocyte (cells that secrete the cartilage matrix, then become embedded there) cultures and human OA cartilage, subchondral bone, and synovial tissue.[41]

Synovial fibroblasts express two ECS endocannabinoids, anandamide and 2-AG, suggesting that the ECS has a role in maintaining joint homeostasis. Research has shown that CB1 and CB2 receptors are expressed on nerve ends that supply the knee with nerves, all suggesting the ECS may play an important role in the development of joint diseases like OA associated with chronic pain.[42]

There's also evidence that cannabinoids have chondroprotective activity (delays OA's progressive joint-space narrowing and improves joint biomechanics), and this may help scientists develop new OA treatments.[43]

Research has shown that cannabinoids, especially CBD, have anti-inflammatory effects and help protect against cartilage degradation in inflamed arthritic joints. Chondrocytes extracted from OA-affected joints were shown to express CB1 and CB2 receptors even in degenerated tissues, demonstrating that these cells could respond to cannabinoids.

---

39 Ibid.
40 Ibid.
41 Ibid.
42 Ibid.
43 Ibid.

Studies have shown that endocannabinoids and synthetic compounds have direct chondroprotective effects, inhibiting proteoglycan (a compound present in connective tissue) breakdown and protecting cartilage. So cannabinoids could help protect against joint degeneration in OA development, the researchers wrote.[44]

The evidence they presented "supports the possibility of using cannabinoids as a novel therapeutic target and/or potential drug in the progression of rheumatic disease states. The question arises as to how to modulate the EC system for the treatment of OA."[45]

They added, "We believe that in light of data investigating the role of the endocannabinoid system in rheumatoid arthritis, its modulation will be a treatment for OA as well. CB1 antagonists [blockers] might reverse the metabolic alterations associated with OA, while activation of CB2 receptors might be beneficial in patients by downregulating [reducing] cytokine production."[46]

Cannabinoids and Reduced Arthritis Pain

Another 2018 study[47] in *Current Opinion in Pharmacology* by M. O'Brien and J. J. McDougall examined the scientific evidence for cannabinoid reduction of osteoarthritis pain.

A growing body of scientific evidence supports the analgesic (pain-reducing) potential of cannabinoids to treat OA pain, which appears as a combination of inflammatory, nociceptive (occurs when sensory neurons called nociceptors detect pain in the body), and neuropathic (nerve-generated) pain, each needing specific kinds of pain relievers.[48]

Commonly used drugs for OA pain are nonsteroidal anti-inflammatory drugs (NSAIDs), acetaminophen (Tylenol), opioids (OxyContin, Percocet, Vicodin, others) and a serotonin-noradrenaline reuptake inhibitor called duloxetine (Cymbalta). But, the researchers wrote, as many as 60 percent of OA patients are unsatisfied with their current pain management, reflecting the need for a better understanding of OA pain mechanisms and more effective analgesics. [49]

---

44 Ibid.

45 Ibid.

46 Ibid.

47 O'Brien, M., and J. J. McDougall. "Cannabis and joints: scientific evidence for the alleviation of osteoarthritis pain by cannabinoids." *Curr Opin Pharmacol* 40:104–9 (https://doi.org/10.1016/j.coph.2018.03.012).

48 Ibid.

49 Ibid.

The body's endocannabinoid system has been shown to improve all these pain subtypes, and ongoing research points to the endocannabinoid system, one of the body's natural pain-reducing systems, as a promising target for new OA therapies.[50]

Researchers have studied ECS presence and function in OA patients in which synovial tissues were found to express the endocannabinoid receptors CB1 and CB2, and synovial fluid contained the ECS endocannabinoids anandamide and 2-AG.[51]

A handful of ongoing clinical trials are exploring the analgesic effects of cannabinoids, with one ongoing trial testing combinations of cannabinoids, opioids, and benzodiazepines (really for anxiety and sleep disorders, but some patients like them for pain[52]) for their pain-relieving effects in a small number of OA patients.[53]

There aren't many OA clinical trials, but the researchers said many more studies have tested cannabinoids in neuropathic and inflammatory pain patients and these results may translate to specific OA populations. A 2011 systematic review of randomized controlled trials examined treating chronic non-cancer pain with cannabinoids.[54]

Eighteen trials met the criteria and included neuropathic pain, fibromyalgia, rheumatoid arthritis, and mixed chronic pain treated with smoked cannabis, nabilone (THC analogue), dronabinol (synthetic THC), nabiximols (Sativex), and another synthetic THC analogue. The study found that more than 80 percent of the trials showed significant pain reduction with cannabinoid use. One study in the review examined the pain-relieving effects of smoked cannabis with a range of THC concentrations (0 to 9.4 percent) in chronic neuropathic pain patients, finding that the high THC doses decreased pain intensity, improved sleep quality, and were well tolerated.[55]

Another study assessed Sativex (1:1 ratio of CBD and THC) in RA patients with inflammatory pain. The sublingual spray significantly reduced pain during movement and rest and improved patients' sleep quality, O'Brien and McDougall wrote. The most commonly reported adverse events in these arthritis patients were mild and included dizziness, dry mouth, and light-headedness.[56]

---

50 Ibid.

51 Ibid.

52 Tennant, F. "Benzodiazepines in pain practice: Necessary but troubling." *Pract Pain Manag* (Editor's Memo): 14(4).

53 O'Brien, M., and J. J. McDougall.

54 Ibid.

55 Ibid.

56 Ibid.

A 2015 study assessed the effectiveness of inhaled cannabis in patients with painful diabetic neuropathy. Low (1 percent THC), medium (4 percent THC), and high (7 percent THC) doses of aerosolized cannabis were administered in a randomized double-blind crossover study. The researchers found a significant dose-dependent reduction in pain, but the highest THC dose impaired cognitive function.[57]

COMPASS (Cannabis for the Management of Pain: Assessment of Safety Study), completed in 2015, explored the safety profile of a cannabis product containing high-dose THC (12.5 percent) for nociceptive and neuropathic pain. The study included patients from seven clinics across Canada and over a year found no difference in the risk of serious adverse events from smoked or ingested medical cannabis versus nonusers. But there was an increased risk for nonserious adverse events, including mild to moderate respiratory irritation.[58]

THC in this study enhanced cognitive function rather than impaired it, possibly due to its positive effect on pain control, sleep quality, and overall mood improvement. Long-term evaluation of the cannabinoid safety profile, including THC

and non-THC-containing products, is still needed, O'Brien and McDougall wrote.[59]

Cannabinoids also have an opioid-sparing effect, the researchers wrote, meaning that in non-cancer patients using morphine or oxycodone, adding vaporized cannabis significantly decreased the amount of opioid required for pain relief, and the synthetic THC agent dronabinol significantly reduced

Clinical Trials: Cannabinoids and Osteoarthritis

Cannabinoid Profile Investigation of Vaporized Cannabis in Patients with Osteoarthritis of the Knee (CAPRI) This randomized, double-blind, placebo-controlled, proof of concept crossover study will determine whether or not vaporized cannabis in forty adults will treat painful osteoarthritis (OA) of the knee. The main objective is to determine the analgesic dose-response characteristics of vaporized cannabinoids with varying degrees of THC:CBD ratios. The study began in June 2015 and ended in June 2019. Study details are available at clinicaltrials.gov/ct2/show/NCT02324777.

57 Ibid.
58 Ibid.
59 Ibid.

pain scores in patients taking opioids for chronic pain. These studies suggest that cannabinoids may be useful additions in OA patients taking opioids to manage chronic pain.[60]

"The complex pharmacodynamics of cannabinoids need to be studied in OA patients so that novel and accurate delivery methods can be developed which circumvent smoking and ingestion as modes of drug administration," O'Brien and McDougall concluded. "Finally, assessment of cannabinoids in discrete OA pain patient subgroups (nociceptive versus inflammatory versus neuropathic) is warranted to identify which population will benefit most from medical cannabis treatment."[61]

Cannabinoids, Rheumatoid Arthritis, and Fibromyalgia

Rheumatoid arthritis (RA) is one of the most prevalent autoimmune diseases and one of the main causes of disability worldwide, causing pain, joint malformation, and joint destruction. Preliminary evidence suggests that cannabinoids have a role in future RA treatment, D. Katz-Talmor and colleagues wrote in a 2018 *Nature Reviews Rheumatology* review paper[62] that discussed cannabinoids and rheumatic diseases.

In one study, the researchers wrote, synovial tissue (the synovium lines the joint's inner surface) from thirteen RA patients undergoing surgery to repair or replace joints expressed the main endocannabinoids—anandamide and 2-AG—and their CB1 and CB2 receptors. Synovial tissue from healthy volunteers showed no endocannabinoids.[63]

The endocannabinoid system protects the body, so endocannabinoids and receptors show up especially where there is damage or insult, like inflammation. That's why it was relevant that receptors and endocannabinoids showed up in RA patients, and that healthy people didn't have or need the endocannabinoid system mobilization.

In a separate study of synovial tissue from RA patients, stimulated synovial cells produced inflammatory signaling molecules called cytokines, and this was weakened by low concentrations of a THC-like chemical that, at high concentrations, inhibited the inflammatory molecules (and because of that, inflammation).

A variety of in vivo (animal) and in vitro (test tube, culture dish) experimental

---

60 Ibid.

61 Ibid.

62 Katz-Talmor, D., I. Katz, B. Porat-Katz, and Y. Schoenfeld. "Cannabinoids for the treatment of rheumatic diseases—where do we stand?" *Nat Rev Rheumatol* 14:488–98 (doi: https://doi. org/10.1038/ s41584-018-0025-5).

63 Ibid.

studies supported the results of the human studies, Katz-Talmor and colleagues wrote. Overall, exposure to the main nonintoxicating cannabinoid CBD or CB2 receptor activators reduced arthritis severity, inflammatory cell infiltration, bone destruction, and production of inflammatory-promoting constituents.[64]

"Although the exact role of the cannabinoid system in RA is not yet clear," the researchers wrote, "these experiments suggest a role for cannabinoids in the treatment of RA."[65]

For pain associated with RA, only one clinical trial has assessed cannabinoid use. In that randomized placebo-controlled study, fifty-eight RA patients were allocated to receive nabiximols (Sativex) or placebo. Compared with placebo, patients treated with nabiximols showed less pain when moving and at rest, and better sleep quality.[66]

Katz-Talmor and colleagues also reviewed clinical results of cannabinoids for fibromyalgia. The disorder is a chronic pain syndrome characterized by diffuse pain, fatigue, and sleep disturbance and by tenderness at specific sites (tender points) on the body.[67]

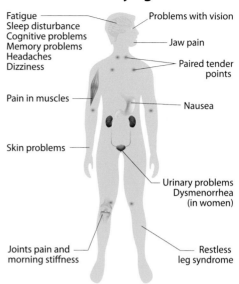

Fibromyalgia

Fatigue
Sleep disturbance
Cognitive problems
Memory problems
Headaches
Dizziness

Problems with vision

Jaw pain

Paired tender points

Pain in muscles

Nausea

Skin problems

Urinary problems
Dysmenorrhea
(in women)

Joints pain and morning stiffness

Restless leg syndrome

Signs and symptoms of fibromyalgia. (From iStock by ttsz)

In the absence of a known pathophysiology or suitable treatment, cannabis, commonly used for its pain-relieving properties, is a natural candidate for treating fibromyalgia, and several countries have approved the use of medical cannabis for fibromyalgia.[68]

To date, the researchers wrote, all clinical trials exploring the effectiveness of cannabinoids as a therapy for fibromyalgia have used nabilone (synthetic THC alone, with no other cannabinoids or terpenes). Two randomized controlled trials

---

64 Ibid.
65 Ibid.
66 Ibid.
67 Ibid.
68 Ibid.

Structural measures

A. Chronic back pain   B. Fibromyalgia

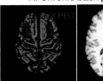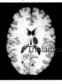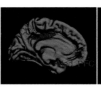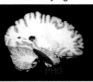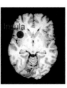

Schematic examples of central nervous system structural changes: Red circles signify decreased gray matter density relative to controls. A. Subjects with chronic back pain show decreases in gray matter density in bilateral dorsolateral prefrontal cortex and right anterior thalamus. B. Fibromyalgia patients show decreases in the cingulate cortex, medial prefrontal cortex, parahippocampal gyrus, and insula. (From Wikimedia Commons, authors Borsook D, Moulton EA, Schmidt KF, Becerra LR. Neuroimaging revolutionizes therapeutic approaches to chronic pain. *Molecular Pain.* 2007 3:25 [doi: 10.1186/1744-8069-3-25]. Licensee BioMed Central Ltd. This file is licensed under the Creative Commons Attribution 2.0 Generic license.)

were included in a Cochrane Database of Systematic Reviews paper addressing this matter.[69]

Both studies showed promising results, with one trial showing that nabilone effectively reduced anxiety, pain, and Fibromyalgia Impact Questionnaire scores, and the other trial showing that nabilone was superior to the antidepressant amitriptyline in resolving sleep disturbance, but with no improvement in quality of life, mood, or pain.[70]

Because the trials had small sample sizes and short durations, the Cochrane review's main conclusion didn't support cannabinoid treatment for fibromyalgia. But a US government-sponsored committee, in the National Academies Press's 2017 *The Health Effects of Cannabis and Cannabinoids: The Current State of Evidence and Recommendations for Research,*[71] reported moderate-grade evidence supporting cannabinoid effectiveness for fibromyalgia.

An observational study that didn't meet Cochrane's inclusion criteria also considered medical cannabis for the disorder. The study population included twenty-eight fibromyalgia patients who used cannabis and twenty-eight who didn't. Evaluating their symptoms before and after cannabis self-administration, the cannabis users reported reductions in pain and stiffness and an increase

69 Ibid.

70 Ibid.

71 National Academies of Sciences, Engineering, and Medicine. 2017. *The Health Effects of Cannabis and Cannabinoids: The Current State of Evidence and Recommendations for Research.* Washington DC: The National Academies Press (https://doi.org/10.17226/24625).

in relaxation accompanied by a rise in somnolence (sleepiness), in feelings of well-being, and in a mental health score two hours after consuming cannabis.[72]

Regardless of promising preclinical findings, Katz-Talmor and colleagues wrote, "the current clinical data simply do not suffice for conclusions to be drawn; therefore, clinicians should not routinely recommend cannabinoids for the treatment of rheumatic diseases. However, in adults with rheumatic diseases, especially in those with fibromyalgia, cannabinoid treatment could be considered in specific cases."[73]

They added, "The increasing legalization of medicinal cannabis emphasizes the need for further research, which should include large-scale clinical trials. In conclusion, although still far from being quantified and standardized therapies, cannabinoids have potential in the management of rheumatic diseases."[74]

Cannabinoids and Inflammatory Bowel Diseases

Inflammatory bowel disease (IBD) is a term for two conditions—Crohn's disease and ulcerative colitis—that are characterized by chronic inflammation of the gastrointestinal (GI) tract. Prolonged inflammation damages the GI tract, according

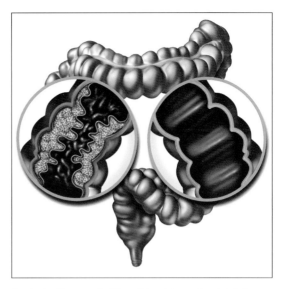

Crohn's disease (left) and healthy colon (right). (From iStock by wildpixel)

to the Centers for Disease Control and Prevention,[75] but there are differences between the disorders.

Crohn's disease can affect any part of the GI tract (mouth to anus), but most often it affects the portion of the small intestine that comes before the large intestine (colon). Damaged areas appear in patches that are next to areas of healthy tissue, and inflammation may reach through the multiple layers of the GI tract wall.[76]

Ulcerative colitis occurs in the large intestine (colon) and the rectum. Damaged areas are continuous (not patchy), usually

---

72 Ibid.

73 Katz-Talmor, D., I. Katz, B. Porat-Katz, and Y. Schoenfeld.

74 Ibid.

75 Centers for Disease Control and Prevention, inflammatory bowel disease, https://www.cdc.gov/ibd/what-is-IBD.htm. Accessed 11/13/18.

76 Ibid.

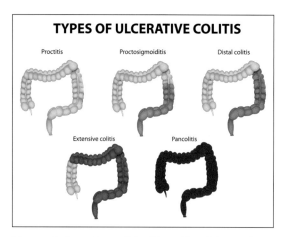

TYPES OF ULCERATIVE COLITIS

Proctitis Proctosigmoiditis Distal colitis

Extensive colitis Pancolitis

Types of ulcerative colitis. (From iStock by ttsz)

starting at the rectum and spreading further into the colon. Inflammation is present only in the innermost layer of the colon lining.[77]

The exact cause of IBD is unknown, but it's the result of a defective immune system, according to CDC. An immune system that's working normally attacks foreign organisms, like viruses and bacteria, to protect the body. In IBD, the immune system responds the wrong way to environmental triggers, which causes GI inflammation.[78]

There may also be a genetic component—someone with a family history of IBD is more likely to develop this abnormal immune response. Some common

IBD symptoms are persistent diarrhea, abdominal pain, rectal bleeding and bloody stools, weight loss, and fatigue.[79]

Several kinds of medications may be used to treat IBD. These include aminosalicylates (for Crohn's disease), corticosteroids (such as prednisone), immunomodulators (regulatory immune system control), and the newest class of drugs approved for IBD, biologics, which are made from or have components of living organisms.[80]

Several vaccinations are recommended for patients with IBD to prevent infections. Those with severe IBD may need surgery to remove damaged parts of the GI tract, but advances in medical treatments mean surgery is less common than it was a few decades ago.[81]

The Endocannabinoid System and the Gastrointestinal Tract

In a 2014 *Digestive Diseases* paper,[82] T. Naftali and colleagues discussed the endocannabinoid system and how elements of the ECS affect the GI tract.

The endocannabinoid system modulates several physiological processes, mainly in the brain, including effects on nociception (sensory nervous system response to harmful stimuli), memory

---

77 Ibid.
78 Ibid.
79 Ibid.
80 Ibid.
81 Ibid.
82 Naftali, T. R. Mechoulam, L. Bar Lev, F. M. Konikoff. "Cannabis for inflammatory bowel disease." *Dig Dis* 32:468–74 (doi: 10.1159/000358155).

processes, plasticity (adaptability), and cell proliferation, the researchers wrote, noting that endocannabinoids play a modulatory role that affects the immune and cardiovascular systems and reproductive endocrine processes, and controls energy metabolism.[83]

The endocannabinoid anandamide can help relieve pain, control motor activity, reduce emesis (vomiting), stimulate appetite, and induce hypothermia. The endocannabinoid 2-AG acts as a messenger molecule in various biological systems, such as the endocrine and immune systems.[84]

In the GI tract, activating prejunctional CB1 receptors (on the nerve terminal's outer surfaces) reduces excitatory enteric (intestinal) transmission and eventually inhibits motility (muscle contractions that mix and move GI tract contents). CB1 activation can inhibit gastric transit and vomiting. CB2 activation counteracts alterations in intestinal motility during inflammatory conditions but not in healthy animals. It also helps control gut inflammation, as seen in mouse models of colitis.[85]

Cannabinoid receptors CB1 and CB2 are present throughout the GI tract, Naftali and colleagues wrote, including liver, pancreas, stomach, and the small and large intestines, and both receptors are found on enteric neurons, nerve fibers, and terminals throughout the enteric nervous system (embedded in the GI system lining).[86]

CB1 receptors were found on the normal and inflamed human colonic epithelium, and both receptors were found in macrophages (white blood cells that remove cellular debris) and plasma cells in the human colon. The pharmacological action of cannabis consumption on the GI tract includes decreased motility, secretion, gastric/colonic emptying, and anti-inflammatory actions, properties that explain why cannabinoids seem to have a beneficial effect on IBD.[87]

In a small study of thirteen patients using inhaled cannabis for IBD over three months, researchers saw a statistically significant increase in subjects' weight, along with an improved disease activity index, perception of general health, and ability to perform daily activities.[88]

---

83 Ibid.
84 Ibid.
85 Ibid.
86 Ibid.
87 Ibid.
88 Ibid.

In 2011, Naftali and colleagues had conducted an observational retrospective study[89] of thirty Crohn's disease patients licensed to use medical cannabis in Israel. Most patients smoked cannabis as joints (0.5 g cannabis per joint) and used one to three joints a day. The Harvey-Bradshaw index (measuring disease severity and potential remission) decreased from an average of about 14 before cannabis consumption to about 7 afterward. The use of other medications (5-aminosalicylic acid, corticosteroids, thiopurines, methotrexate, TNF antagonists, and others) was also significantly reduced after cannabis use.

In 2013, the researchers conducted the first double-blind, placebo-controlled study of THC-rich cannabis inhalation in Crohn's. The study included twenty-one active Crohn's patients. Five of eleven patients in the cannabis group and one of ten in the placebo group achieved complete remission. Ten of eleven in the cannabis group and four of ten in the placebo group showed a clinical response. Three patients in the cannabis group were weaned from steroid dependence. Patients who received cannabis reported improved appetite and sleep, with no significant side effects. Naftali and colleagues wrote that the study was limited by its small size and by a lack of objective measures of disease improvement, like inflammatory markers.[90]

But in their 2014 paper, the researchers wrote, "The cannabinoid system has important regulatory functions throughout the human body, including the GI tract, and a major role in the regulation of inflammatory reactions. Despite the importance of the cannabinoid system, it has stayed 'below the radar' of medical research and we are only beginning to discover its implications."[91]

Accumulating evidence shows that manipulating the endocannabinoid system could have beneficial effects on IBD, but more research is needed before cannabinoids can be declared a medicine, Naftali and colleagues added, noting, "We need to establish the appropriate cannabinoids . . . medical conditions, dose, and mode of administration for cannabinoid use in IBD."[92]

IBD Patients: Turning to Cannabis

Biologicals are first-line alternative treatments now for severe IBD and are powerful tools for changing the course of the disease, but they can cause severe

89 Naftali, T., L. Bar-Lev Schleider, I. Dotan, E. P. Lansky, F. Sklerovsky Benjaminov, and F. M. Konikoff. "Cannabis induces a clinical response in patients with Crohn's disease: a prospective placebo-controlled study." *Clin Gastroenterol Hepatol* 11(10):1276–1280.e1 (doi: 10.1016/j.cgh.2013.04.034) Epub May 4, 2013.
90 Ibid.
91 Naftali, T., R. Mechoulam, L. Bar Lev, F. M. Konikoff.
92 Ibid.

adverse effects like infections, malignancies, and injection or infusion reactions, C. Hasenoehrla and colleagues wrote in a February 2017 *Expert Review of Gastroenterology and Hepatology* paper.[93]

For the antibody treatment vedolizumab (Entyvio), cases of arthritis and sacroiliitis (inflammation of one or both sacroiliac joints) have recently been reported. Conventional treatment is often ineffective, leaving many patients dissatisfied and searching for alternative treatments, including cannabis.[94]

Cannabis was used traditionally thousands of years ago to treat gut inflammation. Today, a growing number of countries have legalized medical cannabis, but clinical studies of cannabis effects in IBD are scarce so far. Here are a few studies the researchers described:

- Questionnaires conducted in Canada, the United States, and Israel showed that patients commonly self-medicate with cannabis to relieve IBD-related symptoms that include abdominal pain, diarrhea, and appetite loss.

- A prospective pilot study with thirteen IBD patients who were told to inhale cannabis when they were in pain concluded that the treatment significantly improved the patients' quality of life.

Hasenoehrla and colleagues observed that most of these clinical studies are statistically underpowered, lack methodological quality, and may not have used the right placebos, given that it's hard to conceal the effects of THC.[95]

The researchers also noted that several preclinical studies have indicated that CBD, the main nonintoxicating cannabinoid, is protective in intestinal inflammation, that CBD could be supportive in maintaining a healthy intestinal barrier, and that another study had recently reviewed CBD's anti-inflammatory potential.[96]

Applying Cannabis in IBD

Medical cannabis is preferably inhaled, with average THC bioavailability levels of about 30 percent, the researchers wrote. Oral THC has been shown to be effective for chemotherapy-induced nausea at

---

93 Hasenoehrla, C., M. Storr, R. Schicho. "Cannabinoids for treating inflammatory bowel diseases: where are we and where do we go?" *Expert Rev Gastroenterol Hepatol* 11(4)329–37. (doi: http://dx.doi.org/10.1080/17474124.2017.1292851).
94 Ibid.
95 Ibid.
96 Ibid.

a dose of 5 mg to 15 mg per body surface area (using body surface area to create a patient-specific dose). Most variations in THC bioavailability are due to differences in individuals, the ratio of THC to other cannabinoids, and differing constituents in cannabis plants.[97]

"These obstacles can be circumvented by using purified ingredients of cannabis or combinations of purified ingredients, as in nabiximols [Sativex], a 1:1 ratio of THC:CBD, applied as a sublingual spray. Each milliliter of nabiximols contains 27 mg THC and 25 mg CBD, and a meta-review summarized the most common maximum dose as 8 sprays per 3 hours, or 48 sprays per 24 hours, in studies of spasticity, pain, nausea, and vomiting," Hasenoehrla and colleagues wrote.[98]

A possible cannabis application for IBD patients is intra-rectal (IR), the researchers said. Preclinical studies in mice have shown an anti-inflammatory effect after IR application of CBD. The IR route could reduce first-pass effects (in which metabolic processes significantly reduce a drug's concentration before it reaches systemic circulation) and would let cannabinoids act locally at endocannabinoid system receptors, which are highly represented in bowel mucosa.[99]

In conclusion, Hasenoehrla and colleagues wrote, experimental data suggest a homeostatic role for the endocannabinoid system in the gut. Some believe enhanced endocannabinoid signaling, as seen through increased levels of endocannabinoids and their receptors and decreased endocannabinoid degrading enzymes, is a response to homeostatic system disturbances and is aimed at restoring balance. Most evidence points to an involvement of CB1 and CB2 receptors, especially in recruiting immune cells.[100]

The researchers wrote, "Further research in this direction, preferably on human IBD material such as explants [cells or tissue transferred to a nutrient medium], cultured biopsies, etc., is highly warranted."[101]

---

97 Ibid.
98 Ibid.
99 Ibid.
100 Ibid.
101 Ibid.

Clinical Trials: Cannabinoids, Crohn's and IBD

Cannabidiol Use as an Adjunct Therapy for Crohn's Disease

This study seeks to pilot a randomized, placebo-controlled trial assessing the efficacy and safety of oral CBD as an adjunct (add-on) therapy in patients with Crohn's disease. The investigators wrote: "With the recent wave of medical cannabis legalization in many states, patients have begun using cannabis or commercially available cannabidiol-containing compounds as an adjunct therapy for their symptoms related to chronic inflammation and pain." The trial has thirty-six adult participants. The study start date was July 2018 and the estimated end date was July 2019. Study details are available at clinicaltrials. gov/ct2/show/NCT03467620.

Combined THC and CBD Drops for Treating Crohn's Disease

This aim of this phase 1 and 2 trial was to investigate the effectiveness of oil containing the cannabinoids THC and CBD given by mouth to induce remission in Crohn's disease. Fifty adults participated in this study. The study date was March 2013 and the end date was March 2015. Study details are available at clinicaltrials.gov/ct2/show/NCT01826188.

Continued on page 212.

Cannabis for Inflammatory Bowel Disease

The aim of this phase 1 and 2 study was to examine in a double-blind placebo-controlled fashion the effect of smoking cannabis on disease activity in twenty adult IBD patients. The study start date was January 2010 and the end date was July 2012. The trial involved smoking cannabis and smoking cigarettes with a placebo. The main outcome measure was to reduce the Crohn's Disease Activity Index by 70 points. The results were published in the October 2013 *Clinical Gastroenterology and Hepatology.*[102] Ten of eleven in the cannabis group and four of ten in the placebo group showed a clinical response. Three patients in the cannabis group were weaned from steroid dependence. Patients who received cannabis reported improved appetite and sleep with no significant side effects. The investigators said the study was limited by its small size and by a lack of objective measures of disease improvement, like inflammatory markers. In conclusion, the researchers wrote, "The cannabinoid system has . . . a major role in the regulation of inflammatory reactions. Despite the importance of the cannabinoid system, it has stayed 'below the radar' of medical research and we are only beginning to discover its implications." Study details are available at clinicaltrials.gov/ct2/show/NCT01040910.

---

102 Naftali, T., L. Bar-Lev Schleider, I. Dotan, E. P. Lansky, F. Sklerovsky Benjaminov, and F. M. Konikoff.

Chapter 12
Cannabinoids, Mood Disorders, and Addiction

Depression (major depressive disorder or clinical depression) is a common but serious mood disorder whose severe symptoms affect how a person feels, thinks, and handles daily activities like sleeping, eating, or working, according to the National Institutes of Health National Institute of Mental Health (NIMH).[1] To be diagnosed with depression, a person must have had symptoms for at least two weeks. Some forms of depression are slightly different or may develop under specific circumstances.

Persistent depressive disorder (dysthymia) is a depressed mood that lasts at least two years. A person diagnosed with this disorder may have episodes of major depression along with periods of less severe symptoms, but symptoms have to last for two years to be considered persistent depressive disorder.[2]

Psychotic depression occurs when someone has severe depression plus some form of psychosis, like having disturbing false fixed beliefs (delusions) or hearing or seeing upsetting things that others can't hear or see (hallucinations). Psychotic symptoms typically have a depressive theme, like delusions of guilt, poverty, or illness.[3]

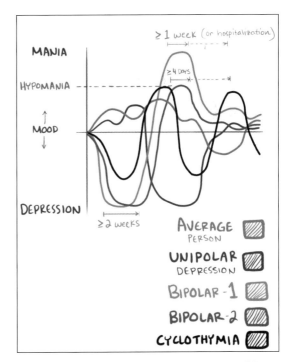

Graphical representation of depressive conditions (From Wikipedia by User:Osmosis. This file is licensed under the Creative Commons Attribution-Share Alike 4.0 International license.)

---

1   National Institutes of Health. National Institute of Mental Health, depression, https://www.nimh.nih.gov/health/topics/depression/index.shtml. Accessed 11/21/18.
2   Ibid.
3   Ibid.

Bipolar disorder is different from depression, but it's included here because someone with bipolar disorder experiences episodes of very low moods that meet the criteria for major depression (called bipolar depression). But a person with bipolar disorder also experiences extreme high—euphoric or irritable—moods called mania, or a less severe form called hypomania.[4]

Other types of depressive disorders added to the diagnostic classification of DSM-5 include disruptive mood dysregulation disorder (diagnosed in children and adolescents) and premenstrual dysphoric disorder.[5]

The Endocannabinoid System in Depression

At the Hotchkiss Brain Institute in Calgary, Alberta, Canada, the primary focus of research in Dr. Matthew Hill's laboratory is to understand the role of the endocannabinoid system in the effects of stress and glucocorticoids (steroid hormones with anti-inflammatory effects).

Within this focus, Hill's research especially involves determining the endocannabinoid system's role in the effects of stress on neuroendocrine function, emotional behavior, energy balance and metabolism, neuroinflammation, and neurodegeneration.[6]

His lab focuses on the role of the endocannabinoid system because they've determined that endocannabinoid signaling is important for terminating the stress response and adapting the stress response after repeated exposure to stress. Hill has also been involved in studies examining endocannabinoid function in psychiatric conditions like depression and PTSD.

"Depression's tricky because it's a very heterogeneous disease," Hill said in a 2017 interview. "My PhD work was much more focused on hypothesizing about the endocannabinoids' role in depression, so the original theory I'd put out there . . . was, there is one subtype of depression called melancholic and this is usually the more severe variant of depression."

The clinical presentation would look like chronic hyperarousal, he explained. People don't sleep a lot and tend not to eat a lot; they're usually more underweight than overweight. There's a high level of anxiety and anhedonia, meaning they don't respond to rewarding stimuli in their environment anymore and they don't have motivation to go for a walk or have sex or do anything they normally

---

4   Ibid.
5   Ibid.
6   Hotchkiss Brain Institute, laboratory of associate professor Dr. Matthew Hill, https://hbi.ucalgary .ca/profiles/dr-matthew-hill. Accessed 5/17/19.

like. They usually have elevated stress hormones.

"People with melancholic depression often wake up at like 3:00 a.m. and lie in bed worrying and having anticipatory anxiety about all the terrible things going on," he said. "It's fundamentally different than a lot of what depression looks like nowadays. What you see more often is usually associated with reduced metabolic function, weight gain, and sleeping a lot, and this is one of the underlying problems in depression—the phenotypes look so different. So making a broad sweeping claim about a biological abnormality that might relate to depression is problematic."

The melancholic depression phenotype is similar to what you would expect to see from an underactive or deficient endocannabinoid system, he added.

"If you give a drug that blocks endocannabinoid signaling for a few weeks, the phenotype, at least in [lab animals], is similar to this," Hill said. "They lose weight, they become highly aroused, they don't have a lot of interest in working to get rewarding stimuli, and they don't eat a lot, so it looks very similar to melancholic depression."

Some studies have looked at gene variants in cannabinoid receptors and found a random gene variant that's not very common in the population. "If you have that gene variant you might not respond to antidepressants, or if you do

a neuroimaging study, your response to smiling faces isn't the same—you don't seem to view that as rewarding. You might have more neuroticism in your personality and you might be a little bit more stress sensitive."

Hill and colleagues have measured endocannabinoids in two female depressed populations and found lower levels of circulating endocannabinoids in depression.

"It's hard to interpret what that necessarily means, but at the time I thought there was enough converging evidence to make a few theories," he said, describing a theory that was similar to his findings in studying PTSD, about how chronic stress degrades or collapses the endocannabinoid system.

"I think this is true for most stress-related psychiatric illnesses," Hill said. "If the system isn't functioning properly a few things will become apparent. Like you might be more sensitive to developing anxiety after stress, you might not recover as quickly from stressful experiences in your life. We know the endocannabinoid system is very important for processing rewarding stimuli, so if it's not working properly you might become more anhedonic."

That's the underlying theory, he explained. "If the system doesn't work right, it might increase your vulnerability to developing an adverse psychiatric illness like depression or anxiety or PTSD after you are exposed to environmental stressors."

Hill added, "Depression usually isn't the same as like PTSD, which very often is an index trauma like a car accident or an assault or a natural disaster where there's a very high trauma load. Depression, if you look at the relationships of life stress, is like compounding things in life—in the year or two preceding, someone close has passed away or a relationship ended or someone lost a job or they moved to a new environment where they didn't have a social network, things like this. Those kinds of stressors are more the ones that relate to depression."

Ultimately, though, the systems involved in PTSD and depression engage the same biological processes in the body, he said. "So our thought, and the hypotheses that we've put out there, is that if the system isn't functioning properly—be it through genetic variants or through individual differences or through environmental effects like chronic exposure to stress compromising the way the system would function—that may then render an individual more vulnerable to developing a psychiatric illness like depression or PTSD."

Hill and colleagues also link depression and stress to inflammation.

Inflammation, he said, "drives the same hormonal stress response elevating cortisol that psychological stress does."

"And we know in the context of chronic psychological stress, cortisol is a big mediator of a lot of the adverse effects on the brain and body that are related to chronic stress," Hill added. "So our reasoning is essentially that, if inflammation is just a different flavor of stressor, it's probably mediating its effects on anxiety and depression in a similar manner as psychological stress because both of them involve recruitment of the same hormonal systems."

Clinical Evidence for the Endocannabinoid System in Depression

Depression is one of the most common mental illnesses, experienced by 15 to 20 percent of a population over their lives. This results in enormous personal suffering and social and economic burden, according to V. Micale and colleagues in a book chapter[7] in *Role of the Endocannabinoid System in Depression: From Preclinical to Clinical Evidence.*

The authors say that those with a major depressive disorder have depressed mood episodes lasting more than two weeks. These often are associated with feelings

---

7   Micale, V., K. Tablova, J. Ruda-Kucerova, and F. Drago. "Role of the endocannabinoid system in depression: From preclinical to clinical evidence," in the book *Cannabinoid Modulation of Emotion, Memory and Motivation*, P. Campolongo and L. Fattore, eds. Springer Science+Business Media (doi: 10.1007/978-1-4939-2294-9_5).

of guilt, decreased interest in pleasurable activities, inability to experience pleasure (anhedonia), low self-esteem and worthlessness, high anxiety, disturbed sleep patterns and appetite, impaired memory, and suicidal ideation. Thirty percent of depressed patients who take conventional antidepressants are resistant to treatment and, treatment resistant or not, antidepressants have to be taken for weeks or months to see clinical benefit.

There's a great need, Micale and colleagues wrote, "to update the current level of knowledge with regard to the pathophysiological mechanisms underlying depressive disorders." To study the problem, they looked into whether an altered endocannabinoid system has a crucial role in the physiological processes associated with depressive disorders, and whether elements of the ECS could offer therapeutic approaches for their treatment.[8]

Multiple lines of evidence have shown that ECS dysregulation is associated with pathological conditions like pain, inflammation, and obesity, and with metabolic, gastrointestinal, hepatic, neurodegenerative, and psychiatric disorders.[9]

Evidence showing that most antidepressants modify CB1 receptor expression and endocannabinoid content in brain regions related to mood disorders supports the endocannabinoid system's role in depression.[10]

The selective serotonin reuptake inhibitor (SSRI) fluoxetine (Prozac) increased CB1 receptor signaling in the limbic region, and the SSRI citalopram (Celexa) reduced CB1 receptor signaling in the hippocampus and hypothalamic paraventricular nucleus, the researchers said, suggesting a region-specific effect of SSRIs on CB1 receptor-mediated signaling.[11]

Tricyclic antidepressants had different effects based on brain region: desipramine (Norpramin) increased hippocampal and hypothalamic CB1 receptor binding, and imipramine (Tofranil) reduced it in the hypothalamus, midbrain, and hypothalamic paraventricular nucleus and increased it in the amygdala.[12]

The monoamine oxidase inhibitor antidepressant tranylcypromine (Parnate) enhanced CB1 receptor binding and levels of the endocannabinoid 2-AG in the prefrontal cortex and hippocampus, and reduced the endocannabinoid anandamide's content in the prefrontal cortex, hippocampus, and hypothalamus.[13]

---

8   Ibid.
9   Ibid.
10 Ibid.
11 Ibid.
12 Ibid.
13 Ibid.

"Despite the conflicting panorama," Micale and colleagues wrote, "these findings suggest that the antidepressants modify endocannabinoid tone in different ways, depending both on the class of drugs and on the different brain regions considered." ECS enzyme elements also may have a role, the researchers wrote, noting that data cited in their paper supports the enzyme FAAH, which breaks down the endocannabinoid anandamide (which in turn increases the amount of anandamide in the brain), as a potential target for identifying new affective disorder treatments.[14]

Based on the hypothesis that reduced endocannabinoid signaling could underlie depressive disorders, it's been seen that acute or repeated treatment with compounds that directly activate cannabinoid receptors, like THC, the endocannabinoid anandamide, and several other CB1 and CB2 agonists, all elicited antidepressant-like effects through CB1 and serotonin receptor or norepinephrine receptor-mediated mechanisms.[15]

Some of the in vivo data didn't give a coherent picture of the role of CB2 receptors in depression, Micale and colleagues wrote, but the molecular data strengthened the rationale for developing selective CB2 receptor agonists as candidates for targeting neurogenesis (stem cell production of neurons), thus bypassing the intoxicating effects of activating CB1 receptors.[16]

Along with this approach to avoiding intoxication, the researchers said plant-derived nonintoxicating, cannabinoids could be used. These include CBD, cannabichromene, cannabigerol, and cannabidivarin, some of which show potential as therapeutic agents in preclinical models of central nervous system disorders.[17]

CBD especially has several positive pharmacological effects in preclinical and clinical studies, giving it attractive therapeutic potential in several diseases. Extensive research has been done into this potential of CBD in anxiety and schizophrenia, but only a few studies have examined its antidepressant-like effects.[18]

In conclusion, Micale and colleagues wrote, current evidence suggests a strong link between the endocannabinoid system and depressive disorders. A deficiency in endocannabinoid tone leads to a depressive-like phenotype (observable characteristics) in animal models of depression, and this is in line with

---

14 Ibid.
15 Ibid.
16 Ibid.
17 Ibid.
18 Ibid.

clinical findings that show depressed patients have reduced levels of endogenous cannabinoids.[19]

But given the complexities of the endocannabinoid system and of modulating the system for certain effects, they added, "only time will tell if targeting the ECS may result in effective pharmacotherapies for major depression and other affective-related disorders."[20]

Cannabinoids and Borderline Personality Disorder

In a 2018 *Journal on the Biology of Stress* paper,[21] K. Wingenfeld and colleagues investigated whether long-term endocannabinoid concentrations are altered in women with borderline personality disorder (BPD).

BPD is a severe psychiatric disorder characterized by intense and rapidly changing mood states and chronic feelings of emptiness, impulsivity, fear of abandonment, and unstable relationships and self-image, and a core feature of non-suicidal self-injurious behavior. BPD patients often suffer from comorbid psychiatric disorders, mainly major depressive disorder, anxiety disorders,

and posttraumatic stress disorder, the researchers wrote.[22]

Endocannabinoids—synthesized by enzymes in the body's cells when they're needed and disassembled by other enzymes when they're not—are involved in affect (the experience of feeling or emotion), pain, and stress regulation. Two important and much-investigated endocannabinoids are anandamide and 2-AG, which may contribute to BPD psychopathology, but more studies on endocannabinoids have been conducted in people with PTSD than those affected by BPD.[23]

One study analyzed endocannabinoids in hair, reflecting long-term endocannabinoid concentrations. In the study, Wingenfeld and colleagues determined long-term endocannabinoid concentrations by measuring anandamide, 2-AG, and a main 2-AG isomer's concentrations in hair, and this represented a cumulative measure over several months or longer, depending on hair length. Based on findings in PTSD patients, the researchers said they expected to find reduced long-term endocannabinoid concentrations in BPD.[24]

---

19 Ibid.
20 Ibid.
21 Wingenfeld, K., L. Dettenborn, C. Kirschbaum, W. Gao, C. Otte, and S. Roepke. "Reduced levels of the endocannabinoid arachidonylethanolamide (AEA) in hair in patients with borderline personality disorder–a pilot study." *STRESS* 21(4): 366–9 (doi: 10.1080/10253890.2018.1451837).
22 Ibid.
23 Ibid.
24 Ibid.

In the study, BPD patients and healthy women (controls) were matched in age, body mass index, and whether they smoked. BPD patients had higher depression and childhood trauma scores, and all fulfilled the *Diagnostic and Statistical Manual of Mental Disorders* (DSM-IV) criteria for BPD. Four also were diagnosed with PTSD, and seven BPD patients met the criteria for current major depressive disorder. Two BPD patients had both comorbidities. The healthy controls were free of psychiatric disorders. Four of the BPD patients were taking medications like atypical antipsychotics and antidepressants (two were taking more than one drug).[25]

The researchers said BPD patients had significantly lower hair anandamide levels than the controls, but there were no differences between BPD patients and healthy controls in hair 2-AG isomer levels. Preliminary data indicated altered long-term secretion of endocannabinoids in female patients with BPD.[26]

In line with their hypothesis, the researchers found decreased hair anandamide concentrations in BPD and noted that anandamide has been reported to reduce depressive and anxious symptoms.

Thus, Wingenfeld and colleagues wrote, "chronically reduced [anandamide] might contribute to psychopathology in BPD such as depressive symptoms or chronic feelings of emptiness." Future studies, they added, should analyze subgroups of BPD patients with comorbid psychiatric disorders like PTSD and major depressive disorder.[27]

The Endocannabinoid System and Psychiatric Illness

"The potential efficacy of cannabinoid treatments in the psychiatric population is an emerging topic of interest that provides potential value going forward in medicine," M. A. Katzman and colleagues wrote in a 2016 *Journal of Clinical Psychopharmacology* review paper.[28] Because of low disorder remission rates and treatments that don't always work, researchers must continually seek new treatments for depressive disorders.

This search has prompted interest in the endocannabinoid system and its potential to improve psychiatric outcomes, just as ECS interactions have improved outcomes in cancers, neuropathic pain, and multiple sclerosis.[29]

---

25 Ibid.
26 Ibid.
27 Ibid.
28 Katzman, M. A., M. Furtado, and L. Anand. "Targeting the endocannabinoid system in psychiatric illness." *J Clin Psychopharmacol* 36(6) (doi: 10.1097/JCP.0000000000000581).
29 Ibid.

Since the ECS was discovered in the early 1990s, its elements have been identified in most of the body's physiological and pathophysiological processes, including psychiatric disease. The ECS's "potential role in the pathophysiology of psychiatric disorders must therefore be considered of primary interest as medicine goes forward through the 21st century," Katzman and colleagues wrote.[30]

In major depressive disorders (MDDs), for example, depression remission rates aren't ideal, even though there's professional consensus on treatment guidelines. More than 50 percent of patients on first-line treatments and about two-thirds on SSRIs don't get better. The ECS has been implicated in the cause of depression, so studies have examined its involvement in the disorder and the effectiveness of targeted treatments, but findings have been contradictory.[31]

The endocannabinoid system has been implicated in mood pathophysiology, but its impact on serotonin, a primary neurotransmitter in mood and antidepressant action, has been sparsely investigated, the researchers wrote. Still, the dorsal raphe, one of the raphe nuclei, the main source of serotonin in the forebrain, has been shown to express the endocannabinoid-degrading FAAH

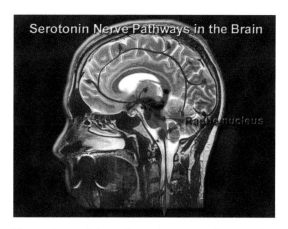

The raphe nuclei are the main source of serotonin in the forebrain. (Courtesy National Institute on Drug Abuse)

enzyme and CB1 receptor mRNA in mice. CB1 receptors also are highly expressed in the prefrontal cortex, which transmits excitatory signals to the dorsal raphe.[32]

The recent discovery that 2-AG is released from midbrain dopamine neurons offers more evidence supporting endocannabinoids' role in psychiatric illness, Katzman and colleagues wrote. Released 2-AG modulates afferent input (from neurons that transmit sensory info to the central nervous system) under physiological synaptic activity and pathological conditions.[33]

Also, the researchers wrote, THC and synthetic CB1 receptor agonists (activators) dose-dependently enhance the firing rate and activity of dopamine

30 Ibid.
31 Ibid.
32 Ibid.
33 Ibid.

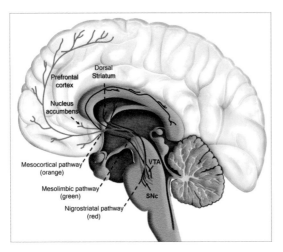

In the brain dopamine plays an important role in regulating reward and movement. As part of the reward pathway (multi-colored lines), dopamine is made in nerve cells in the ventral tegmental area and released in the nucleus accumbens and prefrontal cortex. (From Wikimedia Commons by Oscar Arias-Carrión, Maria Stamelou, Eric Murillo-Rodríguez, Manuel Menéndez-González and Ernst Pöppel. Dopaminergic reward system: a short integrative review, *International Archives of Medicine*. 2010;3:24 doi:10.1186/1755-7682-3-24. This file is licensed under the Creative Commons Attribution 2.0 Generic license.)

neurons in the ventral tegmental area, resulting in increased dopamine release from the prefrontal cortex and nucleus accumbens, regions that play prominent roles in depression.[34]

Dysfunction of the noradrenergic (related to noradrenaline, also called norepinephrine) neurotransmitter system is well established in depression.

Noradrenergic neurons communicate to most brain areas, including the prefrontal cortex, hippocampus, thalamus, hypothalamus, and amygdala, all of which play roles in depressive system development. CB1 receptors have been shown in several of these neural regions and are present on noradrenergic axons and terminals.[35]

The presence of cannabinoids in neurotransmitter systems that play a significant role in depression symptomatology offers more insight into the significance of the endocannabinoid system in treating psychiatric illness.[36]

More large-sample controlled human trials are absolutely needed, but "promising results in this field have been established," Katzman and colleagues concluded. CB1 receptor agonists have shown significant antidepressant effects. The dysfunction is more highly pronounced when anxiety is present, and neural regions associated with anxiety disorders have been shown to target patients treated with CBD.[37]

"Although a significant amount of research in this field is still required to fully elucidate the role of the endocannabinoid system and the effects and safety of treatments targeting it, current results

---

34 Ibid.
35 Ibid.
36 Ibid.
37 Ibid.

are promising," Katzman and colleagues wrote.[38]

"Continued research in this field may provide clinicians with greater treatment options that could potentially enhance patient adherence [to medications] due to both effectiveness and lower rates of adverse events," they added, noting that "cannabinoid products may potentially represent a significant clinical advancement for patients suffering with a variety of psychiatric disorders, and further research is thus imperative."[39]

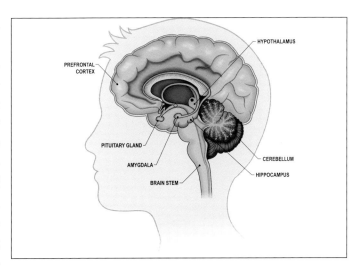

Noradrenergic neurons communicate to most brain areas, including the prefrontal cortex, hippocampus, thalamus, hypothalamus, and amygdala. (From iStock by jambojam)

The ECS, Depression, and a Link with Neurogenesis

In their 2013 *Annual Review of Psychology* paper[40] on the endocannabinoid system and the brain, Mechoulam and Parker wrote that a current hypothesis of depression is that it's linked with neurogenesis, the process by which neural stem cells produce neurons.

This hypothesis is based on downregulation (decrease) of neurogenesis in depressive-like behaviors in animals and upregulation (increase) by antidepressant treatments. Over the past few years, the researchers wrote, much data has indicated that the ECS plays a central role in neurogenesis.[41]

CB1 mRNA is expressed in many regions of the developing brain, CB1 activation is required for the axonal growth response, the ECS drives neural progenitor cell proliferation (differentiating into some neuronal and glial cell types), and cannabinoids actually promote neurogenesis. Reductions in adult neurogenesis were noted in CB1 and CB2 knockout mice, Mechoulam and Parker wrote.[42]

---

38 Ibid.
39 Ibid.
40 Mechoulam, R., and L. A. Parker.
41 Ibid.
42 Ibid.

Clinical Trials: Cannabinoids, Depression and Related Disorders

Effects of Marijuana on Symptoms of OCD

This pilot research study will test whether certain cannabinoids (THC, CBD) may help reduce symptoms in patients with obsessive-compulsive disorder (OCD). Patients enrolled in the study will smoke cannabis containing different concentrations of THC and CBD. Both act on the brain's endocannabinoid system, which is hypothesized to play a role in OCD. The study had twenty participants and began in October 2017. The estimated completion date was March 2019. Details of the study are available at clinicaltrials.gov/ct2/show/ NCT03274440.

Cannabis Observational Study on Mood, Inflammation, and Cognition (COSMIC)

An observational study examines the effects of cannabis on cognition and other domains of function (inflammation, inflammatory response, mood) and whether those effects depend on the product's ratio of THC to CBD. The study began in July 2016 and the estimated completion date is April 2021. The study will have 280 adult participants. Study details are available at clinicaltrials.gov/ ct2/show/NCT03522103.

Effect of Medical Marijuana on Neurocognition and Escalation of Use (MMNE)

This study will use a randomized controlled design to test whether patients who use medical cannabis, compared to a waitlist control group, experience a change in health outcomes (symptom relief [pain, depression, insomnia, and anxiety], or adverse health outcomes like new-onset symptoms of cannabis use disorders, neurocognitive impairments) or brain-based changes. The trial, recruiting 200 adults, began in July 2017 and ends March 2022. Study details are available at clinicaltrials.gov/ct2/show/NCT03224468.

Anxiety, Inflammation, and Stress

An observational study is investigating whether anxiety-relieving and anti-inflammatory effects of cannabis vary with the ratio of CBD to THC to shed light on mixed data linking cannabis use and anxiety. The study start date was April 2018 and the estimated completion date is June 2022. Estimated enrollment will be 210 adults. Details of the study are available at clinicaltrials .gov/ct2/show/NCT03491384.

Other researchers have reported that receptors CB1 and VR1 (also called TRPV1, transient receptor potential vanilloid receptor type 1) are involved in adult neurogenesis. The CB2 receptor has also been shown to promote neural progenitor cell proliferation. Because increased CB2 receptor expression reduces depressive-related behaviors, apparently through a mechanism that differs from that of most antidepressants, the CB2 receptor could be a novel therapeutic target for depression.[43]

The researchers said it would be of interest to establish whether CB2 receptor activity in depression is related to neurogenesis. Because depression decreases neurogenesis, the findings above are particularly exciting because they help researchers understand endocannabinoids' role as the body's endogenous antidepressants and suggest that synthetic endocannabinoid-like compounds may be developed as a novel type of antidepressant drug.[44]

Cannabinoids and Schizophrenia
Schizophrenia is a mental disorder characterized by disrupted thought processes, perceptions, emotional responsiveness, and social interactions. Schizophrenia's course varies among individuals, but it's typically persistent and can be severe and disabling, according to the National Institute of Mental Health (NIMH).[45]

The disorder includes psychotic symptoms like hallucinations, delusions, and thought disorder (unusual ways of thinking), along with reduced expression of emotions, reduced motivation to achieve goals, difficulty in social relationships, and motor and cognitive impairment. Symptoms typically start in late adolescence or early adulthood. Cognitive impairment and unusual behavior sometimes appear in childhood, and the persistence of multiple symptoms represent a later stage of schizophrenia. This pattern may reflect disruptions in brain development and environmental factors like prenatal or early-life stress.[46]

Schizophrenia symptoms fall into three categories: positive, negative, and cognitive. Positive symptoms are psychotic behaviors not usually seen in healthy people. People with positive symptoms may lose touch with some aspects of reality. Symptoms include hallucinations, delusions, thought disorder, and movement disorders.[47]

---

43 Ibid.
44 Ibid.
45 National Institutes of Health. National Institute of Mental Health, schizophrenia, https://www .nimh.nih.gov/health/statistics/schizophrenia.shtml. Accessed 12/4/18.
46 Ibid.
47 Ibid.

Negative symptoms are associated with disruptions to normal emotions and behaviors. Symptoms include flat affect (reduced expression of emotions), reduced feelings of pleasure in everyday life, difficulty beginning and sustaining activities, and reduced speaking.[48]

Cognitive symptoms are subtle for some patients. For others they are more severe, and patients may notice changes in memory or other aspects of thinking. Symptoms include poor executive functioning (the ability to understand information and use it to make decisions), trouble focusing or paying attention, and problems with working memory (the ability to use information immediately after learning it).[49]

Several risk factors contribute to the risk of developing schizophrenia. Scientists have long known that schizophrenia can run in families, but many schizophrenia patients don't have a family member with the disorder, and many people with one or more schizophrenic family members don't develop it themselves.[50]

Many genes may increase schizophrenia risk, but no single gene causes the disorder, and it's not yet possible to genetically predict who will develop schizophrenia. Scientists also think interactions are needed between genes and aspects of a patient's environment for schizophrenia to develop.[51]

An imbalance in the brain's complex, interrelated chemical reactions involving the neurotransmitters dopamine, glutamate, and possibly others play a role in schizophrenia. Some experts also think problems during brain development before birth may lead to faulty connections.[52]

NIMH notes it's hard to get good estimates of schizophrenia prevalence because of the complexity of schizophrenia diagnosis, its overlap with other disorders, and different methods for determining diagnoses.[53]

The best data right now, across studies that use household-based survey samples, clinical diagnostic interviews, and medical records, estimate that prevalence estimates of schizophrenia and related psychotic disorders in the United States are between 0.25 percent and 0.64 percent. The estimate of international schizophrenia prevalence among non-institutionalized people is 0.33 percent to 0.75 percent.[54]

---

48 Ibid.
49 Ibid.
50 Ibid.
51 Ibid.
52 Ibid.
53 Ibid.
54 Ibid.

Cannabinoids and Schizophrenia: Exploring all Approaches

A 2016 *Journal of Clinical Psychopharmacology* review paper[55] by M. A. Katzman and colleagues focuses on the endocannabinoid system and psychiatric illness. In the section on schizophrenia, the researchers noted that a significant amount of research has been conducted in the field, but the disease's cause is still unclear.

Long-term treatment at first consisted mainly of first-generation (chlorpromazine, haloperidol, perphenazine, others) and later mainly second-generation (risperidone, olanzapine, quetiapine, others) antipsychotics. Given remission rates of about 35 percent, and with nearly 75 percent of schizophrenia patients discontinuing medication within eighteen months (mainly because of

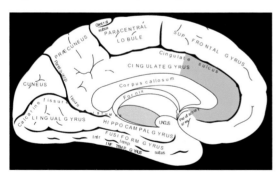

Medial surface of left cerebral hemisphere, with anterior cingulate highlighted (From Wikimedia Commons by Brodmann and Mysid, colored by User:was_a_bee. This file is in the public domain.)

adverse effects), there's a need to explore all potentially efficacious treatment approaches, especially those with better tolerability, the researchers wrote.[56]

A postmortem study in ten schizophrenic patients showed an extensive and homogenous distribution of CB1 receptors in the anterior cingulate cortex, which is involved in decision-making and emotional regulation.[57]

The researchers noted a significant increase in the binding of a synthetic CB1 antagonist (inhibitor) in the schizophrenic group compared with controls. Because the anterior cingulate cortex and CB1 receptors have been hypothesized to play a central role in cognition, motivation, and attention, the core negative features of schizophrenia, including lack of motivation and attention, potentially may be understood in terms of specific changes in the endocannabinoid system in the anterior cingulate cortex.[58]

Researchers also have seen changes in endocannabinoid mediators like anandamide in people with schizophrenia, with data suggesting that anandamide signaling is hyperactive in these patients, the researchers wrote. One study showed that anandamide cerebrospinal fluid levels were about eightfold higher in schizophrenic patients who hadn't yet taken

55 Katzman, M. A., M. Furtado, and L. Anand.
56 Ibid.
57 Ibid.
58 Ibid.

antipsychotics at their first episode compared to healthy controls.[59]

There's evidence of an association between cannabis use and psychosis symptoms, but this causal relationship remains unclear and confounded by variables like genetic contributions. Other findings, Katzman and colleagues wrote, suggest that increased cannabis use may downregulate (decrease) anandamide signaling in schizophrenic patients, and this must be considered when determining the impact of cannabis use on one's mental health.[60]

Determining the strain and content of the cannabis used is essential, they added, in part related to the large variability in cannabinoid content in cannabis and therefore potentially varied outcomes with cannabis use.[61]

Results from a meta-analysis showed cognitive improvements associated with cannabis use in first-episode schizophrenic patients. Eighty-five patients meeting DSM-IV criteria for schizophrenia and presenting with their first psychotic episode were divided into groups—lifetime regular cannabis use and no regular use—and were compared with healthy non-using controls.[62]

Researchers assessed cognitive functioning, and the schizophrenia groups showed expected significant impairments in all cognitive functioning tasks compared to healthy controls. But when comparing the two schizophrenic groups, the non-using group was significantly impaired on fifteen of sixteen tasks, and the cannabis-using group showed only selective impairments on nine tasks.[63]

Interestingly, Katzman and colleagues wrote, the cannabis-using schizophrenic group didn't differ significantly on most cognitive tasks measuring visual memory and planning/reasoning, but the non-using schizophrenic group showed significant impairments. These findings potentially showed cognitive improvements in a schizophrenic population with regular cannabis use. Potential limitations and biases associated with the findings include small sample size and a lack of replicated studies.[64]

Still, as other studies have shown, these findings may point to the value of higher levels of the nonintoxicating cannabinoid CBD in cannabis, which may have been the driving force in relieving psychotic symptoms and improving cognition.[65]

---

59 Ibid.
60 Ibid.
61 Ibid.
62 Ibid.
63 Ibid.
64 Ibid.
65 Ibid.

CBD and Schizophrenia

The same researchers continued their investigation into the CBD in schizophrenic patients in a double-blind randomized clinical trial investigating the effectiveness of CBD versus the second-generation antipsychotic amisulpride in forty-two inpatients suffering from acute schizophrenia symptoms. After an initial screening, in which patients had to be free of antipsychotics for at least three days, they were randomized to receive CBD or amisulpride.[66]

CBD dosing was initiated at 200 mg a day and increased by 200 mg a day to reach a daily dose of 800 mg (200 mg, four times a day). Analyses showed that efficacy was similar in both treatment groups. Katzman and colleagues wrote that this result suggests CBD is as effective in improving psychotic symptoms as the amisulpride.[67]

CBD also was associated with significantly fewer extrapyramidal symptoms (tremor, slurred speech, anxiety, paranoia, and other symptoms mainly associated with improper dosing of antipsychotic medications), less weight gain, and lower prolactin increases (which is known to predict sexual dysfunction) than the amisulpride.[68]

Because many studies have suggested that high-THC cannabis products can induce psychotic symptoms, the researchers wrote, another study assessed whether administering pure CBD before THC treatment can inhibit psychosis and resulting cognitive impairments. Forty-eight healthy participants were randomized to receive CBD (600 mg) or placebo 210 minutes before receiving intravenous THC (1.5 mg), and experimental measures were assessed at baseline, post-CBD/placebo, and post-THC.[69]

Those treated with placebo before THC showed clinically significant positive psychotic symptoms (hallucinations, delusions, thought disorder, movement disorders) compared with the CBD group, and results from a verbal learning task were statistically poorer in the placebo group compared with the CBD group, supporting CBD's inhibiting action on THC-induced psychotic symptoms, Katzman and colleagues wrote. CBD's potential protective action was further shown in 140 cannabis users who were divided into groups based on hair samples as follows: THC only, THC+CBD, and no cannabinoids.[70]

Results showed that the THC-only group had more delusions and other schizophrenia symptoms compared with

---

66 Ibid.
67 Ibid.
68 Ibid.
69 Ibid.
70 Ibid.

the THC+CBD and no cannabinoids groups. This further suggests CBD's potential antipsychotic effects, which may act as a protective barrier against psychotic symptoms induced by THC alone, and makes it even more important to know which cannabinoids people are using.[71]

Overall, Katzman and colleagues wrote, it's imperative to understand the types of cannabinoids people are using to understand the types of effects they're likely to experience. This is unlike what clinicians traditionally do—lump cannabinoids into one category and conceptualize cannabis abuse into a risk factor for psychosis. In doing this, they added, clinicians miss the chance to investigate the exciting potential role of specific cannabinoids, and CBD in particular, in clinical populations.[72]

CBD has shown therapeutic potential as an antipsychotic in schizophrenia, and it can be hypothesized to act through its ability to block CB1 receptor signaling. Further studies are needed to thoroughly assess the therapeutic potential and tolerability of CBD for treating schizophrenia.[73]

The First Placebo-Controlled Trial of CBD in Schizophrenia

In a 2018 *American Journal of Psychiatry* paper,[74] P. McGuire and colleagues discussed their randomized, double-blind, placebo-controlled clinical study that assessed the safety and effectiveness of the nonintoxicating CBD added to current treatments in schizophrenia patients.

The first evidence that CBD might be useful in treating schizophrenia came from a case report about how it improved symptoms in a patient who hadn't responded to the antipsychotic haloperidol. CBD also was reported to reduce psychotic symptoms in patients with Parkinson's disease. The only previous trial of CBD in schizophrenia, described in the segment above by Katzman and colleagues, compared CBD and amisulpride.[75]

Both treatments—haloperidol and CBD—were similarly effective, but CBD had fewer adverse effects. The present study sought to explore CBD safety and effectiveness as an adjunctive (additional) treatment in schizophrenia. In the randomized double-blind trial, patients who'd been partially responsive to antipsychotic medication received CBD or placebo as an add-on treatment for six

---

71 Ibid.
72 Ibid.
73 Ibid.
74 McGuire, P., P. Robson, W. J. Cubala, D. Vasile, P. D. Morrison, R. Barron, A. Taylor, and S. Wright. "Cannabidiol (CBD) as an adjunctive therapy in schizophrenia: A multicenter randomized controlled trial." *Am J Psychiatry* 175:225–31 (doi: 10.1176/appi.ajp.2017.17030325).
75 Ibid.

weeks. McGuire and colleagues examined CBD effects on positive and negative psychotic symptoms, cognitive performance, functioning level, and the treating psychiatrist's clinical impression.[76]

"This is, to our knowledge, the first placebo-controlled trial of CBD in schizophrenia," McGuire and colleagues wrote.[77]

"The data indicate that 6 weeks of treatment adjunctive to antipsychotic medication was associated with significant effects both on positive psychotic symptoms and on the treating clinician's impressions of improvement and illness severity," the researchers added. "There were also improvements in cognitive performance and in the level of overall functioning, although these fell short of statistical significance."[78]

The effect's magnitude on positive symptoms was modest, but it was seen in patients who already were being treated with antipsychotics, so the improvement was over and above antipsychotic treatment, McGuire and colleagues wrote.[79]

Changes in scores on two clinical global impression scales showed an improvement that was evident to the treating psychiatrists and so may be clinically meaningful. The findings were consistent with previous evidence that CBD can reduce psychotic symptoms in schizophrenia, in Parkinson's disease, and in THC-induced psychosis. CBD, the researchers noted, was well tolerated, and adverse event rates were similar between the CBD and placebo groups.[80]

"These findings suggest that CBD has beneficial effects in patients with schizophrenia," McGuire and colleagues wrote. "As CBD's effects do not appear to depend on dopamine receptor antagonism, this agent may represent a new class of treatment for the disorder."[81]

Clinical Trials: Cannabinoids and Schizophrenia

Cannabis, Schizophrenia, and Reward: Self-Medication and Agonist Treatment?

In this translational research proposal, the investigators sought to confirm and expand on pilot data from a previous study suggesting that cannabis and dronabinol (synthetic THC) given in low doses to 240 patients with schizophrenia and co-occurring cannabis use disorder will improve brain reward circuit dysregulation and provide

76 Ibid.
77 Ibid.
78 Ibid.
79 Ibid.
80 Ibid.
81 Ibid.

evidence supporting the role of cannabis as a "self-medication" agent for them. The study start date was July 2014 and the estimated completion date is April 2020. Study details are available at clinicaltrials.gov/ct2/show/NCT01964404.

Cannabis and Thought Disorder in Schizophrenia (CANDI)
The objective of the CANDI study is to assess whether the cannabis use level in fifty patients with schizophrenia modulates the level of thought disorder by modulating functional connectivity between the brain's temporal lobe and putamen. Analyses will be controlled for cannabis composition, in particular the THC:CBD ratio. The start date was October 2018 and the estimated completion date is December 2021. Study details are available at clinicaltrials.gov/ct2/show/NCT03608137.

Evaluation of the Antipsychotic Efficacy of Cannabidiol in Acute Schizophrenic Psychosis
In this study, investigators evaluated CBD effectiveness in treating schizophrenic and schizophreniform psychoses, noting that CBD may be effective in at least a subgroup of these patients and may be expected to reduce anxiety with only minor side effects. The study began in October 2002 and ended in March 2008. In the investigators' 2012 paper[82] on the study, they wrote that results suggested inhibiting anandamide deactivation (thus increasing anandamide activity) may contribute to CBD's antipsychotic effects, potentially representing a new mechanism for treating schizophrenia. Study details are available at clinicaltrials.gov/ct2/show/NCT00628290.

Enhancing Recovery in Early Schizophrenia (CBD)
This study evaluated CBD's effectiveness and safety in maintenance treatment of schizophrenia compared to placebo as an add-on to established treatment with amisulpride, aripiprazole, olanzapine, quetiapine, or risperidone. The study is a twelve-month double-blind, parallel-group, randomized, placebo-controlled clinical trial to gain data on CBD's antipsychotic potential with 180 participants. The study began in April 2017 and the estimated completion date is March 2020. Study details are available at clinicaltrials.gov/ct2/show/NCT02926859.

---

82 Leweke, F. M., D. Piomelli, F. Pahlisch, D. Muhl, C. W. Gerth, C. Hoyer, J. Klosterkötter, M. Hellmich, and D. Koethe. "Cannabidiol enhances anandamide signaling and alleviates psychotic symptoms of schizophrenia." *Transl Psychiatry* 2: e94.

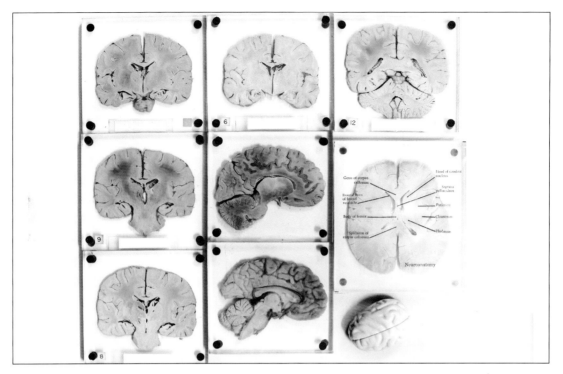

Brain imaging technology has shown addiction to be a brain disease. (From Shutterstock by Atthapon Raksthaput)

Cannabinoids and Addiction

Biological, epidemiological, and social science discoveries of the last three decades offer a detailed understanding of the risks, mechanisms, and consequences of drug abuse and addiction.[83] Scientific advances have transformed the understanding of addiction—from a moral failure to a chronic, relapsing disease.

Scientists have identified brain sites of action where major drugs of abuse—opiates, methamphetamine, cocaine, tobacco, and cannabis—have initial effects. Brain imaging technology has shown addiction to be a brain disease by showing disruptions in addiction's specific brain circuits.[84]

The changes go beyond the brain's reward system to include regions involved in memory, learning, impulse control, stress reactivity, and others. Repeated drug exposure resets the circuits toward compulsive behavior so a person's control over seeking and using

83 National Institutes of Health drug abuse and addiction fact sheet, https://report.nih.gov/nihfact sheets/ViewFactSheet.aspx?csid=38. Accessed 12/7/18.

84 Ibid.

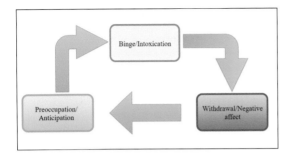

Addiction cycle based on concepts from Koob and Volkow, 2010 (From Wikimedia Commons by User:U3143109. This file is licensed under the Creative Commons Attribution-Share Alike 4.0 International license.)

drugs is compromised, despite negative consequences.[85]

NIH-supported studies of chronic drug exposure, especially in animal models, uncovered the critical role of brain plasticity (adaptability). Addictive drugs modify connection strength between neurons, and this abnormally regulates key brain receptors like glutamate and dopamine. This shows drug addiction as dysfunctional learning that over time can become compulsive behavior.[86]

Addiction is a treatable disease that needs ongoing care and a range of approaches, as do other chronic conditions like diabetes or cardiovascular disease. Treatment includes medications available for nicotine, alcohol, and opioid addiction, and behavioral treatments for these and addictions that have no approved medications.[87]

Emerging medications and treatment will benefit from expanding knowledge of neurobiology and addiction-related brain circuitry. Research has shown that cannabinoids may be promising targets for new medications that treat addiction and health problems like pain.[88]

The Endocannabinoid System's Role in Addiction

Managing the complex disease of addiction makes it critical that scientists identify new therapeutic approaches. One of these novel approaches involves the endocannabinoid system, which plays a crucial role in the neurobiological substrate (layer) underlying drug addiction, J. Manzanares and colleagues wrote in a November 2018 *Biochemical Pharmacology* paper.[89]

First, the researchers describe what scientists know about the substrate. Using opioids, stimulants, alcohol, nicotine, cannabinoids, and other drugs of abuse enhances mesolimbic (central limbic system) dopamine system activity. All these drugs increase dopamine release

85 Ibid.
86 Ibid.
87 Ibid.
88 Ibid.
89 Manzanares, J., D. Cabañero, N. Puente, M. S. García-Gutiérrez, P. Grandes, and R. Maldonado. "Role of the endocannabinoid system in drug addiction." *Biochem Pharmacol* 157:108–21 (doi: https://doi.org/10.1016/j.bcp.2018.09.013).

in the nucleus accumbens by stimulating dopamine neurons from the ventral tegmental area, and this neurochemical response is related to the rewarding effects of abused drugs.[90]

The effects produce a pleasurable experience that is crucial for initiating and maintaining drug use, Manzanares and colleagues wrote. But repeated exposure to such drugs produces changes that lead to weakened dopamine release in the reward circuit, making the reward system less sensitive, and the addict, when using, no longer feels the same degree of euphoria. Repeated drug exposure also changes the extended amygdala's circuitry, enhancing a person's reactivity to stress and causing negative emotions.[91]

The "anti-reward" system includes neurotransmitters involved in stress, and the system becomes overactive in the addicted brain, prompting dysphoric (mental suffering) effects when the drug is gone. These emotional negative consequences are crucial to maintaining drug use, leading to compulsive intake to seek reward and to reduce withdrawal symptoms.[92]

Over time, Manzanares and colleagues wrote, repeated drug exposure leads to decision-making impairment related to changes taking place in the prefrontal cortex, which plays a critical role in executive processes like the capacity for self-regulation, behavioral control, and flexibility. Dysfunction in the dopamine reward system and stress circuits and major changes in cortical areas produce profound behavioral impairments leading to the loss of control, compulsive drug use, and relapse that characterize addiction.[93]

Other neurotransmitter systems are involved in addiction's neurobiological substrate, and one that's widely investigated is the endocannabinoid system, which holds possibilities for novel therapeutic approaches.[94]

The CB1 receptor and endocannabinoids that block or activate it, for example, are expressed through the mesocorticolimbic (reward) pathway and in brain regions involved in decision-making, withdrawal symptoms, and relapse. This distribution makes CB1 critical for establishing addiction to cannabinoid drugs and crucial for neurobehavioral processes that the main drugs of abuse trigger, suggesting that CB1 antagonists (inhibitors) may have potential to treat drug addiction.[95]

---

90 Ibid.
91 Ibid.
92 Ibid.
93 Ibid.
94 Ibid.
95 Ibid.

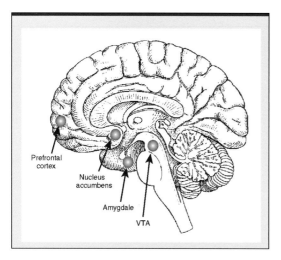

Components of the mesocorticolimbic (reward system) dopamine system and other brain regions affected by stress and its interactions with alcohol and other drugs. (From the National Institute on Alcohol Abuse and Alcoholism by Gary Wand, MD)

Manzanares and colleagues wrote that recent research findings show a potential role for the CB2 receptor in addictive properties of drugs like cocaine and alcohol, presenting a research opportunity to develop possible new therapeutic approaches. The endocannabinoid system "certainly constitutes an excellent source of new possible therapeutic targets for multiple diseases, including drug addiction."[96]

The Endocannabinoid System and Addiction Treatment

In a 2017 *Neuropharmacology* paper,[97] M. E. Sloan and colleagues discussed the endocannabinoid system as a target for several addictions. Despite the toll addictions take on public health, "only a small number of pharmacological treatment strategies are available."

The treatments reduce substance-related mortality but are effective only for a subset of patients, and several substance-use disorders lack a single FDA-approved medication. Many of the drugs just replace the abused drug with one targeting the same receptor system that reduces withdrawal and craving. There's an urgent need, the researchers added, to develop drugs with novel mechanisms of action for patients who don't respond to existing treatments and for those whose drug disorders lack treatments.[98]

Over three decades, compounds that target the endocannabinoid system have been studied as treatments for substance use disorders. Many of the treatments target the CB1 receptor, the main cannabinoid receptor in the central nervous system. CB1 is densely expressed in brain regions (ventral striatum, dorsal striatum, amygdala) involved in developing

96 Ibid.

97 Sloan, M. E., J. L. Gowin, V. A. Ramchandani, L. Yasmin, Y. L. Hurd, and B. Le Foll. "The endocannabinoid system as a target for addiction treatment: Trials and tribulations." *Neuropharmacology* 124:73e83 (http://dx.doi.org/10.1016/j.neuropharm.2017.05.031).

98 Ibid.

and maintaining addictive behavior, and modulating CB1 receptor activity in each region leads to behavioral effects.[99]

CB1 activity, for example, moderates alcohol consumption and alcohol-induced dopamine release in the ventral striatum, affects habit formation in the dorsal striatum, and regulates fear extinction in the amygdala. So compounds that alter endocannabinoid signaling "could be expected to change addictive behavior across substance-use disorders by directly impinging on the neurobiological underpinnings of addiction."[100]

In the following summaries, Sloan and colleagues reviewed evidence from randomized placebo-controlled clinical trials that have investigated whether drugs targeting the endocannabinoid system can help manage substance-use disorders.[101]

Nicotine Use Disorder

A small one-week pilot study that randomized treatment-seeking smokers to a CBD or placebo inhaler found modest reductions in self-reported smoking, but it's unclear which of CBD's pharmacological effects produced the reduction. Further CBD studies are warranted.[102]

Cannabis Use Disorder

Drugs targeting the endocannabinoid system would be a logical strategy for treating cannabis use disorder. Three CB1 agonists (activators) have been studied: dronabinol (synthetic THC in a capsule), nabilone (oral THC analogue) and nabiximols (Sativex), a mouth spray containing about a 1:1 ratio of THC and CBD.

A series of human laboratory trials tested the three medications and found that dronabinol, nabilone, and nabiximols were all effective for cannabis withdrawal, and dronabinol and nabiximols effectiveness for cannabis withdrawal was verified in larger clinical trials involving treatment-seeking participants. Because withdrawal seems to be a factor that leads cannabis-dependent people to relapse, it was hypothesized that prescribing CB1 agonists also could lower relapse rates.

Three randomized controlled trials tested CB1 agonists' relapse prevention effects, and dronabinol alone improved treatment retention. Sativex reduced cannabis withdrawal and increased treatment retention during its administration, but three days later there was no longer a difference in retention. Trials directly comparing dronabinol, nabilone, and Sativex are needed to determine

99 Ibid.
100 Ibid.
101 Ibid.
102 Ibid.

whether any of them produce better clinical outcomes or have better side effect profiles.[103]

Alcohol Use Disorder

Evidence suggests endocannabinoid metabolism can affect alcohol dependence vulnerability and severity, so treatments targeting this system may be effective. Given that CBD has shown early signs of effectiveness in other addictions and recently was found to reduce alcohol consumption in mice, investigating "its effects on human alcohol use is also warranted. Much work remains to be done if we are to elucidate whether the endocannabinoid system is a viable treatment target for alcohol use disorder."[104]

Opioid Use Disorder

All medications now used to prevent opioid-use relapse target the mu-opioid receptor, one of four kinds of opioid receptor.

Dronabinol (synthetic THC in a capsule) has been studied as a clinical opioid withdrawal treatment based on the finding that CB1 blockers reduce some withdrawal symptoms in rodents. One clinical trial randomized opioid-dependent participants to dronabinol or placebo while they were undergoing an eight-day inpatient detoxification with naltrexone (ReVia, Vivitrol). Dronabinol reduced opioid withdrawal symptoms compared

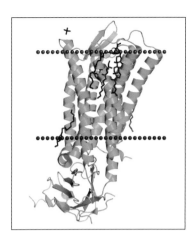

The mu-opioid receptor is one of four kinds of opioid receptor. (From Orientations of Proteins in Membranes database, Lomize Group, College of Pharmacy, University of Michigan, used with permission)

to placebo but the trial didn't compare dronabinol to an active treatment.

In a second human laboratory trial, regular opioid users were admitted to an inpatient unit for five weeks, maintained on oxycodone (semisynthetic codeine derivative), and then withdrawn from it to experimentally induce withdrawal in seven test sessions. Oxycodone but not dronabinol weakened physical withdrawal symptoms. The 20 mg and 30 mg dronabinol doses induced rapid heart rate. When using opioid withdrawal scales rather than direct physiological measures, the 20 mg and 30 mg dronabinol doses reduced withdrawal compared to placebo but were much less effective than oxycodone.

103 Ibid.
104 Ibid.

Pilot data reported in a recent review suggest that CBD may blunt cue-induced craving in opioid dependent people after a period of abstinence. This is being studied in a larger number of participants. More safety data and results from human lab studies are needed before CBD is ready for clinical testing.[105]

Cannabinoids and Alternative Opioid Addiction Treatments

In their 2018 *Cannabis and Cannabinoid Research* paper,[106] B. Wiese and A. R. Wilson-Poe wrote that despite decades of research on how best to treat opioid-use disorder, overdose deaths are at an all-time high and relapse is pervasive. FDA-approved opioid replacement therapies and maintenance medications aren't risk free and don't work for everyone. Legal and logistical bottlenecks make it hard to get traditional opioid replacement therapies like methadone or buprenorphine, and demand far outweighs supply and access.

New treatments or add-ons to traditional drugs are needed, and cannabinoids may have potential to prevent opioid misuse, ease opioid withdrawal symptoms, and decrease relapse. The compelling nature of these data and the relative safety profile of cannabis warrant further exploration of cannabis as an adjunct or alternative opioid use disorder treatment.[107]

Interactions Between Cannabis and Opioids

The endocannabinoid and opioidergic (directly affect opioid systems) systems interact in lots of ways, from their receptor distribution to cross-sensitization of their behavioral pharmacology, Wiese and Wilson-Poe wrote.[108] (In cross-sensitization, sensitization to a stimulus [oxycodone, for example] is generalized to a related stimulus [THC, for example] and this boosts responses to both.)

CB1 receptors and mu opioid receptors are distributed in many of the same brain areas, including the periaqueductal gray, locus coeruleus, ventral tegmental area, nucleus accumbens, prefrontal cortex, raphe nuclei, and others. The extent of this overlapping expression and frequent co-localization of CB1 and mu opioid receptors offer a clear underpinning for interactions between the receptor systems in reward and withdrawal, the researchers wrote.[109]

105 Ibid.
106 Wiese, B., and A. R. Wilson-Poe. "Emerging evidence for cannabis' role in opioid use disorder." *Cannabis Cannabinoid Res* 3.1 (doi: 10.1089/can.2018.0022).
107 Ibid.
108 Ibid.
109 Ibid.

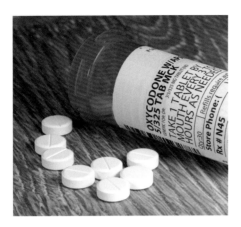

Oxycodone is a semisynthetic, morphine-like opioid alkaloid with pain-relieving activity, according to the NIH PubChem website. Oxycodone exerts its pain-reducing activity by binding to mu-receptors (opioid receptors) in the central nervous system and mimicking the effects of endogenous [biosynthesized in human cells] opioids. (From Shutterstock by Steve Heap)

Cannabis Rather than Opioids for Pain

The main use for prescription opioids and cannabis is to reduce pain. Up to 90 percent of patients in state-level medical cannabis registries list chronic pain as their qualifying condition for the medical program, Wiese and Wilson-Poe wrote.[110]

In an exhaustive 2017 review, the National Academies of Sciences, Engineering and Medicine[111] confirmed the effectiveness of cannabis for chronic pain in adults.

When given access to cannabis, people using opioids for chronic pain decrease their use of opioids by 40 percent to 60 percent and report that they prefer cannabis to opioids. Patients in these studies reported fewer side effects with cannabis than with their opioid medications (including improved cognitive function) and a better quality of life with cannabis than with opioids.

Cannabis is consistently shown to reduce the opioid dose needed to reduce pain. For CBD, pilot clinical studies have shown that in people recently off heroin, CBD reduces heroin craving, Wiese and Wilson-Poe added.[112]

This effect occurs as soon as one hour after CBD administration and lasts up to seven days. As an adjunct (added to another drug), CBD seems safe and tolerable—400 mg and 800 mg oral CBD doesn't intensify the effects of intravenous fentanyl or create adverse effects. CBD also isn't intoxicating or rewarding and has a very large therapeutic window and an impressive safety profile, so using CBD to inhibit opioid craving has great therapeutic potential, they concluded.[113]

---

110 Ibid.
111 National Academies of Sciences, Engineering, and Medicine.
112 Wiese, B., and A. R. Wilson-Poe.
113 Ibid.

Clinical Trials: Cannabinoids and Addiction

MEMO—Medical Marijuana and Opioids Study

This study will examine how medical cannabis use affects opioid analgesic (pain-relieving) use over time, with attention to THC/CBD content, HIV outcomes, and severe adverse events. The study began in September 2018 and will end in June 2022. Participants are 250 adults with chronic pain who are certified for medical cannabis in New York. Study details are available at clinicaltrials.gov/ct2/show/NCT03268551.

Opioid and Cannabinoid Interactions

This study will examine the effects of doses of cannabis and placebo and doses of opioid and placebo, alone and in combination. Primary outcomes are related to pharmacodynamic measures (subjective ratings of drug liking and other abuse-related effects; physiological outcomes) to determine the interaction effects of the compounds. Participants are 105 adults in this randomized, double-blind, placebo-controlled study. The study began in December 2018 and the estimated completion date is December 2021. Study details are available at clinicaltrials.gov/ct2/show/NCT03705559.

Cannabidiol Pharmacotherapy for Adults with Cannabis Use Disorder

Investigators aim to determine Epidiolex's promise as a pharmacotherapy for cannabis use disorder. Investigators hypothesize that Epidiolex (plant-extracted CBD with other cannabinoids), when added to medical management, will produce greater reductions in cannabis use compared to placebo as measured by quantitative THC levels and self-report. In this randomized, double-blind, placebo-controlled trial, sixty cannabis-dependent adults received medical management over six weeks, with half receiving Epidiolex and half receiving placebo. The study began in February 2016 and the estimated study completion date was January 2018. Results and study details are available at clinicaltrials .gov/ct2/show/NCT03102918.

Chapter 13
Cannabinoids and Cancer

Cancer is a group of more than 100 types of related diseases, according to the National Institutes of Health National Cancer Institute (NCI).[1]

In normal circumstances, human cells grow and divide to form new cells when the body needs them. When cells get old or damaged, they die and new cells take their place, but cancer disrupts the process. As cells become more abnormal, old or damaged cells live when they should die and new cells form when they're not needed. The extra cells can divide continuously and some form tumors.[165]

As tumors grow, cancer cells can break off and travel to distant places in the body (metastasis) through the blood or lymph system and form new tumors far from the original. Benign tumors don't spread to or invade nearby tissues, but they can be large. When they're removed, they usually don't grow back as malignant tumors sometimes do. But benign brain tumors can be life threatening.[2]

Cancer cells differ from normal cells in ways that let them grow out of

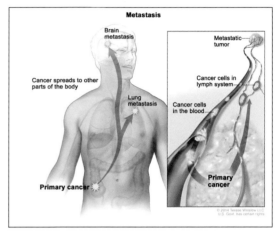

In metastasis, cancer cells break away from where they first form and travel through the blood or lymph system. They form new (metastatic) tumors elsewhere in the body, and these tumors are of the original cancer type. (Courtesy NIH National Cancer Institute by Terese Winslow LLC)

control and become invasive. Normal cells mature into cell types with specific functions and cancer cells don't, which is one reason cancer cells can continuously divide. Cancer cells also aren't affected by signals that tell cells to stop dividing or that start a process called programmed cell death (apoptosis) that the body uses to get rid of unneeded cells.[3]

---

1   National Institutes of Health, National Cancer Institute's Understanding Cancer, https://www .cancer.gov/about-cancer/understanding/what-is-cancer. Accessed 12/18/18.
2   Ibid.
3   Ibid.

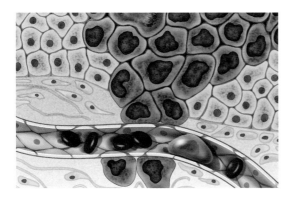

Growing cancer cells (purple) are surrounded by healthy cells (pink), showing a primary tumor spreading to other parts of the body through the circulatory system. (Courtesy NIH National Human Genome Research Institute, by Darryl Leja, NHGRI)

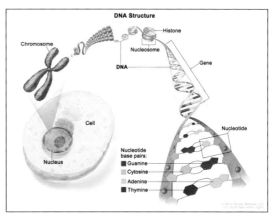

Structure of DNA (Courtesy NIH National Cancer Institute by Terese Winslow LLC)

Cancer cells also can influence normal cells, molecules, and blood vessels that surround and feed a tumor. They can also evade the immune system—a network of organs, tissues, and specialized cells that protects the body from infections and other challenges.[4]

Cancer is a genetic disease caused by changes to genes that control the way cells work, especially how they grow and divide. These genetic changes can be inherited from parents, or they can arise because of errors in cell division or DNA damage caused by environmental exposure to chemicals in tobacco smoke and radiation like ultraviolet rays from the sun, among others.[5]

Each person's cancer has a unique combination of genetic changes, and more occur as the cancer grows. Even within the same tumor, different cells can have different genetic changes. Cancer cells generally have more genetic changes, like DNA mutations, than normal cells do, and some changes may be the cancer's result, not its cause.[6]

Cannabinoids and Cancer in the Clinic | Dr. Donald Abrams

Dr. Donald I. Abrams is an oncologist at Zuckerberg San Francisco General Hospital, an integrative oncologist at the University of California–San Francisco (UCSF) Osher Center for Integrative Medicine, and a professor of clinical medicine at UCSF. He was also a member of the sixteen-person professionally diverse committee that produced the 486-page volume *The Health Effects of*

4   Ibid.
5   Ibid.
6   Ibid.

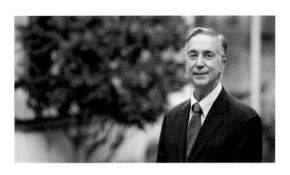

Dr. Donald I. Abrams is an oncologist at Zuckerberg San Francisco General Hospital, an integrative oncologist at the University of California-San Francisco (UCSF) Osher Center for Integrative Medicine, and professor of clinical medicine at UCSF. (Courtesy Dr. Donald I. Abrams)

Cannabis and Cannabinoids: The Current State of Evidence, a 2017 update on the topic from the National Academies of Sciences, Engineering and Medicine.[7]

"I've been an oncologist in San Francisco for thirty-six years now, and I venture to say that most of the cancer patients I've taken care of have used cannabis," he said in a May 3, 2019, interview. "But there isn't a day that goes by where I don't see a cancer patient with loss of appetite, nausea, vomiting, insomnia, pain, depression, or anxiety, and if I have one medicine that can decrease nausea and vomiting, enhance appetite, decrease pain, and improve sleep and mood, I consider that to be a valuable intervention. Instead of writing prescriptions for five or six pharmaceuticals that all could interact with each other or the chemotherapy I prescribe, I can recommend one very safe botanical."

When Abrams was a medical intern and resident in 1970s San Francisco, many people used cannabis, including young people with cancer. He started an oncology fellowship at UCSF in 1980, a time when cannabis was still popular and there weren't many effective anti-emetics (drugs that help nausea and vomiting).

"We had prochlorperazine, or Compazine, and Tigan [trimethobenzamine hydrochloride] . . . but they weren't very good," Abrams said, "and young people getting young-people cancers, such as Hodgkin's disease or testicular cancer, told us, 'You know what? Cannabis is an effective anti-nausea therapy, better than your prescription meds.'" Abrams thinks that's what led the National Institutes of Health National Cancer Institute and several pharmaceutical companies to investigate synthetic delta-9 THC as a potential anti-nausea medication.

"A number of studies were conducted in the '70s and '80s that allowed both dronabinol [synthetic THC in a capsule] and nabilone [oral THC analogue] to be approved in 1985 for treatment of chemotherapy-induced nausea and vomiting. I'm not sure how much of that I used for patients in those days," he added, "but in 1992 the FDA expanded the indication

---

7   National Academies of Sciences, Engineering, and Medicine.

for use of dronabinol to treat anorexia associated with weight loss in patients with HIV."

That's when he first really started with dronabinol, Abrams said, "because I became an AIDS doctor after my training to be a cancer specialist, and that's when I started to really prescribe a lot of dronabinol. And patients said, 'You can keep it. I prefer to smoke cannabis because [dronabinol] takes too long to kick in and when it does I get too zonked.'" Delta-9 THC in sesame oil is a very different medicine from whole-plant cannabis, Abrams said, "and that's what I learned in my first clinical trial."

In the mid-1990s and now, the National Institute on Drug Abuse is the only official source of cannabis for clinical trials, and NIDA has a congressional mandate to fund only studies investigating substances of abuse as substances of abuse and not as therapeutic agents, Abrams said.

"So they could never fund a study that I was trying to do—to show that cannabis benefitted patients with AIDS wasting—but they could fund a study to see if it was safe for HIV patients on protease inhibitors to inhale cannabis, so that study ultimately got funded." It was his first NIH-funded cannabis study. A third of the patients took dronabinol, 2.5 mg three times a day, a third smoked a whole-plant NIDA cigarette, and a third took a dronabinol placebo.

"The patients were each in our General Clinical Research Center for twenty-five days, during twenty-one of which they took the dronabinol or smoked the cannabis. And it was very clear to me which patients were on dronabinol because they were in bed pretty much all day long, totally wiped out. Whereas the cannabis patients were up and dancing, cleaning their rooms, and very much more activated. So yeah," Abrams said, "I think it's definitely a different medicine."

One thing that's fairly dramatic in his experience with cancer patients, Abrams added, is that "a lot of cancer patients at the end of their lives are put on opiates by well-meaning oncologists who are trying to ease their pain and suffering, both physical and emotional. And the patients say, 'This doesn't allow me to communicate with my family because I'm way too stoned.' So they wean off of opiates and just use cannabis, and they like that a lot better."

Abrams said medical cannabis has been legal in California for twenty-three years and recreational for two years, but in the days when a medical recommendation was needed, Abrams would write a letter that patients would take to the dispensary, and that would allow them to obtain cannabis for a year.

"But I didn't say take this strain, this much, this many times a day," he said. "I don't think cannabis is a medication that needs a package insert. Most people can probably figure out how to use it. Every patient is different, every strain is different—I think the best recommendation is 'start low, go slow.' That's become quite a mantra." And Abrams thinks the pharmaceuticalization of cannabis is wrong.

"I think we should regard it as a botanical therapy that's been around for 5,000 years and has significant benefits," the oncologist said. "But to try to say that it's a medicine using a pharmaceutically dominated paradigm might not be correct. I think it should be treated like saw palmetto and echinacea but regulated like tobacco and alcohol, and let responsible adults use it as they see fit."

The Landscape of Medical Cannabis and Cancer

In a 2018 *Cannabis and Cannabinoid Research* perspective article[8] on using cannabis to manage symptoms of those seriously ill with cancer, Dr. Manuel Guzmán, professor of biochemistry and molecular biology at Complutense University of Madrid in Spain, discusses the landscape of medical cannabis, what he calls the "living laboratory" of medical cannabis users.

He also addresses the nearly complete lack of knowledge about the effectiveness and safety profiles of medical cannabis preparations and their most appropriate doses and administration routes.[9]

In the paper he names Israel, led by Professor Raphael Mechoulam, as one of the most prominent countries in scientific and clinical cannabis research. The Israeli Ministry of Health began authorizing medical cannabis in 2007, and more than 30,00 patients there use cannabis, especially for cancer symptoms.[10]

In a March 2018 *European Journal of Internal Medicine* paper, Guzmán writes, Bar-Lev Schleider and colleagues offered insight into about 3,000 of those cancer patients who used prescribed cannabis to manage malignancy-associated symptoms. Just over 60 percent responded to the study, and of these, 95.9 percent reported a significant or moderate improvement in their condition. Only 18.8 percent reported good/very good quality of life before treatment but 69.5 percent did so after the six-month cannabis treatment.[11]

Among the group, cannabis was generally well tolerated, and most side effects reported—dizziness, dry mouth, drowsiness—could be considered mild, Guzmán wrote, especially in the advanced-cancer patient population. The study had

---

8   Guzmán, M. "Cannabis for the Management of Cancer Symptoms: THC Version 2.0?" *Cannabis Cannabinoid Res* 3.1 (doi: 10.1089/can.2018.0009).
9   Ibid.
10 Ibid.
11 Ibid.

limitations but provided precious information about using medical cannabis for managing cancer symptoms.[12]

Based on current knowledge of the cannabinoid mechanism of action, the therapeutic activity of THC-rich preparations for treating classical cancer symptoms is probably due to THC's CB1 receptor activation on precise anatomical sites, Guzmán wrote. Therapeutic activity includes inhibiting nausea and vomiting, stimulating appetite, attenuating cachexia/energy expenditure, and reducing pain, in which effects mediated by CB2 receptors also could be involved.[13]

Beyond THC, Guzmán wrote, it's increasingly accepted that CBD, aside from exerting its own therapeutic activity, buffers the intoxicating risk of cannabis. So THC/CBD-balanced preparations, if well produced and standardized, could be considered a therapeutically safer option than the synthetic, purified THC-like drugs dronabinol and nabilone, whose therapeutic windows tend to be narrow.[14]

Other cannabis constituents (absent in synthetic, purified THC), especially terpenes (myrcene, a-pinene, and beta-caryophyllene), have been proposed to exert synergic therapeutic actions (entourage effect) with plant cannabinoids. The question remains: For each patient in each pathological status, what is the best cannabis chemotype and THC:CBD ratio?[15]

Guzmán says that because *Cannabis sativa* has a complex composition, it's essential to define its precise chemotypes for specific patients as valid therapeutic options. Medical-grade cannabis preparations that could be personalized would improve therapeutic interventions through use of different THC:CBD ratios, activating versus sedating cannabis strains, and slow (oral oils) versus fast (vaporized inflorescences [flower heads]) delivery routes.[16]

But he added that rigorous clinical studies are warranted to move from scattered anecdotal evidence to clinical knowledge. Nowadays, Guzmán wrote, "on practical grounds, interpretation of empirical [based on observation] records on medical cannabis use combined with a rational application of our current understanding of the mechanism of cannabinoid action, as well as some 'trial and error,' may be the only way to delineate which cannabis preparations may adjust best (in terms of efficacy and tolerability)

12 Ibid.
13 Ibid.
14 Ibid.
15 Ibid.
16 Ibid.

to the specific needs of each patient at each disease stage."[17]

Cannabinoids and Antitumor Effects

In a 2018 *British Journal of Pharmacology* review paper[18] about the endocannabinoid system and cancer, A. Fraguas-Sánchez and colleagues wrote, "In the last few decades, the endocannabinoid system has attracted a great deal of interest in terms of its applications to clinical medicine. In particular, its applications in cancer probably represent one of the therapeutic areas with most promise."

On one hand, endocannabinoid system (receptor) expression is altered in numerous tumor types compared to healthy tissue, and this aberrant expression has been related to cancer prognosis and disease outcome, suggesting a role for the endocannabinoid system in tumor growth and progression that depends on cancer type.[19]

On the other hand, Fraguas-Sánchez and colleagues wrote, cannabinoids exert anticancer activity by inhibiting cancer cell proliferation and migration and tumor angiogenesis (when new blood vessels grow to feed tumors).[20]

In a 2018 *Drugs* review paper[21] about the medical use of cannabinoids in different kinds of cancer, Fraguas-Sánchez and Torres-Suárez wrote that an altered endocannabinoid system in cancer indicates the ECS may be a potential target for anticancer treatments, noting that in lab and animal models of cancer, many cannabinoid compounds have been shown to inhibit tumor growth, and cannabinoid receptors mediate some of these effects.

Cannabinoids, Gliomas, and Glioblastomas

Gliomas are brain cancers that begin in glial cells that surround and support nerve cells. Glioblastomas are malignant Grade IV (fast-growing and spreading) tumors in which a large number of tumor cells are reproducing and dividing at any given time.[22]

In the 2000s, Fraguas-Sánchez and Torres-Suárez wrote, the Guzmán group's work on gliomas reported a wide application of cannabinoids as anticancer treatments in these neoplasms (new abnormal

---

17 Ibid.
18 Fraguas-Sánchez, A. I., C. Martín-Sabroso, and A. I. Torres-Suárez. "Insights into the effects of the endocannabinoid system in cancer: a review." *Br J Pharmacol* 175:13 (https://doi.org/10.1111/bph.14331).
19 Ibid.
20 Ibid.
21 Fraguas-Sánchez, A. I., and A. I. Torres-Suárez. "Medical use of cannabinoids." *Drugs* 78:1665–1703 (https://doi.org/10.1007/s40265-018-0996-1).
22 National Institutes of Health, National Cancer Institute's Understanding Cancer.

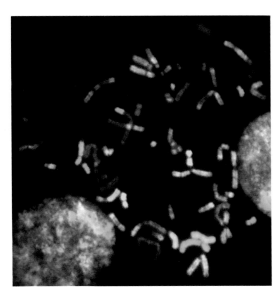

Chromosomes from glioblastoma cells; new research suggests men and women respond differently to glioblastoma treatments. (Courtesy National Cancer Institute)

Some researchers have reported that levels of the endocannabinoid anandamide were lower in gliomas compared with non-tumor tissue, but others detected higher levels of anandamide in gliomas and meningiomas (primary central nervous system tumors that begin in the brain or spinal cord), Fraguas-Sánchez and Torres-Suárez wrote. They cited researchers who reported that the other main endocannabinoid, 2-AG, was upregulated in both kinds of brain tumor.[24]

Cannabinoids also have shown anti-tumor activity in brain cancer, they added, noting that several authors have reported that anandamide inhibited in vitro proliferation of several glioma cells by inducing programmed cell death. Anandamide decreased the cells' migration and invasion; anandamide, 2-AG, and other endocannabinoids reduced the proliferation of C6 glioma cells (a glioma cell line for lab experiments); and these effects were mediated through cannabinoid receptors.[25]

CBD and THC, alone or in combination, have shown anti-proliferative effects, including apoptosis, on several glioma cell lines with CB2 receptor participation, the researchers wrote.[26]

tissue growth). Recent studies have shown that CB1 receptors are overexpressed in glioblastomas and in pediatric low-grade gliomas, where higher CB1 levels have been related to tumor involution (shrinking) because activating CB1 receptors helps generate programmed cell death and arrests the cell cycle. CB2 receptors also are highly expressed in glioblastomas and astrocytomas (astrocyte tumors) and related to tumor grade.[23]

23 Fraguas-Sánchez, A. I., and A. I. Torres-Suárez.
24 Ibid.
25 Ibid.
26 Ibid.

Cannabinoids, Glioblastomas, and Chemotherapy

In a 2018 *Frontiers in Molecular Neuroscience* review paper,[27] C. A. Dumitru and colleagues reported on cannabinoids and their benefits in patients with glioblastoma, one of the most malignant tumors. Cannabinoids' therapeutic effects, they wrote, are based on reducing tumor growth by inhibiting tumor proliferation and angiogenesis (growth of tumor-feeding blood vessels) and inducing tumor cell death.

Cannabinoids also have been shown to inhibit the invasiveness and stem-cell-like properties of glioblastoma tumors. Recent phase 2 clinical trials indicated positive results for survival of glioblastoma patients undergoing cannabinoid treatment, and antitumor cannabinoid effects have been investigated in other studies.[28]

A pilot phase 1 clinical trial for treating glioblastoma patients had a good safety profile for THC, Dumitru and colleagues wrote, and intra-tumor THC administration in nine patients with growing recurrent glioblastoma decreased tumor cell proliferation and induced apoptosis. Cannabinoids also promoted the survival of healthy glial cells in the brain and neurons. A tumor-specific "cytotoxic effect of cannabinoids would therefore have great relevance for the treatment of glioblastoma."[29]

Beneficial effects of THC:CBD preparations in preclinical models led to a placebo-controlled phase 2 clinical trial investigating a THC:CBD mixture given with dose-intense temozolomide (an oral chemotherapy drug) in glioblastoma patients, the researchers wrote. GW Pharmaceuticals reported positive results in treating glioblastoma in their orphan-drug-designated study (clinical trial NCT01812603).[30]

Participants were twenty-one adults with confirmed glioblastoma, receiving orally a maximum of twelve sprays a day delivering 100 ml of Sativex (containing 27 mg/ml THC and 25 mg/ml CBD). The control group received temozolomide only and had a 44 percent one-year survival rate. The Sativex plus temozolomide group had an 83 percent one-year survival rate with median survival over 662 days compared with 369 days in the control group.[31]

Dumitru and colleagues wrote, "These first results of clinical investigations are promising and point to the importance of

---

27 Dumitru, C. A., I. E. Sandalcioglu, and M. Karsak. "Cannabinoids in glioblastoma therapy: New applications for old drugs." *Front Mol Neurosci* 11:159 (doi: 10.3389/fnmol.2018.00159) eCollection 2018.
28 Ibid.
29 Ibid.
30 Ibid.
31 Ibid.

cannabinoid translational research leading to clinically relevant studies."[32]

They added, "Ultimately, these findings might foster the development of improved therapeutic strategies against glioblastoma and perhaps other diseases of the nervous system."[33]

Cannabinoids and Other Cancer Tumors

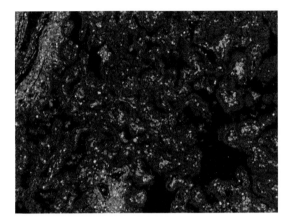

A multiplex spectrally unmixed immunofluorescence image of a lung-cancer tissue stained with seven biomarkers. (Courtesy NIH National Cancer Institute by Houssein A. Sater, NCI)

Cannabinoids also have shown anticancer activity in other kinds of tumors, Fraguas-Sánchez and Torres-Suárez wrote.[34] In lung cancer tumors, for example, it was reported for the first time in 1975 that several cannabinoids (including THC)

could inhibit tumor growth, and that CBD slows lung cancer cell proliferation.

In hepatocarcinoma (the most common primary liver tumor), CB1 and CB2 receptors were overexpressed compared with healthy liver, and this overexpression has been associated with better free-survival rates (the length of time after primary treatment ends that the patient lives with no cancer symptoms). The endocannabinoid anandamide also showed anti-proliferative activity in liver tumors independent of cannabinoid receptors. CB1 and CB2 agonists also have been shown to hinder hepatocarcinoma cell invasion.[35]

"The aforementioned studies suggest the participation of the endocannabinoid

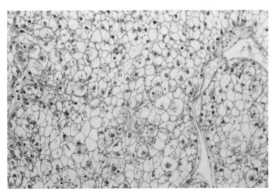

This clear cell variant of hepatocellular carcinoma is a rare entity, occurring at a frequency of less than 10% of hepatocellular carcinoma, associated with hepatitis C and cirrhosis. (From iStock by OGphoto)

---

32 Ibid.
33 Ibid.
34 Fraguas-Sánchez, A. I., and A. I. Torres-Suárez.
35 Ibid.

system in cancer disease and the potential antitumor activity of cannabinoids, perhaps as combined therapy with other antitumor drugs," Fraguas-Sánchez and Torres-Suárez wrote.[36]

But, they added, "the possible use of cannabinoids as chemotherapy is not as clear and depends on cancer type. Among all cannabinoids, THC and CBD appear to be the most promising. The combination of several cannabinoids also could be beneficial, owing to their entourage effect."[37]

CBD, Other Cannabinoids, and Antitumor Effects

In a 2006 *Journal of Pharmacology and Experimental Therapeutics* paper,[38] A. Ligresti and colleagues reported on their investigation of antitumor activities of plant cannabinoids other than THC, which has antitumor effects on different kinds of cancer cell types but whose usage is limited by its psychoactivity.

For the study they used CBD, cannabigerol (CBG), cannabichromene (CBC), cannabidiolic acid (CBDA), and tetrahydrocannabinolic acid (THCA) (precursors to CBD and THC that exist in the plant as acids and become CBD and THC only when exposed to heat or light).[39]

The researchers also assessed the difference in antitumor activity between cannabis extracts enriched in CBD or THC over pure (single) cannabinoids. CBD-rich and THC-rich extracts contained about 70 percent of CBD or THC, and lesser amounts of other cannabinoids.[40] (See chapter 5.)

For the laboratory part of the research, the researchers studied cannabinoid effects using a panel of tumor cell lines: cell lines from human breast carcinoma cells, human prostate carcinoma cells, human colorectal carcinoma cells, human gastric adenocarcinoma (non-small cell lung cancer) cells, rat glioma cells, rat thyroid cells, and rat basophilic leukemia (a rare form of acute leukemia) cells.[41]

Results clearly indicated that of the five natural compounds tested, CBD was the most potent inhibitor of cancer cell growth, with much lower potency in non-cancer cells, Ligresti and colleagues reported. The CBD-rich extract was just as potent as CBD alone, followed

---

36 Ibid.
37 Ibid.
38 Ligresti, A., A. S. Moriello, K. Starowicz, I. Matias, S. Pisanti, L. De Petrocellis, C. Laezza, G. Portella, M. Bifulco, and V. Di Marzo. "Antitumor activity of plant cannabinoids with emphasis on the effect of cannabidiol on human breast carcinoma." *J Pharmacol Exp Ther* 318:1375–87 (doi: 10.1124/jpet.106.105247).
39 Ibid.
40 Ibid.
41 Ibid.

by cannabigerol and cannabichromene. CBD and the CBD-rich extract inhibited the growth of tumors in a mouse model of human breast carcinoma tumors and rat thyroid epithelial cells, and reduced lung metastases from rat-model highly invasive human breast cancer cells.[42]

Their data, Ligresti and colleagues concluded, "indicate that CBD, and possibly cannabis extracts enriched in this natural cannabinoid, represent a promising nonintoxicating antineoplastic [antitumor] strategy. In particular, for a highly malignant human breast carcinoma cell line, we have shown here that cannabidiol and a cannabidiol-rich extract counteract cell growth both in vivo [animal model] and in vitro [test tube, culture dish] and tumor metastasis in vivo."[43]

Cannabinoids and Other Kinds of Cancers

As early as 2003 it was known that the endocannabinoids anandamide and 2-AG inhibited cancer cell proliferation by acting at cannabinoid receptors. Researchers were already examining potential effects of modulating the endocannabinoid system to affect different kinds of cancer.

Endocannabinoids and Colorectal Cancer

Writing in the September 2003 *Gastroenterology*,[44] A. Ligresti and colleagues described their study, which was based on reports of THC's antitumor activity in the lab and in animal models, the anti-proliferative effects of anandamide and 2-AG in breast and prostate cancer cells in the lab, and others. They decided to investigate whether endocannabinoids, their receptors, and FAAH (an enzyme that breaks down anandamide and, under certain experimental conditions, 2-AG[45]), were present, and with what biologic function in colorectal carcinomas and colorectal adenomatous polyps that are known to progress to colorectal carcinoma.

In the study, Ligresti and colleagues obtained healthy and cancerous tissue by biopsy during colonoscopy from twenty-one patients and then compared levels of anandamide, 2-AG, CB1, CB2, and FAAH in normal colon mucosa to those in transformed mucosa (adenomas and carcinomas).[46]

In their results, Ligresti and colleagues showed that endocannabinoids

---

42 Ibid.

43 Ibid.

44 Ligresti, A., T. Bisogno, I. Matias, L. De Petrocellis, M. G. Cascio, V. Cosenza, G. D'Argenio, G. Scaglione, M. Bifulco, I Sorrentini, and V. Di Marzo. "Possible endocannabinoid control of colorectal cancer growth." *Gastroenterology* 3(125):677–87.

45 Di Marzo, V., and M. Maccarrone. "FAAH and anandamide: is 2-AG really the odd one out?" *Trends Pharmacol Sci* 29(5):229–33 (doi: 10.1016/j.tips.2008.03.001) Epub April 18, 2008.

46 Ibid.

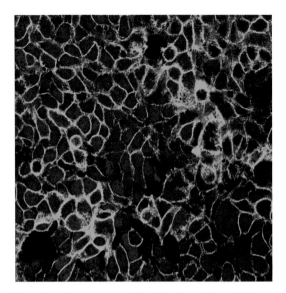

Human colon cancer cells with the cell nuclei stained red and the protein E-cadherin stained green. E-cadherin is a cell adhesion molecule whose loss signals a process where cells acquire the ability to migrate and become invasive. (Courtesy NIH National Cancer Institute Center for Cancer Research by Urbain Weyemi, Christophe E. Redon, William M. Bonner)

expressed in colorectal mucosa and colorectal carcinoma cells, they added.[47]

"Endocannabinoids can be regarded as potential endogenous tumor-growth inhibitors [and] possible markers for cancer cells," they wrote, noting that metabolically stable substances that act by directly stimulating cannabinoid receptors could have anticancer actions in colorectal carcinoma and other tumors. They suggested substances that further enhance tumor levels of anandamide and 2-AG, like inhibitors of the endocannabinoids' cellular uptake and enzymatic breakdown (endocannabinoid system enzymes), might be a more effective and tolerable treatment strategy against colorectal carcinoma and other kinds of cancer.[48]

The Endocannabinoid System and Breast Cancer

In their 2019 *International Journal of Molecular Sciences* review paper,[49] T. Kisková and colleagues wrote that cannabinoids from the cannabis plant provide relief for tumor-associated symptoms (nausea, anorexia, neuropathic pain) in the palliative treatment of cancer patients, and that cannabinoids also may decelerate tumor progression in breast cancer patients. THC, CBD, and other

are overproduced in cancerous and especially precancerous (adenoma) colon tissue, and wrote that, "they have a growth-inhibitory effect on colorectal carcinoma cells in culture, in which the extent of their action and levels seems to depend on the degree of differentiation [and malignancy/invasiveness] of these cells." Endocannabinoid anti-proliferative effects are largely exerted by stimulating cannabinoid receptors that are

47 Ibid.
48 Ibid.
49 Kisková, T., F. Mungenast, M. Suváková, W. Jäger, and T. Thalhammer. "Future aspects for cannabinoids in breast cancer therapy." *Int J Mol Sci* 20:1673–94 (doi:10.3390/ijms20071673).

cannabinoids inhibited disease progression in breast cancer models.

In breast cancer, CB1 expression is moderate but CB2 expression is high and related to tumor aggressiveness. Cannabinoids block cell-cycle progression and cell growth, and induce cancer-cell apoptosis, or programmed cell death, by inhibiting certain pro-oncogenic signaling pathways. They reduce angiogenesis (blood vessel growth that feeds tumors) and tumor metastasis in animal models of breast cancer.[50]

Cannabinoids are active against estrogen receptor-positive and estrogen-resistant breast cancer cells. In human epidermal growth factor receptor 2-positive and triple-negative breast cancer cells, blocking protein kinase B- and cyclooxygenase-2 (COX-2)-signaling via CB2 prevents tumor progression and metastasis. Selective estrogen receptor modulators (SERMs), including tamoxifen, bind to cannabinoid receptors, and this process may contribute to the growth-inhibitory effect of SERMs in cancer cells lacking the estrogen receptor.[51]

In summary, the researchers wrote in their abstract, "cannabinoids are already administered to breast cancer patients at advanced stages of the disease, but they might also be effective at earlier stages to decelerate tumor progression."[52]

Cannabinoid Receptors, Endocannabinoids, and Prostate Cancer

CB1 and CB2 receptor expression is higher in prostate cancer than in normal prostate tissue, Fraguas-Sánchez and Torres-Suárez wrote,[53] and CB1 overexpression has been associated with a major Gleason score (grading system for prostate cancer aggression) and metastasis incidence, serving as a negative marker for prostate cancer outcome.

Other studies have reported cannabinoid anti-proliferative activity in prostate tumors, and anandamide inhibits the cell proliferation and primary cultures of prostate cancer via CB1 receptors. THC and CBD anti-proliferative activity doesn't involve cannabinoid receptors.[54]

Endocannabinoids decrease prostate cancer cell invasion, and 2-AG has been suggested as a potential inhibitor of androgen prostate tumor invasion with the involvement of CB1 receptors. The increase of 2-AG levels through MAGL enzyme inhibition also interfered with cancer progression (MAGL inhibits 2-AG breakdown).[55]

50 Ibid.
51 Ibid.
52 Ibid.
53 Fraguas-Sánchez, A. I., and A. I. Torres-Suárez.
54 Ibid.
55 Ibid.

Cannabinoids in Cancer Treatment

In a 2017 *Advances in Pharmacology* paper,[56] R. Ramer and B. Hinz wrote that the endocannabinoid system has become a target for drug therapy approaches to treating many diseases. Besides the palliative (treating pain but not the disease's cause) effects of cannabinoids used in cancer treatment, plant cannabinoids, synthetic agonists, and substances that boost endocannabinoid levels have attracted interest as potential systemic cancer treatment agents (which spread throughout the body to treat cancer).

Cannabinoid compounds have been reported to inhibit tumor growth and spreading in many rodent models, and the underlying mechanisms include inducing apoptosis, autophagy (the cell's natural process for breaking down and clearing damaged cells), cell-cycle arrest in tumor cells, and inhibiting tumor-cell invasion and angiogenic (forming new blood vessels) features of endothelial cells (which cover inside and outside surfaces of the body and organs).[57]

Cannabinoids also have been shown to enhance tumor immune surveillance, support chemotherapy effects on drug-resistant cancer cells, and suppress epithelial-to-mesenchymal transition,[58] the process that turns epithelial cells into mesenchymal cells. In this process, according to the mechanobiology website MBINFO,[59] epithelial cells (which line the body's hollow structures, like the gut) lose the ability to, for example, migrate, proliferate, and begin the process of metastasis.

Ramer and Hinz wrote that the significance of drugs that help inhibit metastasis is that almost all fatal progressions of malignant diseases are associated with metastasis. Specific options for counteracting metastasis are barely available, so there's an urgent need for new therapeutics that target these processes. Based on preclinical findings, cannabinoids may serve as anti-metastatics to improve clinical prospects for treating advanced-stage cancer diseases.[60]

"Cannabinoids may support the future armamentarium for treatment of cancer diseases beyond their palliative use as inhibitors of cancer growth," the researchers concluded, "as cytostatic boosters, as anti-metastatics and as inhibitors of tumor neovascularization [new blood vessel formation], given that clinical studies will [one day] exceed case

56 Ramer, R., and B. Hinz. "Cannabinoids as Anticancer Drugs." *Adv Pharmacol* 80(12):397–436 (doi: http://dx.doi.org/10.1016/bs.apha.2017.04.002).

57 Ibid.

58 Ibid.

59 MBINFO: Defining Mechanobiology, https://www.mechanobio.info/development/what-is-the-epithelial-to-mesenchymal-transition-emt/. Accessed 1/21/19.

60 Ramer, R., and B. Hinz.

reports and will provide evidence for considerable systemic benefits."[61]

CBD and Cancer in the Clinic

In a 2018 *Anticancer Research* paper,[62] J. Kenyon and colleagues assessed the effects of pharmaceutical-grade synthetic CBD on a range of cancer patients. The investigators analyzed data routinely collected as part of their treatment program in 119 cancer patients over four years and saw clinical responses in 92 percent of the 119 cases with solid tumors.

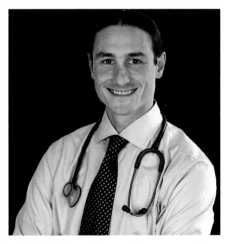

Dr. Dustin Sulak is an integrative osteopathic physician and medical cannabis expert whose clinical practice has focused on treating refractory conditions in adults and children with cannabis and other integrative techniques since 2009. (Courtesy Dr. Dustin Sulak)

This included "a reduction in circulating tumor cells in many cases, and in other cases a reduction in tumor size as shown by repeat scans.

"No side effects of any kind were observed when using pharmaceutical grade synthetic cannabidiol," they added. Among the patients who clearly improved using the synthetic CBD were a seventy-two-year-old prostate cancer patient, a sixty-eight-year-old breast cancer patient with bone metastasis, a sixty-five-year-old female with esophageal cancer, a sixty-five-year-old patient with breast cancer, a sixty-two-year-old patient with breast cancer, and a sixty-seven-year-old patient with lobular breast cancer.[63]

"The fact that we have been able to document improvement in cancer in a few patients strongly supports further studies of CBD-based products in cancer patients who have exhausted standard treatments. Our primary data in a murine [mice and other rodents] glioma model showing enhanced sensitivity to radiotherapy without any side effects suggests this would be an ideal clinical trial to initiate in the first instance."[64]

---

61 Ibid.
62 Kenyon, J., W. Liu, and A. Dalgleish. "Report of objective clinical responses of cancer patients to pharmaceutical-grade synthetic cannabidiol." *Anticancer Res* 38:5831–5 (doi:10.21873/anticanres. 12924).
63 Ibid.
64 Ibid.

Cannabinoids and Cancer in the Clinic | Dr. Dustin Sulak

When working with cancer patients, Dr. Dustin Sulak says,[65] cannabis treatment efforts often take two distinct paths—using cannabis to reduce symptoms and improve treatment tolerability, or using cannabis, typically in high doses, to help kill the cancer. The goals aren't mutually exclusive, he adds, but each requires a different approach to dosing.

Sulak is an integrative osteopathic physician and medical cannabis expert whose clinical practice has focused on treating refractory conditions in adults and children with cannabis and other integrative techniques since 2009. He is the founder of Integr8 Health, a medical practice in Maine that follows more than 8,000 patients using medical cannabis, and Healer.com, a medical cannabis education resource. He sits on the board of directors of the Society of Cannabis Clinicians, has published in the peer-reviewed literature, and lectures to healthcare providers internationally on the clinical applications of cannabis.[66]

The following information is adapted, with permission, from Sulak's Healer.com educational website, where he offers a range of programs about medical cannabis and a medical cannabis training and certification program for physicians, other health professionals, and consumers.[67]

Cannabis to Relieve Cancer Symptoms and Treatment Side Effects

When used properly, cannabis can be a safe, effective treatment for cancer patients with chronic pain, insomnia, and chemotherapy-induced nausea and vomiting. Animal studies have shown that cannabinoids can prevent the development of neuropathic pain, a common chemotherapy side effect that can limit a patient's chemo dose or course. Even after achieving cancer remission, many patients are left with debilitating neuropathic pain that can be permanent.[68]

"Patients can often achieve significant improvements in quality of life with minimal side effects, using very low doses of cannabinoids in the range of 10 mg to 60 mg per day," Sulak writes in his course materials. "A combination of THC, CBD, and other cannabinoids in various ratios can be used to fine-tune the benefits and minimize the side effects of cannabinoid treatment."[69]

---

65 Sulak, D.
66 Ibid.
67 Ibid.
68 Ibid.
69 Ibid.

Medical cannabis can help patients tolerate conventional cancer treatments like chemo and radiation, and can be used along with these treatments with a low likelihood of drug interaction. This means there is seldom a reason to avoid combining cannabis with conventional cancer treatments, with a few exceptions noted in the educational materials. For patients with terminal cancer, cannabis offers many benefits in palliative care at the end of life.[70]

Sulak adds, "It's an incredibly useful addition to conventional treatments in hospice medicine."[71]

Cannabis to Fight Cancer and Promote Healing

Along with symptom relief and improved quality of life in cancer patients, cannabinoids also have shown anticancer effects in many cell and animal experimental models, and a large body of anecdotal evidence suggests that human cancers also respond to cannabinoid treatment, Sulak writes. Several patients have reported slowing or arresting tumor growth, and others have experienced full remission of aggressive cancers while using cannabis extracts.[72]

To achieve these powerful anticancer effects, most patients need a higher dose than is needed for symptom relief—often 200 mg to 2,000 mg of cannabinoids a day, or the equivalent of one to two ounces of herbal cannabis a week. This treatment level may be cost effective if the cannabis is grown outdoors, but buying this amount of medicine from a medical cannabis retailer could be expensive.[73]

At these high doses, Sulak says, "a knowledgeable medical provider must monitor the treatment to prevent side effects and interactions with conventional cancer treatment. Patients must carefully titrate up to reach these high doses without significant adverse effects. Surprisingly, doses in the range of 2,000 mg/day can be well tolerated."[74]

Any medical treatment carries certain risks, he adds, but even high-dose cannabis is nonlethal and much safer than conventional chemotherapy, though the effectiveness of high-dose cannabis for cancer hasn't been studied in people. Some patients reaching very high doses report global improvement in symptoms and better quality of life. Others find that at ultrahigh doses the cannabis stops helping with symptoms like pain, anxiety, and sleep disturbance—benefits

---

70 Ibid.
71 Ibid.
72 Ibid.
73 Ibid.
74 Ibid.

they easily achieved at lower doses. Still others fail to build tolerance to the adverse effects of high cannabis doses and find themselves stoned, groggy, and uncomfortable.[75]

No Cookie-Cutter Solutions

Sulak says patients and students should beware of anyone who claims to have a cookie-cutter solution to cannabis dosing for cancer. The internet is full of ratios, doses, and other treatment plans for specific cancer types, but many of these claims are based on the success of a single patient or on partially relevant findings from the preclinical literature (cell and animal studies).

Cancer is incredibly complex, Sulak writes, and "even the same type of cancer in two different individuals can respond very differently to standard or alternative treatments. Because they're abnormal cells, cancers do unusual things—like overexpress or fail to express cannabinoid receptors," he adds. "Each individual's inner physiologic environment, genetics, diet, and other factors produce a unique case. Good results from one case or one study can't be broadly applied—at best they can be used as guides. A cancer treatment plan also must take into account an individual's goals and personal preferences."[76]

Cannabinoids fight cancer through different mechanisms of action, including triggering cell death, preventing cell growth and division, preventing the growth of blood vessels that feed tumors, and preventing cancer cells from migrating to other areas of the body. Most individual accounts of success using cannabis to kill cancer involve high doses, the clinician adds, but several stories describe patients who have experienced profound reductions in cancer burden while taking low-to-moderate doses.[77]

"Unlike conventional chemotherapy treatments," he writes, "we know that cannabinoids are nontoxic to normal cells. In conventional chemotherapy, the strategy is usually to use a drug that's more toxic to cancer cells than it is to healthy cells, and to give the patient as much as he or she can tolerate. Intolerable side effects, like peripheral neuropathy or malnutrition from nausea and vomiting, often are the limiting factors in treatment.[78]

"Cannabis dosing may be limited by side effects," Sulak said, "but not by toxicity that will lead to long-term limitations."[79]

---

75 Ibid.
76 Ibid.
77 Ibid.
78 Ibid.
79 Ibid.

Clinical Trials: Cannabinoids and Cancer

A Study of Sativex for Pain Relief in Patients with Advanced Malignancy (SPRAY)
The study sought to determine the effective dose range and demonstrate a non-effective dose range of Sativex in 360 adults with advanced cancer who experienced inadequate pain relief on optimized chronic opioid therapy. The study start date was November 2007 and the end date was January 2010. Results were published in the May 2012 *Journal of Pain*. The investigators said 263 patients completed the study. Analysis of average daily pain showed the proportion of patients reporting pain relief was greater for Sativex than placebo overall, specifically in low- and medium-dose groups. For adverse events, only the high-dose group compared unfavorably with placebo. The investigators wrote that the study supports Sativex efficacy and safety at the two lower doses and provides important dose information for future trials. Study details are available at clinicaltrials.gov/ct2/show/NCT00530764.

A Safety Study of Sativex Compared with Placebo (both with dose-intense temozolomide) in Recurrent Glioblastoma Patients
This randomized, parallel-assignment study was an open-label phase to assess the frequency and severity of adverse events in recurrent glioblastoma patients receiving Sativex in combination with dose-intense temozolomide. The study start date was September 2014 and it was completed in June 2016. The investigators wrote, "This randomized study provides preliminary evidence that 1:1 CBD:THC offers some efficacy in patients with recurrent GBM when used as an adjunct to dose-intense temozolomide and confirms the safety and feasibility of individualized dosing." Study details are available at clinicaltrials .gov/ct2/show/NCT01812616.

Safety and Efficacy of Smoked Cannabis for Improving Quality of Life in Advanced Cancer Patients
This study tested whether advanced cancer patients who use inhaled medical cannabis (PPP001, 280 mg dried cannabis pellet with 9 percent THC and 2 percent CBD per pellet) with palliative care management would experience improved quality of life, and whether the drug would relieve uncontrolled pain, providing safety conditions. Participants were 946 adults; the study start date

was September 2018 and the estimated end date was December 2018. Study details are available at clinicaltrials.gov/ct2/show/NCT03339622.

A Study of the Efficacy of Cannabidiol in Patients with Multiple Myeloma, Glioblastoma Multiforme, and GI Malignancies
This study is a randomized, double-blind, placebo-controlled, parallel multicenter study to assess the efficacy of BRCX014 (CBD) combined with standard-of-care treatment in 160 adult subjects with glioblastoma multiforme, multiple myeloma, and gastrointestinal malignancies. The investigators wrote that several studies have shown a potential antitumor role for cannabinoids. The study seeks to show that combining chemotherapy with BRCX014 will have greater antitumor and anti-proliferative activity when compared to standard of care alone. The estimated start date was January 2019 and the estimated end date is June 2020. Study details are available at clinicaltrials.gov/ct2/show/NCT03607643.

Keep checking clinicaltrials.gov for new studies. Start by searching for the disease name and the terms cannabis *and* cannabinoids.

Resources

Medical Cannabis-related Organizations

Project CBD: Medical Marijuana and Cannabinoid Science

https://www.projectcbd.org/

Project CBD is a California-based nonprofit established in 2010 and dedicated to promoting and publicizing research into the medical uses of cannabidiol (CBD), the main nonintoxicating element in cannabis, and other components of the plant. The organization also provides educational services for physicians, patients, industry professionals, and the public.

Multidisciplinary Association for Psychedelic Studies (MAPS)

http://www.maps.org/

Founded in 1986, MAPS is a 501(c)(3) nonprofit research and education organization that develops medical, legal, and cultural contexts for people to benefit from the careful uses of psychedelics and cannabis.

NORML: Working to Reform Marijuana Laws

http://www.norml.org

The mission of the National Organization for the Reform of Marijuana Laws (NORML), established in 1970, is to move public opinion enough to legalize the responsible use of cannabis by adults.

Marijuana Policy Project: We Change Laws

https://www.mpp.org/

MPP, founded in 1995, is the largest organization in the United States focused only on ending marijuana prohibition.

National Conference of State Legislatures

http://www.ncsl.org/research/health/state-medical-marijuana-laws.aspx

Medical cannabis laws by state.

Cannabis Resources for Patients

Patients Out of Time: Protecting Patients and Reducing Harm

http://patientsoutoftime.org/

A medical cannabis nonprofit organization and patient rights group established in 1995.

Realm of Caring

https://www.theroc.us

The nonprofit RoC Foundation, established in 2012, empowers members to take control of their health and enhance their quality of life by providing cannabinoid research initiatives and educational programs and services.

Americans for Safe Access: Advancing Legal Medical Marijuana Therapeutics and Research

http://www.safeaccessnow.org

The ASA, founded in 2002, seeks to ensure safe and legal access to cannabis for therapeutic use and research.

Web Resources

Leafly: Find Cannabis Strains, Dispensaries, and News

http://www.leafly.com

Leafly, according to its website, is the world's largest cannabis information resource, empowering people in legal cannabis markets to learn about the right products for their lifestyle and wellness needs, find those products safely and efficiently, and buy them from licensed and regulated dispensaries.

High Times

https://hightimes.com/

High Times calls itself the definitive resource for all things cannabis. From cultivation and legalization, to entertainment and culture, to hard-hitting news exposing the War on Drugs, *High Times* has been the preeminent source for cannabis information since 1974.

Merry Jane

https://merryjane.com/

Rapper Snoop Dogg launched this cannabis-focused digital media platform in 2015, with media entrepreneur Ted Chung. The website has editorial content on the cannabis industry, original video series, a database for identifying cannabis strains, and dispensaries.

Medical Jane

https://www.medicaljane.com/

The Medical Jane website offers free medical cannabis education and lots of resources to patients who deserve a better quality of life.

DOPE Magazine

https://dopemagazine.com/

DOPE (for Defending Our Plant Everywhere), founded in 2011, has a monthly print magazine, digital platform, social media handles, and events.

Leaf Science

https://www.leafscience.com/

Leaf Science, founded in 2014, is an online media company offering health and science information to cannabis consumers and professionals. The website has hundreds of free articles on cannabis-related health and science topics.

Online Medical Cannabis User Manuals

Project CBD User's Guide

https://www.projectcbd.org/how-to/
cbd-user-guide

Americans for Safe Access Patient's Guide to Medical Cannabis

https://www.safeaccessnow.org/
patients-guide

National Council for Aging Care

The Complete Guide to Medical Marijuana for Seniors

http://www.aging.com/the-complete-guide-to-medical-marijuana-for-seniors/

Index

A

Abrams, D. I., 54, 243–246
Abuhasira, R., 190, 193
acupuncture, 81–82
AD. *See* Alzheimer's disease (AD)
Adams, Mike, 98
addiction, 36, 59, 73–74, 233–241
AEA. *See* arachidonoyl ethanolamide (AEA)
aging, 140–145, 190–193
alcohol consumption, 83
alcohol use disorder, 238
allodynia, mechanical, 40–41
ALS. *See* amyotrophic lateral sclerosis (ALS)
Alzheimer's disease (AD), 39, 41, 84,
    142–157, 166, 185–186, 193
Americans for Safe Access (ASA), 96
amphioxus, 8
amputation, 127–128
amygdala, 125–126
amyloid plaque, 38, 41, 145–146, 148,
    153–155
amyotrophic lateral sclerosis (ALS), 39,
    141–142, 144–145, 168–176, 193
anandamide, 7, 25, 28, 46, 81–83,
    122–123, 144
antidepressants, 217
anti-inflammatory, 52, 54, 73
anxiety, 48–49, 75, 80, 115, 224
arachidonoyl ethanolamide (AEA), 17, 28–29
arachidonoylglycerol (2-AG), 17–19, 25, 28–
    29, 32, 42, 46, 81, 123, 144, 170, 200, 202,
    217, 219–221, 253, 255
arthritis, 107, 115, 118, 195–196. *See also*
    osteoarthritis (OA); rheumatoid arthritis
    (RA)
ASA. *See* Americans for Safe Access (ASA)
Assyria, 11–12
astrocytes, 30–31
atherosclerosis, 110–111
Aymerich, M. S., 46, 62, 169–170, 172, 185–186

B

Bar-Lev Schleider, L., 246
basal ganglia, 158–159, 162
Ben-Shabat, Shimon, 13, 29, 76
beta-amyloid. *See* amyloid plaque
beta-caryophyllene, 5, 72–74
Bilkei-Gorzo, A., 55
bipolar disorder, 214
blood-brain barrier, 31, 144–145
Bonner, Tom, 15
Booth, J. K., 4
borderline personality disorder (BPD),
    219–220
Bost, Jeff, 102
BPD. *See* borderline personality disorder
    (BPD)
brain trauma, 134–140
breast milk, 81
bronchodilation, 52

C

caffeine, 83
California, 92, 101
Cameron, M., 178, 180
cancer
    breast, 67, 254–255
    cannabichromene and, 68
    cannabigerol and, 67
    colorectal, 253–254
    limonene and, 75
    liver, 251
    lung, 251
    metastasis of, 242
    myrcene and, 74
    prostate, 67–68, 255–257
    side effects, 258–259
    symptoms, 258–259
    THCA and, 53
CandacePert, Candace, 109
Cannabaceae, 8

cannabichromene (CBC), 68–69
cannabidiol (CBD), 5, 10, 56–64
    extracts *vs.* purified, 63–64
    Farm Bill and, 62–63
    molecule, 56
    neuroprotective properties of, 57–58,
        102–103, 154
    receptors and, 32–33
    THC and, 44, 61
    THC synergy with, 51–52
cannabidiolic acid (CBDA), 59, 139
cannabidiophorol (CBDP), 66
cannabigerol (CBG), 67–68
cannabinoid receptors, 15–17, 29–42
cannabinoids, 3, 5
    outside endocannabinoid system, 42–45
cannabinol (CBN), 19–20, 65–67
cannabis resin, 3–4
cannabis use disorder, 237–238
Canna-Tsu, 105
carboxyl group, 51
cardiovascular disease, 37, 110–111, 234. *See
    also* stroke
Casarejos, M. J., 151
Cascio, M. G., 70
Castillo, P. E., 29
Catlow, B., 162, 167
CB1 receptor, 8, 15, 24–25, 29, 32–38
    addiction and, 235
    amyotrophic lateral sclerosis and, 171, 174
    arthritis and, 198–199
    depression and, 217
    gastrointestinal tract and, 207
    glioblastoma and, 249
    Huntington's disease and, 162–163
    neurogenesis and, 223
    Parkinson's and, 71
    posttraumatic stress disorder and, 121,
        123–124
    psychiatric illness and, 221
    receptors and, 32
    schizophrenia and, 227
    tetrahydrocannabivarin, 69
    THCA and, 53
CB2 receptor, 8, 15, 29, 31–32, 38–42
    addiction and, 236

Alzheimer's and, 146
amyotrophic lateral sclerosis and, 170–174
arthritis, 198–199
beta-caryophyllene and, 73
gastrointestinal tract and, 207
glioblastoma and, 249
Huntington's disease and, 163
neurogenesis and, 225
Parkinson's and, 71
tetrahydrocannabivarin, 69
THCA AND, 53
traumatic brain injury and, 136
CBC. *See* cannabichromene (CBC)
CBD. *See* cannabidiol (CBD)
CBG. *See* cannabigerol (CBG)
CBN. *See* cannabinol (CBN)
cell structure, 22
central sensitization, 87
China, 11, 92
cholesterol, 70
chronic traumatic encephalopathy (CTE),
    137–138
Citti, C., 66
Coates, Joan R., 172–173
cognition, 55–56, 156, 224
Comprehensive Drug Abuse Prevention and
    Control Act, 91, 100
Consroe, Paul, 181
Controlled Substances Act, 62, 91, 112–113
cortisol, 114–115
Crohn's disease, 193, 205–206, 208, 211
CTE. *See* chronic traumatic encephalopathy
    (CTE)

D
decarboxylation, 51
depression, 86–87, 115–118, 193–195, 213–219.
    See also mood
Devane, William, 14, 20
dexanabinol, 136
diabetes, 44, 69–70, 195, 201
diacylglycerol lipases (DAGLs), 18–19
dietary supplements, endocannabinoid
    system and, 80–81
Di Marzo, Vincenzo, 46–49, 78, 94, 96,
    140–141, 176

dopamine, 43–44, 158, 221–222, 234–235

dopamine pathways, 43

Dravet syndrome, 61

dronabinol, 112, 150–151, 238, 245

Drug Supply Program, 93–94

Dumitru, C. A., 250

dysthymia, 213. *See also* depression

E

ECS. *See* endocannabinoid system (ECS)

electroacupuncture, 81–82

Elixinol, 107

Elphick, Maurice, 7–8, 15, 37

ElSohly, Mahmoud, 5, 65

Endoca, 108

endocannabinoid deficiency, 84–87, 126–128

endocannabinoid enzymes, 46–48

endocannabinoids, 6, 17–18, 25–26, 28–31
   role of, 48–49

endocannabinoid system (ECS), 6–27
   acupuncture and, 81–82
   in addiction, 234–236
   aging and, 140–145
   alcohol consumption and, 83
   in balance, 78–87
   in depression, 214–219, 223–225
   depression-pain and, 193–195
   dietary supplements and, 80–81
   early-life dietary considerations and, 81
   exercise and, 82–83
   gastrointestinal tract and, 206–208
   lifestyle modifications and, 82–84
   modulation of, 79–84
   omega 3 supplements and, 80
   osteoarthritis and, 200
   osteopathic manipulation and, 82
   pain-depression and, 193–195
   pharmaceuticals and, 79–80
   prebiotics and, 81
   probiotics and, 80–81
   psychiatric illness and, 220–232
   signaling collapse, 115–119
   smoking and, 83
   teaching, 95–97
   tone, 47, 126–127
   weight loss and, 82

entourage effect, 63–64, 76–77

enzymes, 18–19, 46–48

Epidiolex, 61–62, 94, 136, 186

epilepsy, 61–62

Espay, A. J., 159

evolution, 8–10

exercise, endocannabinoid system and, 82–83

F

Farm Bill, 62–63, 101

fatty acid amide hydrolase (FAAH), 18, 46–47,
   79, 122, 124, 186, 194, 218, 221, 253

Fernández-Ruiz, J., 70, 137, 143–145, 152,
   164, 174–175, 187

Fernández-Trapero, M., 173–174

fibromyalgia, 85, 87, 194, 202–205

Finn, David, 119

Fitzgibbon, M., 194

Fraguas-Sánchez, A., 248, 251–252

G

GABA. *See* gamma-aminobutyric acid (GABA)

gamma-aminobutyric acid (GABA), 35–36

Gaoni, Yehiel, 13–14, 65

Garcia, A. B., 34–36

Gerdeman, Greg, 21–26, 37, 110–111, 121,
   123–125, 138–139

glioblastomas, 248–251, 261–262

gliomas, 248–251

glutamate, 25, 135

glycine, 43–44

Golgi, Camillo, 21–22

Gottlieb, Scott, 62–63

Gowers, William, 167

GPCRs. *See* G protein-coupled receptors
   (GPCRs)

G protein-coupled receptors (GPCRs), 15–16,
   34, 45

graft-*versus*-host disease (GvHD), 58

Gupta, Sanjay, 59–60

Guy, Geoffrey, 182

Guzmán, Manuel, 246–247

GvHD. *See* graft-*versus*-host disease (GvHD)

H

Hanus, Lumir, 17

Harle-Tsu, 105
Hasenoehrla, C., 209–210
HD. *See* Huntington's disease (HD)
Healer.com, 96
helplessness, learned, 124–125
Hergenrather, Jeffrey, 148
Hill, Matthew, 114–119, 125–126, 130–132,
    214–216
Hinz, B., 256
Howlett, Allyn, 14
HU-211, 136
Huntington's disease (HD), 39, 142, 144,
    160–162, 164

I
IACM. *See* International Association for
    Cannabis as Medicine (IACM)
IBD. *See* inflammatory bowel disease (IBD)
IBS. *See* irritable bowel syndrome (IBS)
ICCI. *See* International Cannabis and
    Cannabinoids Institute (ICCI)
inflammation, 35, 37, 39–42, 113–115,
    117–119, 224
inflammatory bowel disease (IBD), 205–212.
    See also irritable bowel syndrome (IBS)
International Association for Cannabis as
    Medicine (IACM), 97
International Cannabis and Cannabinoids
    Institute (ICCI), 96–97
irritable bowel syndrome (IBS), 86–87. *See
    also* inflammatory bowel disease (IBD)
isoprene, 71

J
Jadoon, K. A., 69
Jetly, R., 131

K
Karl, T., 154–156
Katzman, M. A., 220–223, 228–229
Katz-Talmor, D., 202–203
Kenyon, J., 257
Kisková, T., 254
Korem, N., 120–121

L
law, medical cannabis and, 91–99
learned helplessness, 124–125
Lee, Martin A, 14, 56, 59, 101, 104
legal status, 93–94, 100–101
Lennox-Gastaut syndrome, 61
Levine, Rachel, 98
Ligresti, A., 252–253
limonene, 5, 75
linalool, 75
Lindblad-Toh, Kerstin, 172
LSD, 109–110

M
MacCallum, Caroline, 102–103
Mackie, Ken, 9–10
Malek, N., 197
Malinowska, B., 47
Manzanares, J., 234–236
Marcu, Jahan, 6, 34, 58, 69, 71, 73–74
Marijuana Tax Act, 91
Maroon, Joseph, 102
McDougall, J. J., 199–202
McGuire, P., 230–231
McPartland, John, 77, 81, 83
mechanical allodynia, 40–41
Mechoulam, Raphael, 6, 13–14, 19–20, 35,
    39, 52, 78, 156, 246
melancholic depression, 214–215. *See also*
    depression
memory, 36–37, 120, 123, 129
metastasis, 242
methicillin-resistant *Staphylococcus aureus*
    (MRSA), 67
Micale, V., 216–218
microglial activation, 40, 153
migraine, 85
monoglyceride lipase (MAGL), 18–19
mood, 85, 117–119. *See also* anxiety;
    depression
morphine, 45
MRSA. *See* methicillin-resistant *Staphylococcus
    aureus* (MRSA)
MS. *See* multiple sclerosis (MS)
multiple sclerosis (MS), 39, 45, 94, 118,
    141–142, 176–184, 193

Munro, Sean, 15
Musty, Richard, 181
myrcene, 74

N
nabilone, 112, 131, 180–181
N-acylphosphatidylethanolamine-
    phospholipase D (NAPE-PLD), 19
Naftali, T., 206–208
namacizumab, 46–47
NAPE-PLD. *See*
    N-acylphosphatidylethanolamine-
    phospholipase D (NAPE-PLD)
neurodegeneration, 39, 140, 164. *See also*
    Alzheimer's disease (AD); amyotrophic
    lateral sclerosis (ALS); Huntington's
    disease (HD); multiple sclerosis (MS);
    Parkinson's disease (PD)
neurofibrillary tangles, 145
neurogenesis, 52, 148, 156, 164, 223–225
neuropathic pain, 25, 39–41, 73
Nichols, David E., 110
nicotine use disorder, 237
norepinephrine, 45, 68, 84, 159, 222–223

O
OA. *See* osteoarthritis (OA)
O'Brien, M., 199–202
obsessive-compulsive disorder (OCD), 224
omega 3 supplements, 80
opioids, 54–55, 128, 188–189, 239–240
opioid use disorder, 238–239
opium, 11–12
Oregon, 92
osteoarthritis (OA), 196–199. *See also* arthritis
osteopathic manipulation, 82

P
Page, Jonathan, 3, 72
pain, 240
    arthritis and, 199–202
    chronic, 54, 82–83, 87, 188–195
    depression and, 193–195
    neuropathic, 25, 39–41, 73
    in Parkinson's, 168
    phantom-limb, 127–128

THC and, 54–55
Papaver somnieferum, 11–12
Parker, L. A., 34–35, 39, 156, 223
Parkinson's disease (PD), 39, 53, 70–71, 84,
    103, 142–145, 158–160, 162, 164–168,
    193–194, 230
PD. *See* Parkinson's disease (PD)
Pennsylvania, 97–99
Pennywise, 105
peroxisome proliferator-activated receptor
    (PPAR), 32, 44, 70, 186
persistent depressive disorder, 213
Pertwee, Roger, 14–15, 28, 52, 68, 181–182
phantom-limb pain, 127–128
pinene, 5
posttraumatic stress disorder (PTSD), 85, 87,
    117, 120–133, 216, 220
PPAR. *See* peroxisome proliferator-activated
    receptor (PPAR)
prebiotics, 81
prices, 106
probiotics, 80–81
protective, cannabinoids as, 24–26
psychiatric illness, 220–232. *See also*
    depression
psychotic depression, 213. *See also* depression
PTSD. *See* posttraumatic stress disorder
    (PTSD)
public health, 100–103
public opinion, 93
pyramidal neurons, 155

R
RA. *See* rheumatoid arthritis (RA)
Ramer, R., 256
Ramón y Cajal, Santiago, 21–22
raphe nuclei, 221
reactive oxygen species (ROS), 146–147
Rein, Judith, 181
research, 94–95, 112
resin, 3–4
retrograde signaling, 23–25, 116
rheumatoid arthritis (RA), 193, 196–197,
    202–205. *See also* arthritis
Rice, J., 178, 180
Ringo's Gift, 105

Roitman, P., 130
Romero-Sandoval, E. A., 189
ROS. *See* reactive oxygen species (ROS)
Russo, Ethan, 5–6, 25, 27–29, 33–34, 38, 47,
     58, 60–61, 67–68, 71, 73–74, 84–87, 94–95,
     103, 108–110, 127–128, 137, 146–147

S
Sanchez-Ramos, J., 162, 167
Schedule I, 91–92, 100, 112–113
schizophrenia, 121, 225–232
Schleiden, Matthias, 22
Schwann, Theodor, 22
sea squirt, 7–8
Seau, Junior, 139
Seligman, Martin, 124
sensitization, central, 87
serotonin, 43–44, 221
serotonin pathways, 43
serotonin receptors, 68, 70
Sharpless, Ned, 63
Skaper, S. D., 78
sleep, 129
Sloan, M. E., 236
smoking, 83, 237
Sour Tsunami, 105
Spalding, David, 105–106
sports, 137–138
Starowicz, K., 197
Stephen Hawking Kush, 105
stress, 49, 81, 115–117, 224. *See also*
     posttraumatic stress disorder (PTSD)
stroke, 134–137
Sugiura, Takayuki, 17–18
Sulak, Dustin, 54, 59, 138, 257–260
Sweet and Sour Widow, 105

T
tau kinases, 145
TBI. *See* traumatic brain injury (TBI)
terpenes, 4–5, 64, 71–75
tetrahydrocannabinol (THC), 5, 13, 52–56
     CBD and, 44, 61
     CBD synergy with, 51–52

cognition and, 55–56
in industrial hemp, 105
molecule, 53
pain and, 54–55
PPAR and, 44
receptors and, 32–33, 37–38
tetrahydrocannabinolic acid (THCA), 53–54,
     139, 149, 166
tetrahydrocannabiphorol (THCP), 66
tetrahydrocannabivarin (THCV), 69–71, 186
THC. *See* tetrahydrocannabinol (THC)
The Medical Cannabis Institute (TMCI), 96
Tillery, Whitney, 181
TMCI. *See* The Medical Cannabis Institute
     (TMCI)
Toczek, M., 47
Torres-Suárez, A. I., 248–249, 251–252
transient receptor potential vanilloid 1
     (TRVP1), 30, 32, 45, 225
trauma, brain, 134–140
traumatic brain injury (TBI), 135–136
trichomes, 3–5
TRPV1. *See* transient receptor potential
     vanilloid 1 (TRVP1)
tumor necrosis factor alpha (TNF-a), 54

U
ulcerative colitis, 205–206
US Pharmacopeia, 12

V
Virchow, Rudolph, 22

W
Wade, Claire, 172
Wang, M., 51
Watt, G., 154–156
weight loss, 82
white willow, 109
Whittle, Brian, 182
Wiese, B., 238, 240
Wilson-Poe, A. R., 238, 240
Wolf, Tom, 97, 99
Woodhams, S. G., 188